Aging in Sub-Saharan Africa

Recommendations for Furthering Research

Panel on Policy Research and Data Needs to Meet the
Challenge of Aging in Africa

Barney Cohen and Jane Menken, *Editors*

Committee on Population

Division of Behavioral and Social Sciences and Education

NATIONAL RESEARCH COUNCIL
OF THE NATIONAL ACADEMIES

THE NATIONAL ACADEMIES PRESS
Washington, D.C.
www.nap.edu

THE NATIONAL ACADEMIES PRESS •500 Fifth Street, NW •Washington, DC 20001

NOTICE: The project that is the subject of this report was approved by the Governing Board of the National Research Council, whose members are drawn from the councils of the National Academy of Sciences, the National Academy of Engineering, and the Institute of Medicine. The members of the committee responsible for the report were chosen for their special competences and with regard for appropriate balance.

This study was supported by Contract No. N01-OD-4-2139, TO#119 between the National Academy of Sciences and the National Institutes of Health and the National Institute of Aging. Any opinions, findings, conclusions, or recommendations expressed in this publication are those of the author(s) and do not necessarily reflect the views of the organizations or agencies that provided support for the project.

International Standard Book Number-10: 0-309-010281-2
International Standard Book Number-13: 978-0-309-010281-0

THE NATIONAL ACADEMIES
Advisers to the Nation on Science, Engineering, and Medicine

The **National Academy of Sciences** is a private, nonprofit, self-perpetuating society of distinguished scholars engaged in scientific and engineering research, dedicated to the furtherance of science and technology and to their use for the general welfare. Upon the authority of the charter granted to it by the Congress in 1863, the Academy has a mandate that requires it to advise the federal government on scientific and technical matters. Dr. Ralph J. Cicerone is president of the National Academy of Sciences.

The **National Academy of Engineering** was established in 1964, under the charter of the National Academy of Sciences, as a parallel organization of outstanding engineers. It is autonomous in its administration and in the selection of its members, sharing with the National Academy of Sciences the responsibility for advising the federal government. The National Academy of Engineering also sponsors engineering programs aimed at meeting national needs, encourages education and research, and recognizes the superior achievements of engineers. Dr. Wm. A. Wulf is president of the National Academy of Engineering.

The **Institute of Medicine** was established in 1970 by the National Academy of Sciences to secure the services of eminent members of appropriate professions in the examination of policy matters pertaining to the health of the public. The Institute acts under the responsibility given to the National Academy of Sciences by its congressional charter to be an adviser to the federal government and, upon its own initiative, to identify issues of medical care, research, and education. Dr. Harvey V. Fineberg is president of the Institute of Medicine.

The **National Research Council** was organized by the National Academy of Sciences in 1916 to associate the broad community of science and technology with the Academy's purposes of furthering knowledge and advising the federal government. Functioning in accordance with general policies determined by the Academy, the Council has become the principal operating agency of both the National Academy of Sciences and the National Academy of Engineering in providing services to the government, the public, and the scientific and engineering communities. The Council is administered jointly by both Academies and the Institute of Medicine. Dr. Ralph J. Cicerone and Dr. Wm. A. Wulf are chair and vice chair, respectively, of the National Research Council.

www.national-academies.org

PANEL ON POLICY RESEARCH AND DATA NEEDS TO MEET THE CHALLENGE OF AGING IN AFRICA

JANE MENKEN (*Chair*), Institute of Behavioral Science and Department of Sociology, University of Colorado

ALEX EZEH, African Population and Health Research Center, Nairobi, Kenya

EDWELL KASEKE, School of Social Work, University of Zimbabwe

BARTHÉLÉMY KUATE-DEFO, Department of Demography, University of Montreal, Canada

DAVID LAM, Department of Economics, University of Michigan

ALBERTO PALLONI, Department of Sociology, Institute for Environmental Studies, University of Wisconsin at Madison

STEPHEN TOLLMAN, School of Public Health, University of the Witwatersrand, Johannesburg, South Africa

ROBERT J. WILLIS, Institute for Social Research, University of Michigan

BARNEY COHEN, *Director, Committee on Population*
ANTHONY S. MANN, *Senior Project Assistant*

COMMITTEE ON POPULATION

Acknowledgments

This report adds to the empirical and conceptual knowledge of the situation of older people in sub-Saharan Africa and makes practical suggestions for further research in this area. The report is based on a workshop organized by the Committee on Population in collaboration with the Health and Population Division, School of Public Health, University of the Witwatersrand in Johannesburg, South Africa, in July 2004. The report draws on a number of papers commissioned for the workshop, on the comments made by a panel of distinguished discussants, and on the discussion by workshop participants.

Many people made generous contributions to the workshop's success. We are grateful to our colleagues, Alex Ezeh, Edwell Kaseke, Barthélémy Kuate-Defo, David Lam, Alberto Palloni, Stephen Tollman, and Robert Willis, who served on the panel that was charged with organizing the workshop and preparing a document that outlined the priority research areas in relation to aging in sub-Saharan Africa. Belinda Bezzoli, deputy vice-chancellor for research of the University of the Witwatersrand, and Richard Suzman, of the National Institute on Aging, supported the planning of the workshop and participated throughout. We are also especially grateful to the various authors and discussants who prepared papers or presentations in advance of the meeting: Mary Amuyunzu-Nyamongo, African Population and Health Research Center; Ayaga Bawah, Navrongo Health Research Center; Peter Byass, Umeå University; Samuel Clark, University of Colorado at Boulder and University of Washington; Gloria Chepngeno, University of Southampton; Mark Collinson, University of the Witwatersrand; Myles Connor, University of the Witwatersrand; Rob Dorrington, University of Cape Town; Alex Ezeh, African Population and Health Research Center; James Fairburn, University of KwaZulu-Natal; Michel Garenne, French Institute for Research and Development (IRD); Victoria Hosegood, London School of Hygiene & Tropical Medicine; Gillian Hundt, University of Warwick; Kathleen Kahn, University of the Witwatersrand; Benoit Kalasa, United Nations Population Fund; Edwell Kaseke, University of Zimbabwe; Abdhalah Ziraba Kasiira, African Population and Health Research Center; Paul Kowal, World Health Organization; Barthélémy Kuate-Defo, University of Montreal; Rodreck Mupedziswa, University of the Witwatersrand; Randall Kuhn, University of Colorado at Boulder; David Lam, University of Michigan; Murray Leibbrandt, University of Cape Town; Frances Lund, University of KwaZulu-Natal; M. Giovanna Merli, University of Wisconsin; Tavengwa Nhongo, HelpAge International; Alberto Palloni, University of Wisconsin; Karen Peachey, consultant; Dorrit Posel, University of KwaZulu-Natal; M. Omar Rahman, Independent University, Bangladesh; Vimal Ranchhod, University of Michigan; Kalanidhi Subbarao, The World Bank; Negussie Taffa-Wordofa, African Population and Health Research Center; Ian M. Timaeus, London School of Hygiene & Tropical Medicine; Margaret Thorogood, University of Warwick; Stephen Tollman, University of the Witwatersrand; Eric Udjo, Human Sciences Research Council; Servaas van der Berg, University of Stellenbosch; Victoria Velkoff, U.S. Census Bureau; Robert Willis, University of Michigan; Martin Wittenberg, University of Cape Town; and Zewdu Woubalem, African Population and Health Research Center.

The Committee on Population was extremely fortunate to be able to enlist the help and cooperation of the staff and faculty of the Health and Population Division, School of Public Health, University of the Witwatersrand, in Johannesburg, South Africa. Particular thanks are due to Stephen Tollman for his invaluable assistance facilitating the meeting and to Dereshni Ramnarain for her assistance in ensuring that the meeting ran smoothly and successfully.

In Washington, DC, several members of the staff of the National Academies made significant contributions to the report. We thank Kirsten Sampson Snyder for her help guiding the report through review, Christine McShane for her skillful editing, and Yvonne Wise for managing the production process. The project took place under the general direction of Jane L. Ross and Barney Cohen. On behalf of the panel, we thank them for their efforts.

This report has been reviewed in draft form by individuals chosen for their diverse perspectives and technical expertise, in accordance with procedures approved by the National Research Council's Report Review Committee. The purpose of this independent review is to provide candid and critical comments that will assist the institution in making the published report as sound as possible and to ensure that the report meets institutional standards for objectivity, evidence, and responsiveness to the study charge. The review comments and draft manuscript remain confidential to protect the integrity of the deliberative process.

We wish to thank the following individuals for their participation in the review of the report: Ronald Angel, Department of Sociology, University of Texas at Austin; Channing Arndt, Department of Agricultural Economics, Purdue University; Yael Benyamini, School of Social Work, Tel Aviv University; Peter Byass, Department of Public Health and Clinical Medicine, Umeå University; Benjamin Campbell, Department of Anthropology, Boston University; David Canning, Department of Population and International Health, Harvard School of Public Health; Julia Dayton, consultant; Gary V. Engelhardt, Center for Policy Research, Syracuse University; Bibi Essama, Westat; Monica Ferreira, The Albertina and Walter Sisulu Institute of Ageing in Africa, University of Cape Town, South Africa; Gary Fields, Department of Economics, Cornell University; Kathleen Ford, Department of Epidemiology, University of Michigan; Lucy Gilson, School of Public Health, University of the Witwatersrand; Mark Gorman, Department of Economic and Social Affairs, HelpAge International; William T.S. Gould, Department of Geography, University of Liverpool; Ellen Idler, Institute for Health, Rutgers, State University of New Jersey; Benoit Kalasa, advisor, United Nations Population Fund; Peter Lloyd-Sherlock, Faculty of Social Sciences, University of East Anglia; Monde Makiwane, Child, Youth, Family and Social Development, Human Sciences Research Council, Pretoria, South Africa; Douglas L. Miller, Department of Economics, University of California, Davis; Akim Mturi, School of Development Studies, University of KwaZulu-Natal; Sendhil Mullainathan, Department of Economics, Harvard University; Laura Rudkin, Department of Preventive Medicine and Community Health, University of Texas; Joshua Salomon, Department of Population and International Health, Harvard University; Gigi Santow, independent researcher; Doreen Tempo, Department of Social Policy and Social Work, University of Oxford; Joseph R. Troisi, II, Department of Psychology, Saint Anselm College; Etienne van de Walle, Department of Sociology, University of Pennsylvania; Stig Wall, Department of Public Health and Clinical Medicine, Umeå University; Alan Whiteside, Health Economics and HIV/AIDS Research Division, University of KwaZulu-Natal; Alun Williams, Centre for Human Ageing, University of Queensland, Australia; Martin Wittenberg, School of Economics, University of Cape Town; Zewdu Woubalem, African Population and Health Research Center; and Zachary Zimmer, Policy Research Division, Population Council.

Although the reviewers listed above have provided many constructive comments and suggestions, they were not asked to endorse the conclusions or recommendations nor did they see the final draft of the report before release. The review of this report was overseen by Allan G. Hill, Department of Population and International Health, Harvard School of Public Health. Appointed by the National Research Council, he was responsible for making certain that an independent examination of this report was carried out in accordance with institutional procedures and that all review comments were carefully considered. Responsibility for the final context of this report rests entirely with the authoring committee and the institution.

Jane Menken, *Chair*
Panel on Policy Research and Data Needs to
Meet the Challenge of Aging in Africa

Barney Cohen, *Director*
Committee on Population

Contents

Executive Summary

Economic security, health and disability, and living conditions in old age are policy concerns throughout the world, but the nature of the problem differs considerably from continent to continent and between and within countries. In sub-Saharan Africa older people make up a relatively small fraction of the total population, and traditionally their main source of support has been the household and family, supplemented in many cases by other informal mechanisms, such as kinship networks and mutual aid societies. Although very little careful empirical research has been undertaken on long-term trends in the welfare of older people, there are a number of reasons to believe that traditional caring and social support mechanisms in sub-Saharan Africa are under increasing strain.

Located on the least developed and poorest continent, African economies are still heavily dependent on subsistence agriculture, and average income per capita is now lower than it was at the end of the 1960s. Consequently, the region contains a growing share of the world's poor. In addition, reductions in fertility and child mortality have meant that, despite the huge impact of the HIV/AIDS epidemic across much of the region, both the absolute size and the proportion of the population age 60 and over have grown and will continue to grow over the next 30 years.

In sub-Saharan Africa, older people have traditionally been viewed in a positive light, as repositories of information and wisdom. And while African families are generally still intact, development and modernization are closely connected with social and economic changes that can weaken traditional social values and networks that provide care and support in later life. Formal education, for example, leads to greater independence and au-

1

tonomy and weakening traditional social ties and obligations, factors that tend to undermine traditional extended family systems.

In parts of sub-Saharan Africa, however, these changes pale in comparison to the effects of the HIV/AIDS pandemic. Sub-Saharan Africa has long carried a high burden of disease, including from malaria and tuberculosis; today it is home to more than 60 percent of all people living with HIV—some 25.8 million in 2005. The vast majority of those affected are still in their prime wage-earning years, at an age when, normally, they would be expected to be the main wage earners and principal sources of financial and material support for older people and children in their families. Many older people have had to deal with the loss of their own support while absorbing the additional responsibilities of caring for their orphaned grandchildren. Increasingly, then, it appears that African societies are being asked to cope with population aging with neither a comprehensive formal social security system nor a well-functioning traditional care system in place.

It is against this backdrop that, in 2004, the National Institute on Aging (NIA) asked the National Academies' Committee on Population to organize a workshop on advancing aging research in sub-Saharan Africa. NIA was interested in exploring ways in which to promote U.S. research interests and to augment sub-Saharan African governments' capacity to address the many challenges posed by population aging.

KEY THEMES

Five key themes emerged from the workshop and the discussion. The first is the lack of basic, agreed-upon definitions crucial to the study of aging in sub-Saharan African societies. Most fundamentally, who is considered an older person in sub-Saharan Africa? Do the definitions used in industrialized societies have the same meaning for sub-Saharan Africa? And in the African context, with its complex and extended family structures, what constitutes the household, the usual unit within which older people are studied? Research can adequately assess the situation of older people in sub-Saharan Africa only if it is conducted in a framework that can allow for a full range of actors and impacts on their well-being. A second theme and persistent lament throughout the workshop is the lack of careful empirical research and the dearth of comprehensive data needed to rectify this situation. Third is the participants' belief that the situation of older people in sub-Saharan Africa is changing fairly rapidly. Fourth is the need to recognize the considerable diversity across sub-Saharan Africa with respect to a wide range of indicators. The final central theme is the need to support the development of local research capacity and facilitate research.

KEY AREAS FOR FUTURE RESEARCH

Five key areas of research—all closely interrelated—emerged as essential to the advancement of understanding of the situation of older people in sub-Saharan Africa and as necessary precursors to the development of sound aging policy in the region. These are (1) income, wealth, and expenditure; (2) health and well-being; (3) the nature of family support and social networks; (4) the changing roles and responsibilities of older people as a function of the AIDS crisis; and (5) the nature and role of various kinds of formal and informal social protection schemes.

RECOMMENDATIONS

The panel's recommendations fall into three groups: (1) recommendations for a research agenda, (2) for enhancing research opportunity and implementation, and (3) for translation of research findings.

Research Agenda

There can be little doubt that, as a function of the emerging fertility transition in sub-Saharan Africa, the changing macroeconomic climate, and the impact of the devastating HIV/AIDS epidemic, researchers are paying increasing attention to the social, economic, and demographic dimensions of aging in sub-Saharan Africa. The five key areas listed above and described in detail in this report constitute an agenda of needed research on aging in sub-Saharan Africa. To carry out this agenda, we recommend the following:

1. Increase Research on Aging in Sub-Saharan Africa

Increased attention can be turned into action only with increased funding directed to this arena. Funders should consider mechanisms—existing or new—to enable the research agenda identified in this report to be carried out.

2. Explore Ways to Leverage Existing Data Collection Efforts to Learn More About Older People in Sub-Saharan Africa

National governments will need both to invest more in basic research and to develop mechanisms to establish common definitions that will facilitate the harmonization of data collection across countries. Improving understanding of the situation of older people will also require a better picture of the simultaneous interplay among multiple factors, including health, economic, and social characteristics. Hence, the development and use of multidisciplinary research designs will be essential in the development and production of any new data on aging in sub-Saharan Africa.

Enhancing Research Opportunity and Implementation

3. Improve Support for Library Infrastructure and Dissemination Tools to Create a More Integrated Body of Knowledge in Sub-Saharan Africa

There is a need for more support for library and information services as well as a need for greater information sharing and professional networking, perhaps through the sponsorship of more local or regional conferences. Given the rapid takeoff of electronic journal retrieval systems, such as JSTOR, increased investment in Internet access—both to high-speed Internet itself and to rights to use resources available on the Internet—may be one of the most effective means of closing the gap between continents in terms of access to existing research.

4. Improve Archiving of Past Censuses and Surveys

Data handling and storage technology are advancing so rapidly that the burden of making data available in a useful format cannot rest with individual researchers. There is a need for a more systematic archiving of African microdata.

5. Improve Access to Ongoing Data Collection Efforts

If investments in new data are to be realized, better mechanisms will need to be put in place to improve storage, retrieval, and access to aging data. Much of the best research undertaken to date has been made possible only by the establishment of international research partnerships between researchers in the developed and the developing world. These partnerships are quite complex to establish and maintain, since they involve negotiating such thorny issues as fair allocation of research roles, balance in infrastructure investments, and fairness in ascribing authorship and related credits. The challenge will be to strengthen these partnerships in ways that both support local institutions and increase timely access to data.

6. Strengthen International Collaboration and Capacity-Building in the Short Term

More and better research on various dimensions of aging in sub-Saharan Africa cannot happen without an increase in the funding for research, more well-trained local researchers, and improvements in administrative procedures that currently hinder the execution of research projects. Because it is unlikely that sub-Saharan African governments are going to increase their level of research funding substantially in the near future, foreign financial and technical assistance will remain essential in the short term to the development of local universities and the strengthening of local research capacity.

7. Remove Barriers to Implementation of Research

Collaborative research with sub-Saharan African institutions requires approvals by all collaborating institutions, frequently involving more than one review board for the ethical conduct of research as well as government offices and officials in the country in which data collection takes place. If research on these important subjects is to be carried out in timely fashion, it is essential that institutions, review boards, and government bodies at all relevant levels establish procedures and processes that make speedy review possible, without repetitive reviews of scientific merit.

8. In the Long Term, Sub-Saharan African Governments Must Give Reasonable Priority to Aging Research and Strengthen Local Research Capacity

In the long run, the importance of foreign-supported research in the region must be reduced. It will be up to sub-Saharan African national governments to prioritize aging as a focal area and to find the resources needed to be able to drive the region's research agenda on aging. Numerous related processes are already under way in Africa aimed at strengthening research institutes and building research capacity. Nevertheless, sub-Saharan African governments generally need to place a greater value on the role of higher education and find funding to rebuild and strengthen local universities. In many countries, pay scales will need to be adjusted in order to attract and retain the best researchers.

Translation of Research Findings

9. Improve Dialogue Between Local Researchers and Policy Makers

Researchers need to do a better job of drawing out the main policy and programmatic implications of their work, and policy makers need to better articulate what information they most need for more effective planning and program design. Otherwise, the danger is that local programs and policies will be only marginally based on a solid understanding of local needs and conditions, while research will continue to be undervalued by policy makers and therefore underfunded.

Part I

Report

1

Aging in Sub-Saharan Africa: Recommendations for Furthering Research

Economic security, health and disability, and living conditions in old age are policy concerns throughout the world, but the nature of the problems differs considerably from continent to continent and between and within countries. In industrialized countries, old age support comes to a great extent from large public or private pension and health systems. These systems are becoming increasingly strained as population aging has increased the proportion of older people. At the same time, in much of the industrialized world (Russia being a major exception), the health of the older population is, at a minimum, remaining steady and, in many places, it is improving rapidly.

By contrast, throughout most of the developing world, providing support for older people is still primarily a family responsibility. Traditionally in sub-Saharan Africa,[1] the main source of support has been the household and family, supplemented in many cases by other informal mechanisms, such as kinship networks and mutual aid societies. With the notable exceptions of Botswana, Mauritius, Namibia, and South Africa, formal pensions (whether contributory or not) or other social welfare schemes are virtually nonexistent and, when they do exist, tend to pay minimal benefits and cover only a small fraction of the elderly population (Gillian, Turner, Bailey, and Latulippe, 2000). Population aging is only beginning and, because fertility is falling, it is occurring during a temporary phase of declining dependency

---

[1]Unless otherwise specified, "Africa" refers to sub-Saharan Africa throughout this chapter.

9

burdens (see the paper by Velkoff and Kowal in this volume). Older people make up a relatively small fraction of the total population, which is expected to increase slowly, although their numbers are increasing rapidly. There are also major differences in the principal health challenges in sub-Saharan Africa compared with industrialized countries. In much of sub-Saharan Africa, gains in life expectancy that were achieved throughout the latter half of the 20th century have been eroded by the HIV/AIDS pandemic (see Chapter 2). Yet little is known about the health and disability of older people and patterns of change. In addition, traditional caring and social support mechanisms now appear to be under increasing strain (Apt, 1996; Dhemba, Gumbo, and Nyamusara, 2002; Kasente, Asingwire, Banugire, and Kyomuhenda, 2002; Mchomvu, Tungaraza, and Maghimbi, 2002; Mukuka, Kalikiti, and Musenge, 2002; Williams, 2003; Williams and Tumwekwase, 2001).

Reasons for this strain include a series of profound economic and social changes associated with development and modernization. In sub-Saharan Africa, older people have traditionally been viewed in a positive light, as repositories of information and wisdom. To date, sub-Saharan African families have shown a great deal of resilience and are generally still intact. Changes associated with development and modernization can, however, combine to weaken traditional social values and networks that stress the important role of older people in society and that reinforce traditions of intergenerational exchange and reciprocity. These changes include increasing formal education and the migration of young people from rural to urban areas, leaving older family members behind. Far more is known about the impact of these changes in other regions of the world, particularly Asia (see Hermalin, 2002), compared with sub-Saharan Africa. Yet their effects pale, in parts of sub-Saharan Africa, in comparison to the effects of the HIV/AIDS pandemic.

Sub-Saharan Africa has long carried a high burden of disease, including from malaria and tuberculosis; today it remains at the center of the HIV/AIDS pandemic. The Joint United Nations Programme on HIV/AIDS and the World Health Organization estimate that more than 60 percent of all people living with HIV are in sub-Saharan Africa—some 25.8 million in 2005 (Joint United Nations Programme on HIV/AIDS, 2006). The lives of older people may be affected by their own illness, but it is more likely, given the age structure of the pandemic, that they are affected by sickness and death of their adult children. Not only do these older people face the loss of a child or children who may well have been a vital source of support and caregiving, but many are also then faced with additional obligations and responsibilities for grandchildren and other members of their extended families.

Finally, AIDS and other social changes are occurring against a backdrop of persistent poverty and deprivation. Sub-Saharan Africa remains the least developed and least urbanized region in the world. Approximately two-thirds of the population of sub-Saharan Africa still live in rural areas and rely largely on near subsistence agriculture or traditional pastoralism for their livelihoods. In such settings, families have to be very self-reliant. Chronic poverty becomes a critical risk factor for the well-being of older people, and more than two of every five of the continent's inhabitants remain trapped in debilitating poverty (United Nations, 2006). In addition, while the continent has witnessed a decline in the number of armed conflicts since the early 1990s, persistent violence and in some cases seemingly intractable conflicts compound the region's problems and present critical obstacles to development in some countries (Marshall and Gurr, 2005; Porter, Robinson, Smyth, Schnabel, and Osaghae, 2005).[2]

Researchers in sub-Saharan Africa are only now beginning to ask how all of these factors—trends in socioeconomic conditions, changing cultural norms and values, changing levels of formal and informal social support, ongoing poor health conditions, and the AIDS crisis—are combining to affect the well-being of older people. African gerontology has expanded in recent years, much of the work based on anthropological approaches (see, for example, Makoni and Stroeken, 2002). Elsewhere—in Europe and Asia, for example—major research programs focused on older people are under way, and longitudinal studies now provide a great deal of information on economic well-being, health, and family processes (see, for example, Börsch-Supan et al., 2005; Hermalin, 2002). Comparable efforts are only beginning in sub-Saharan Africa; instead, much of what is known today comes either from censuses, which often are not particularly reliable or particularly detailed, or from small cross-sectional surveys, which often suffer from problems of nongeneralizability.[3]

---

[2]According to the most recent Global Internally Displaced Persons Survey, there are currently more than 12 million such persons in Africa (Internal Displacement Monitoring Center, 2006). In addition, at least 3 million refugees have fled their own countries to seek refuge in neighboring countries (United Nations High Commission for Refugees, 2006).

[3]The World Health Organization included 18 sub-Saharan African countries among the 72 in which World Health Surveys (WHS) were conducted in recent years (see Üstün et al., 2003). Data from these surveys are expected to be available shortly after the publication of this report. A further effort, the WHO Study on Global Aging (SAGE), is under way in six countries, two of which (Ghana and South Africa) are in sub-Saharan Africa. SAGE is planned to follow up respondents to the WHS over a 5-10 year period in order to, among other goals, study the determinants of health and health-related outcomes (see http://www.who.int/healthinfo/systems/sage/en/index3.html).

WORKSHOP ON AGING IN AFRICA

It is against this backdrop that in 2004 the National Institute on Aging asked the National Academies' Committee on Population to organize a workshop on advancing aging research in Africa. The workshop was to explore ways to promote U.S. research interests in aging in developing countries and to increase the capacity of sub-Saharan African governments and institutions to address the many challenges posed by the changing position of older persons in an era of AIDS. The workshop provided an opportunity for leading scientists from a variety of relevant disciplines to come together and review the evidence on economic security, health, and living conditions of older people and the ways in which critical changes are affecting their well-being.

The Committee on Population appointed an eight-member panel comprised of U.S. and African researchers. The panel had two charges: to develop the two-day workshop and to identify, subsequently, a research agenda aimed at gathering new data that would enable policy makers to better anticipate existing and changing needs of older people and to better assess the viability and potential impact of various public policy options.

In advance of the workshop, the panel commissioned 12 papers by prominent researchers to gather together recent research findings relevant to the goals of the workshop. These papers covered important domains of research on aging, including the changing demography of sub-Saharan Africa (Velkoff and Kowal), demographic impacts of the HIV epidemic on older people (Clark, Merli and Palloni, and Hosegood and Timaeus), formal and informal social security systems (Kaseke), health (Kahn et al., Kuhn et al., and Kuate-Defo), measurement (Kuhn et al.), the impact of social pensions (Lam et al. and Posel et al.), the situation of older people in urban areas (Ezeh et al.), living arrangements (Kuate-Defo and Ezeh et al.), and policy (Peachey and Nhongo). The primary focus of the workshop was to present and discuss recent studies using high-quality data from the region on the situation of older people. Selected papers from the workshop were revised and edited for inclusion in this volume. The workshop also included a focused discussion on data needs and future research directions. Thus, the principal inputs into this report are the panel's interpretation of the literature consulted,[4] the presentations of the commissioned papers, and the rich interactive discussion that occurred at the workshop.

---

[4]This report is not intended to be an exhaustive literature review of the entire field of aging. Rather it draws on a selected subset of the literature that relates to the material covered by the workshop papers and additional literature known to the primary authors of the report.

KEY THEMES

Five key themes emerged from the panel's original planning meeting, the workshop papers, and the workshop discussion. The first is the lack of basic, agreed-upon definitions crucial to the study of aging in sub-Saharan African societies. Most fundamentally, who is elderly in sub-Saharan Africa? Do the definitions used in industrialized societies have the same meaning for sub-Saharan Africa? And, in the African context, with its complex and extended family structure, what constitutes a household, the usual unit in which older people are studied (van de Walle, 2006)? Research can adequately assess the situation of older people in sub-Saharan Africa only if it is conducted in a framework that can allow for a full range of actors and impacts on the well-being of older people.

A second theme and persistent lament throughout the workshop is the lack of careful empirical research and the dearth of comprehensive data needed to rectify this situation. Third is the participants' belief that the situation of older people in sub-Saharan Africa is changing fairly rapidly. Fourth is the need to recognize the considerable diversity across sub-Saharan Africa with respect to a wide range of indicators. The final central theme is the need to support the development of local research capacity and facilitate research. Each of these themes is amplified below.

Definitions

When asked who is old, participants in recent focus group interviews in Nairobi claimed that old people can be identified in a variety of ways: by their physical attributes or appearance (e.g., gray hair, wrinkles, obvious frailty), by their life experiences (e.g., their reproductive history), or by the roles that they sometimes play in their community (see the paper by Ezeh et al. in this volume). Consequently, chronological age—which in any event may not even be known in sub-Saharan Africa—may be a poorer indicator of being elderly than social standing. Chronological age may also differ markedly from functional age, which can be the most important dimension of aging in a rural subsistence agricultural context. In general, it is important to recognize that in some sub-Saharan African settings, people who are younger than 60 may be considered old because they exhibit morbidity profiles and take on status roles more usually associated with people over the age of 60 in other settings.

Similar definitional problems surround the meaning of the term household (van de Walle, 2006). Due to the extended-family system, households are more likely to be larger, multigenerational, and less nuclear than in Western societies. For example, a recent study of household composition in Gabon found that about half of all households in Libreville and Port-Gentil contained at least one guest who had some sort of kinship tie to the family but who did not belong to the nuclear family (Rapoport, 2004). A similar situation can be found in a large number of sub-Saharan African countries. Households can also be split across geographic locations, with families maintaining both a rural home and an urban home. This situation frequently occurs when households decide to allocate their labor resources between rural and urban areas in order to diversify risk, maximize incomes, or both (Agesa, 2004; Lucas and Stark, 1985; Stark, 1991, 1995). Sub-Saharan African family structures complicate the study of older people's well-being, and basic definitional questions must be resolved before comparative analysis can take place easily.

Lack of Data

As stated above, research on aging in sub-Saharan Africa is still very much in its infancy. The current situation of older people in sub-Saharan Africa is, in fact, quite poorly known, and micro-level data are available only for a limited number of countries. The World Health Surveys and the follow-up Study on Global Aging (SAGE) will improve availability of data on health for some countries. Very little information is readily available for Francophone or Lusophone (Portuguese-speaking) Africa. In addition, the range of topics addressed at the workshop illustrates the need for multidisciplinary work that cuts across traditional research domains. In Asia, by contrast, a decade of in-depth and wide-ranging research on multiple aspects of peoples' lives has generated considerable insight into the situation of older people in that region (see, for example, Hermalin, 2002), which may well be able to inform the design and implementation of similar research in sub-Saharan Africa (Knodel, 2005).

The Changing Situation of Older People

Despite the lack of longitudinal studies, many observers believe that older people are worse off than they were in the past. There are a number of reasons why this might be the case, although there is currently very little empirical research that documents whether older people are worse or better off on most measures of welfare. Three dimensions of change that have bearing on the well-being of older persons were repeatedly raised throughout the two days of the workshop: demographic change, modernization and development, and the impact of HIV/AIDS.

Based on the demographic changes taking place, both the absolute size and the relative proportion of the population age 60 and over are projected over the next 25 years to grow faster than at all younger ages (Table 1-1,

TABLE 1-1 Demographic Indicators of Sub-Saharan Africa, Selected Years 1965-2030

	1965	1985	2005	2030	Change[a]		
					1965-1985	1985-2005	2005-2030
Population (in thousands)	255,825	448,051	751,273	1,248,262	2.8	2.6	2.0
Under age 15	113,333	204,441	326,715	462,431	2.9	2.3	1.4
Age 60 and over	12,513	20,961	36,594	71,033	2.6	2.8	2.7
Age 80 and over	652	1,211	2,626	6,550	3.1	3.9	3.7
Percentage of the Population							
Under age 15	44.3	45.6	43.5	37.0	2.9	-4.6	-14.9
Age 60 and over	4.9	4.7	4.9	5.7	-4.1	4.3	16.3
Age 80 and over	0.3	0.3	0.3	0.5	0.0	0.0	66.7
Median Age	17.9	17.1	18	21.2	-4.5	5.3	17.8
Total Fertility Rate[b]	6.8	6.7	5.5	3.6	-1.9	-17.7	-34.0
Life Expectancy at Birth[b]	41.4	48.6	45.9	55.4	17.4	-5.6	20.7
Male	39.9	46.9	45.2	54.5	17.5	-3.6	20.6
Female	42.9	50.2	46.6	56.2	17.0	-7.2	20.6
Dependency Ratio	89.7	94.3	87.2	69.0	5.1	-7.5	-20.9
Child dependency	84.1	88.7	81.4	62.6	5.5	-8.2	-23.1
Old age dependency	5.7	5.6	5.8	6.4	-0.7	3.1	10.4

[a]Change figures represent the annualized growth rate per 100 people between population estimates and projections and the percent change among all other indicators.

[b]Estimated for 5-year periods ending in the year indicated.

SOURCE: United Nations (2005).

and see Chapter 2). The increase in the population age 75 and over will be particularly noticeable.

Modernization and development have led to broad social and economic changes that put in doubt the continued viability of traditional arrangements for the care and support of older people. For example, formal education and modernization are generally associated with weakening traditional social ties and obligations and greater independence and autonomy, factors that tend to undermine traditional extended family systems. Similarly, economic development is associated with young people migrating from rural to urban areas, leaving older family members geographically isolated.[5] Once established in urban areas, migrants tend to form new nuclear households. Although children may remit money and goods, such flows are typically irregular and may not be enough to provide much in the way of real economic security. These changes have combined to alter, probably permanently, the nature of the relationship between generations.

The HIV/AIDS epidemic has severely affected many communities across sub-Saharan Africa, with multiple impacts on older people. The vast majority of the estimated 25.8 million people living with HIV are still in their prime wage-earning years—that is, at ages at which normally they would be expected to be not only wage earners but also the principal sources of financial and material support for older people and children in their families (Joint United Nations Programme on HIV/AIDS, 2006).

There is a substantial amount of uncertainty about the future course of the pandemic. While some positive news about gradual, modest declines in HIV prevalence are emerging from East Africa and Zimbabwe, HIV prevalence has soared in Southern Africa in recent years (Asamoah-Odei, Garcia Calleia, and Boerma, 2004; Joint United Nations Programme on HIV/AIDS, 2006). In some antenatal clinics in urban areas of Southern Africa, HIV prevalence rates as high as 25 percent have been recorded, whereas they were only around 5 percent in 1990. Very high HIV prevalence—almost 40 percent of pregnant women found to be HIV positive—has been recorded recently in Botswana and Swaziland (Asamoah-Odei et al., 2004). Increasingly, because of the HIV/AIDS epidemic, older people are being asked to provide emotional and economic support both to their own children, the immediate victims of the HIV/AIDS epidemic, and to their grandchildren (Makiwane, Schneider, and Gopane, 2004; Nyambedha, Wandibba, and Aagaard-Hansen, 2003; Williams and Tumwekwase, 2001).

While modernization theory has been the most prominent theoretical

---

[5]For more information on cohort-specific rural-urban migration in Africa, see Becker and Grewe (1996).

framework used to explain the ongoing changes in family support to older people in Africa, some African gerontologists have criticized the theory, arguing that it is overly deterministic and simplistic (see, for example, Ferreira, 1999). Recently, contemporary African researchers have adopted alternative theoretical frameworks to better understand how ongoing economic and social changes are affecting older people.

For example, some researchers have suggested an alternative explanation for a possible decline in material support for older persons: rising economic hardship (Aboderin, 2004; Nyambedha et al., 2003). Sub-Saharan Africa faces a greater set of development challenges than any other major region of the world, and, on average, income per capita is now lower than it was at the end of the 1960s (World Bank, 2006a, 2006b). Although the region's per capita gross national income has grown at a rate of around 3 percent per year for the past two years, it still stands at only $600 per year. An estimated 516 million people in the region are forced to survive on less than $2 a day, and 303 million on less than $1 a day (World Bank, 2006a, 2006b). In contrast to such countries as China and India, where substantial progress has been made over the past 5 years in combating poverty, the number of extremely poor people in sub-Saharan Africa has almost doubled since 1981 (World Bank, 2005). Consequently, sub-Saharan Africa is home to a growing share of the world's absolute poor (United Nations, 2006). Thus, rather than emphasizing weakening filial obligations, some researchers have argued that declines in support for older people may simply reflect a growing incapacity on the part of the younger generation (see, for example, Aboderin, 2004). Increasingly, it appears that sub-Saharan African societies are being asked to cope with population aging and a catastrophic health crisis with neither a comprehensive formal social security system nor a well-functioning traditional care system in place.

Diversity Across the Region

The second largest and the second most populous continent in the world, the diversity across sub-Saharan Africa is apparent in the region's physical geography and climate, in its plurality of cultural heritages, official and native languages, traditions, beliefs, religions, and value systems, in its modes of production and levels of economic development, and in its diverse social and political structures. Differences across countries and cultures make generalization from small-scale studies quite problematic, and the current lack of long-term comparable data from multiple sites hinders the ability to make meaningful cross-country comparisons. This heterogeneity also implies that cross-country comparisons are never going to be possible without careful longitudinal and multidisciplinary research designs. At the same time, because many countries are now in the early stages of adapting to their changing population age structures and because current and prospective policy responses are likely to differ among countries, it may be possible to take advantage of this diversity to design a number of natural experiments enabling countries to learn from other's experiences (see for example, Knight and Sabot, 1990). Thus, sub-Saharan African countries that are beginning to experience population aging may learn from those whose demographic shift began earlier. Similarly, the experiences of African governments that implement some form of social protection scheme can inform others contemplating a similar program.

Need to Develop Local Research Capacity and Facilitate Research

A current list of local hurdles to research includes lack of access to adequate funding for research and lack of highly skilled local researchers to do the work, as well as sometimes difficult administrative barriers to carrying out research. Even in industrially advanced countries, amassing the resources required to undertake multifaceted research endeavors can be extremely complicated and time-consuming, but these difficulties are multiplied many-fold in sub-Saharan Africa. Many universities in the region have been badly neglected for decades. Their limited budgets are spent predominantly on (entirely inadequate) salaries, leaving few resources for maintaining facilities or equipment, purchasing computers or other basic office supplies, or initiating and sustaining a long-term research program. Consequently, much of the best research on aging in sub-Saharan Africa has been undertaken only with technical cooperation and foreign assistance from the international community. In the long run, it is essential to help sub-Saharan African countries develop their own research capacity by strengthening their universities and by augmenting the skills of their researchers.

The current dependence on international partners is not without its own controversies. While many donor agencies emphasize the importance of capacity building, the net result of their investments in this area in the past has often been quite modest (Commission for Africa, 2005). External researchers and funding agencies may design research projects that may not align closely with the priorities of national governments. They may also design them on a fairly short (2-year) time frame, which, while appropriate for accomplishing immediate research objectives, may not be sufficient to build sustainable in-country research capacity. Furthermore, while most people would agree that collaborations involving scientists from both the north and the south are vital to making sustained scientific progress, there is still a great deal of debate and uncertainty as to what constitutes "fair scientific partnerships" (Tollman, 2004). Essentially this refers to the way that different scientists and institutions allocate the benefits and obligations of collaborative ventures, including allocation of funds, division of research roles, extent of data sharing, and method of ascribing authorship and related credits.

Even with good collaboration and adequate funding for research, investigators frequently are confronted with unwieldy procedures for obtaining permission to carry out the research. These may take the form of institutional review boards that are unfamiliar with social science research or government agencies that are slow to respond to requests for approval or multiple agencies that must be convinced of the value of the work to be undertaken and which may have agendas that do not give high priority to aging research.

KEY AREAS FOR FUTURE RESEARCH

The aging of individuals and populations and the changing position and well-being of older people in sub-Saharan Africa present a set of key challenges for African nations to begin to address. Yet evidence and a strong knowledge base of information on the nature and dynamics of poverty, health, social support networks, and the changing roles and responsibilities of older people and their implications are lacking. To fill this gap and provide information vital to the development of appropriate policies and programs, there is urgent need for an enhanced research effort on aging in sub-Saharan Africa, pursuing a variety of data collection strategies and analytic approaches.

Five key areas of research—all closely interrelated—emerged as essential to the advancement of understanding of the situation of older people in sub-Saharan Africa and as necessary precursors to the development of sound aging policy in the region. These are (1) income, wealth, and expenditure; (2) health and well-being; (3) the nature of family support and social networks; (4) the changing roles and responsibilities of older people as a function of the AIDS crisis; and (5) the nature and role of various kinds of formal and informal social protection schemes. Some discussion of each of these topics is provided below. In each case, a rationale for why a particular theme was included is provided, along with a discussion of measurement problems and selected findings from recent research on each topic, including findings from the papers included in this volume.

Income, Wealth, and Expenditure

Critical to assessing the impact of programs intended to assist older persons in poverty is the ability to measure living standards and to monitor how they change over time. Even in the poorest sub-Saharan African agrarian economies in which the great majority of the population is absolutely poor, inequality can be considerable, so that some households are substantially better off than others (House, 1991; House and Phillips-Howard, 1990; de Savigney et al., 2005). In such economic systems, the household is typically conceived of as the decision-making unit whose principal input is the labor of household members and the principal objective is to achieve self-sufficiency in basic food production (see Chayanov, 1925).

Although several countries have participated in the World Bank's Living Standards Measurement Study or conducted other forms of ad hoc cross-sectional surveys of income, expenditure, and consumption to provide a snapshot of household living standards at a given point in time (see, for example, National Bureau of Statistics [Tanzania], 2002; National Statistics Office [Malawi], 2005), virtually no sub-Saharan African country regularly collects nationally representative household-level survey data to monitor trends in household income and expenditure over time. More typically, the period between surveys is 10 years or more, and in some sub-Saharan African countries there has not been a large-scale, nationally representative household survey for decades.

The measurement of the economic well-being of older people in sub-Saharan Africa is complicated by a number of conceptual and practical issues. Economists have traditionally relied on income as the most important indicator of economic status at a point in time. Measuring individual or household income in sub-Saharan Africa can be very challenging, however, particularly in communities in which a significant fraction of the population is still engaged in subsistence agriculture.[6] In most surveys of income and expenditure, rates of nonresponse to questions related to earnings tend to be high and nonrandom, and sources of income that are infrequent (such as crops that are harvested only in periods of drought or cash remittances from distant family members) can easily be missed or underreported.

Further compounding these measurement problems, older people in sub-Saharan Africa typically do not live alone; they live with other family members (see van de Walle, 2006, and the papers by Lam et al. and Ezeh et al. in this volume). Households containing only older people constitute a very small percentage of households in sub-Saharan Africa (Kakwani and Subbarao, 2005). Resources that come into households are typically shared in some fashion among various household members, and it is often extremely difficult, if not impossible, to determine how these resources are divided (Deaton and Paxson, 1992). A common supposition in the development literature is that prime-age adults who bring money into a household

---

[6]It should also not be forgotten that nomadic pastoralism remains an important subsistence system in many parts of Africa. For a discussion of the social and economic organization of pastoral societies, see Deng (1984) and McCabe (2004).

receive better treatment than older people or others who make only in-kind contributions to household well-being, but there is little empirical evidence to support this conjecture (Behrman, 1997; Deaton and Paxson, 1992). In many cases, surveys simply take the household as the unit of observation in which case any analysis of differential treatment of certain members in the household becomes impossible.

A further problem with using current income as a measure of economic well-being is that it may not be closely correlated with total wealth, which may be a better indicator of economic security or future consumption. Yet obtaining accurate information about wealth can be even more challenging than measuring current income. In many sub-Saharan African settings, household wealth can be gauged only in terms of possessions of basic household items (such as tables, chairs, beds, mosquito nets, shoes), housing type (i.e., the type of construction materials used to build the house), or the number of animals or amount of landholdings. In practice, these measures have not always been good predictors of consumption per adult (Montgomery, Gragnolati, Burke, and Paredes, 2000).

In sub-Saharan Africa, attention is often focused less on levels of household income and inequality than on the proportion of households that fail to surpass a certain poverty threshold. This is not as straightforward an assessment as one might first expect because, among other things, it requires a well-accepted definition of poverty. An enormous amount of work has been undertaken over the years to conceptualize and measure poverty. Perhaps the main controversy that has arisen over how to identify the poor relates to the issue of whether poverty should be considered an absolute or a relative measure. A common approach, the origins of which can be traced back to Rowntree's study of the population of York, England, at the turn of the 20th century, is to identify a poverty line on the basis of nutritional standards, a basic diet, and the opinions of the potentially poor themselves as to their minimum requirements for expenditure on nonfood items (Rowntree, 1901). This "basic needs" approach has been widely adopted in studies on poverty in sub-Saharan Africa (see, for example, National Bureau of Statistics [Tanzania], 2002). But for policy-building purposes, it is also important to be able to deconstruct the various dimensions of poverty and to determine the prevalence of each of these among older people.

Kakwani and Subbarao (2005) recently investigated differences in the prevalence of poverty by household composition. Drawing on available recent household survey information collected over the period 1998-2001, the authors present a profile of older people in 15 low-income sub-Saharan African countries. The sample included countries in East and West Africa, Francophone and Anglophone countries, and countries with various levels of HIV prevalence and incidence. The sample countries can be taken as broadly representative of the region. The authors found that households containing older persons only or older persons and children only have higher income shortfalls than households with no older people, and the differences are statistically significant in most cases (Kakwani and Subbarao, 2005). Furthermore, the size of the gap among households headed by older people is much higher than those not headed by older people. There are also significant rural-urban differences, with a much higher proportion of single older people who are poor in rural areas compared with urban areas in every country.

In summary, evidence on income, wealth, and expenditure in sub-Saharan Africa that is derived from (small-scale) household survey data currently has important limitations of coverage and content when used as a gauge of the economic status of older people (Barrientos, Gorman, and Heslop, 2003). Qualitative studies, such as those sponsored by the World Bank and others in the late 1990s and early 2000s, provide a basic picture of household living standards, but they do not focus explicitly on the condition of older people. When investigations have included older people, they reveal that poverty in old age is associated with poor access to paid work, basic services, and social networks, and there is a close relationship between older people's ability to contribute to traditional roles and responsibilities and their ability to access support (Barrientos et al., 2003).

Income and expenditure studies also typically find that women have lower incomes than men, and that female-headed households are more prone to poverty than male-headed households. Building on that finding, the paper by Kuate-Defo in this volume uses unique data from Cameroon to examine the extent and nature of gender inequalities in health in later life and the extent to which these inequalities can be explained by differences in the socioeconomic characteristics and living arrangements of older women and men. Documenting important gender differences in self-rated health and functional limitations, the author found a strong association between poor health and low socioeconomic status. But more research is needed on the health and socioeconomic status of elderly women, particularly those who are widowed and childless, who may be especially vulnerable to poverty.[7] Parts of sub-Saharan Africa are still heavily patriarchal, and in such societies the status of women can be very low. Women may lack certain rights of ownership to property, and inheritance is through the male side of the family (Toulmin, 2006). Consequently, upon their husband's death, widows are at risk of dispossession of their house and land by their dead husband's kin.

---

[7]Because women tend to marry men who are older and because they remarry less frequently upon divorce or the death of their spouse, the percentage of women widowed at any given age tends to be higher than the corresponding statistic for men.

Health and Well-Being

In sub-Saharan Africa, good health and nutrition are often emphasized as critical components of basic needs. In 1978, African delegates joined the representatives of other nations in endorsing the Declaration of Alma Ata, which committed all governments throughout the world to the common goal of achieving health for all by the year 2000. This goal included ensuring a life that was both long and free of a heavy burden of illness. It is well known that mortality rates increase at older ages, along with functional limitations and chronic conditions. But given the extremely limited resources available for health services in sub-Saharan Africa, most public health programs on the continent are far more concerned with eradicating or at least controlling preventable childhood diseases, such as measles and diarrhea, than they are with treating chronic diseases or managing the health care of the frail elderly. This is hardly surprising given that more than one out of every six children in sub-Saharan Africa dies before their fifth birthday (Lopez et al., 2006) and that the vast majority of these deaths are preventable with very low-cost interventions such as oral rehydration salts and vaccinations that cost just a few cents each. Furthermore, the HIV/AIDS pandemic continues to take an extremely heavy toll on the young adult population. In Southern Africa, for example, life expectancy at birth has fallen from 62 to 48, and it is projected to decrease further to 43 over the next decade (Joint United Nations Programme on HIV/AIDS, 2006). For most sub-Saharan African ministries of health, the challenges prior to old age are simply overwhelming.

Despite efforts in a number of sub-Saharan African countries to decentralize their health care budgets and realign health care expenditures to emphasize prevention rather than care, most countries still spend a significant fraction of their total health care budgets treating adult illness (Feachem et al., 1992; Poullier, Hernandez, and Kawabata, 2003; Tollman, Doherty, and Mulligan, 2006). The average sub-Saharan African country spends approximately 5.5 percent of gross domestic product on health care, of which perhaps half is spent on hospital care (Poullier, Hernandez, Kawabata, and Savedoff, 2003). Given that some African countries achieve substantially better population health outcomes than others on similar budget constraints, there is reason to believe that a substantial proportion of health resources in some countries could be better programmed (Murray and Evans, 2003; Laxminarayan, Chou, and Shahid-Salles, 2006). But in order to improve the allocation of resources, it is first necessary to understand the nature of health problems that given age groups face and how they are evolving over time.

From comprehensive assessments of the changing global burden of disease, sub-Saharan African governments can anticipate that, as their populations age, the observed pattern of disease will change: noncommunicable diseases, such as depression and heart disease, and injuries will become more important, and infectious diseases and malnutrition will become proportionately less important causes of disability and premature death (Lopez et al., 2006; Omram, 1971). In 2001, communicable, maternal, perinatal, and nutritional conditions accounted for 70 percent of the burden of disease in sub-Saharan Africa, while noncommunicable diseases and injuries accounted for 21 and 8 percent, respectively (Lopez et al., 2006). On the basis of 1990 data, Murray and Lopez (1996) predicted that communicable diseases will decline to around 40 percent of the burden of disease (as measured in disability-adjusted life-years) by 2020 in Africa, while noncommunicable diseases and injuries will grow. However, life expectancy in sub-Saharan Africa was 6 years lower in 2001 than it was in 1990 (Lopez et al., 2006), reinforcing the point that a considerable degree of uncertainty surrounds the estimates of the burden of disease there (see Cooper, Osotimehin, Kaufman, and Forrester, 1998; Mathers et al., 2006) and, in any event, may not reflect conditions that prevail among the poorest deciles of the population (Gwatkin, Guillot, and Heuveline, 1999). Furthermore, scholars are still divided on the extent to which sub-Saharan Africa's health transition will traverse a unique path. In their paper in this volume, Kahn et al. document the rising burden of chronic disease and associated risk factors affecting older persons simultaneously, with worsening infections and illness affecting younger adults. Consequently, there is growing recognition that classic epidemiological transition theory is inadequate to explain the patterns of health and disease emerging in rural sub-Saharan Africa. The study of health in later life should also include understanding the changing physical and cognitive functioning of older people and its implications on the demand for health care services.

While there is a need to describe and monitor patterns of ill health and disability among older people in sub-Saharan Africa as well as monitor the health of other household members who may be under the care of older people and to better understand the relationships between health and poverty, there are numerous challenges to measuring health status in social surveys (see Thomas and Frankenberg, 2002, and the paper by Kuate-Defo in this volume for a more complete treatment of these issues). Assessing an individual's health in the field can be difficult and add considerable expense to any survey, particularly if it involves the use of trained medical professionals. There may also be thorny ethical issues to overcome if blood or any other biological measures are to be collected, analyzed, and stored. Because they tend to be easy and inexpensive to collect and because they have been found in numerous contexts to be quite useful predictors of future mortality, self-reported responses to questions about health status tend to be the mainstay of health status measurement in social surveys in other parts of the world.

One problem with self-reported health, however, is that it can be sensitive to the cultural context in which it is collected, so that cross-country comparisons of the relative extent of ill health in two different communities can lead to false conclusions. For this reason, over the past 10 years, researchers have attempted to increase the comparability of self-reported health status measures by the use of anchored vignettes (Murray et al., 2002, 2003; Salomon, Tandon, and Murray, 2003). Anchored vignettes may enable researchers to create a common metric to enable more reliable analysis of cross-cultural variations in ill health, thereby strengthening the reliability and usefulness of self-reported measures of health as a measure of well-being. (See the paper by Kuhn et al. in this volume for a further discussion of the pros and cons of using self-reported measures of health in social surveys.)

A potential challenge to using self-reported measures of health in sub-Saharan Africa has to do with the fact that illness and disease can be viewed as both cultural and as biomedical constructs. Consequently, there is a wide range of ways that people perceive and treat different illnesses in sub-Saharan Africa. For example, a recent analysis of Mozambican refugees' understanding of stroke-like symptoms found that such symptoms are considered to be both a physical and a social condition (SASPI Team, 2004). Consequently, most people with stroke-like symptoms in that community seek treatment both from Western-trained doctors and from healers or prophets (SASPI Team, 2004).

Finally, in order to understand the determinants of health and disability among older people, health care researchers in sub-Saharan Africa not only need to understand the general socioeconomic, cultural, and environment conditions, but they also need to understand how patterns of health care utilization are changing over time. Sub-Saharan African governments typically struggle to provide health care services to older people in rural areas who still tend to have far poorer access to any kind of service relative to urban dwellers. Furthermore, in many sub-Saharan African communities, traditional medicine is often the only affordable and even the only available source of health care to large sections of the population. Across sub-Saharan Africa, traditional healers outnumber allopathic medical practitioners by more than 50 to 1 (Addae-Mensah, 2005).

The above discussion highlights the need for a better understanding of the magnitude and underlying causes of ill health and morbidity among older people in sub-Saharan Africa, how these patterns are evolving over time, and the implications of those changes for older people, their families, and patterns of health care utilization over time.

The Nature of Family Support and Social Networks

The projected increase in the absolute numbers of older people in sub-Saharan Africa, particularly the projected rise in the oldest old, as well as the projected growth in the proportion of the general population over age 60 are likely to have profound implications for families and kin networks. Hence a major question for policy makers is whether the traditional family in sub-Saharan Africa can cope successfully with the demographic, health, social, and economic changes that are taking place and can continue to provide older people with the range of support that they need. At the moment, traditional support systems, based on family and kinship ties, represent a way of life for most people in sub-Saharan Africa. Economically active adults in the family or kinship network provide support to children, older people, and others who are unable to care for themselves. Social protection is the natural outcome of commonly shared principles of solidarity, reciprocity, and redistribution in an extended family.

As discussed earlier, economic development and modernization are also associated with a range of economic and social changes that combine to weaken social networks that traditionally provide care and support in later life. Migration of young people from the rural areas to the towns, for example, can leave older family members geographically and socially more isolated. Formal education also provides a major counterpoint to the family in the socialization of the young. Schools have enormous potential to influence the values, expectations, and behaviors of the young and tend to weaken traditional social ties and obligations and place greater emphasis on independent thinking and autonomy, factors that tend to undermine traditional extended family systems (National Research Council and Institute of Medicine, 2005). In addition, the AIDS epidemic has placed enormous strains on traditional institutions.

To examine changes in societal arrangements for the support of older people, one starting point, albeit imperfect, that demographers have used extensively in other settings is trends in living arrangements. Such analyses can be particularly complex in sub-Saharan Africa due to the variety of household structures, including resident and nonresident household members and multiple household memberships (see van de Walle, 2006). Zimmer and Dayton (2005) examined data from Demographic and Health Surveys conducted in 24 countries and found substantial variation in household composition. The authors found that 59 percent of older adults in sub-Saharan Africa live with a child and 46 percent with a grandchild. The authors also found that older adults are more likely to be living with orphans in countries with high AIDS-related mortality (Zimmer and Dayton, 2005).

The net implications of economic development on the welfare of older persons in sub-Saharan Africa are extremely difficult to determine. The general view among African researchers working in this area is that the situation of older people is getting worse. Although there are a number of reasons why this might be the case, not all social changes are necessarily detrimental. It therefore is an empirical question as to whether the situation of older people has improved or worsened. Migration and urbanization, for example, are frequently charged with leading to a breakdown of traditional family structures that weaken the position of older people. But in a largely subsistence agriculture economy with surplus labor, the absence of a family member due to migration may be a net loss or a net benefit to household welfare. Conventional microeconomic models of rural-urban migration are based on the premise that migration is an individual response to a higher expected urban income (Todaro, 1969). However, in sub-Saharan Africa labor migration may also be the outcome of a family or household-level decision to diversify sources of household income, lower total household risk, or a rational response to imperfect rural credit markets (see, for example, Stark, 1991, 1995). Work on intergenerational remittances in Botswana, for example, supports the view that migrants can sometimes be considered as members of a single household that is spatially split between two locations (Lucas and Stark, 1985).

More work is needed that builds on new as well as existing analytical frameworks in order to develop testable hypotheses related to the pathways and mechanisms by which the forces of modernization and change are affecting traditional social relations.

Changing Roles and Responsibilities of Older People in an Era of AIDS

No analysis of the situation of older people in sub-Saharan Africa would be complete without acknowledgment of the fact that the region is experiencing a very severe HIV/AIDS pandemic with important implications for older people. The region is home to more than 60 percent of all people living with HIV, around 25.8 million in 2005 (Joint United Nations Programme on HIV/AIDS, 2006). And since the start of the epidemic, HIV/AIDS has infected roughly 50 million Africans, of whom more than 22 million have already died. Even if new transmissions were halted today, millions of Africans who are currently infected would still develop AIDS and die over the next 5 to 10 years. As noted above, in some southern African countries, life expectancy has fallen from 62 years in 1990-1995 to 48 years in 2000-2005 and is projected to decrease further to 43 years over the next decade (United Nations, 2005).

While it is important to remember that HIV/AIDS prevalence remains quite variable across the region, where it is prevalent, the epidemic can affect the lives of older people in many different ways. Knodel et al. (2003)

have developed a framework to examine a broad range of potential pathways through which AIDS can adversely affect the well-being of parents of adult children with AIDS and their possible demographic, psychological, economic, or social consequences (see Table 1-2). Although developed based on the authors' experience with AIDS in Asia, it offers a useful starting point for formulating the issues in an African setting. Older people most directly affected by the epidemic are likely to be either infected by the virus themselves or parents of infected adult-age children. Not only do parents of adult children with AIDS have to face the pain of seeing their own children suffer and die, but they can also face serious economic hardship, both in the short term due to unforeseen medical expenses and funeral costs and in the long term due to being deprived of one of their primary sources of economic support in old age. In addition, older people, particularly elderly women, are also frequently left to care for grandchildren. Thus these older people face the double burden of having to replace lost sources of income while supporting additional family members.

Older people may also suffer indirect health consequences, such as the mental and physical fatigue associated with caregiving, additional labor force participation, exposure to TB or other opportunistic infections brought into the household by the person with HIV, and stigmatization and isolation following the death of household members due to AIDS (Dayton and Ainsworth, 2004; Knodel et al., 2003; World Health Organization, 2002). AIDS is also likely to have important indirect impacts on society in general, such as the demand and availability of health services, per capita income growth, and macroeconomic performance (National Research Council, 1996).

Finally, older people may be directly affected by the virus themselves. Approximately 6 percent of officially reported AIDS cases in Africa in 1999 affected people age 50 or older (Knodel et al., 2003). (The official number of AIDS cases worldwide is widely acknowledged to represent merely the tip of the iceberg with regard to the true extent of the epidemic, but it is the only readily available source of data for comparing caseloads by age.) But with more than 1 in every 10 adults in Africa estimated to be HIV positive, far more older people in Africa are being affected indirectly by sickness and death among the younger generation, which can have many direct and indirect consequences for their material well-being.

While most of the attention to date has focused on how the pandemic affects persons with HIV and their surviving orphans, greater recognition needs to be given to the consequences of the pandemic for older people, who in many cases are playing critical roles as caregivers for the sick and guardians for orphaned grandchildren left behind. There is still very little research on the impact of HIV/AIDS on older people in sub-Saharan Africa. The papers by Clark, Merli and Palloni, and Hosegood and Timaeus use a variety of research strategies to help fill this gap. The chapter by Hosegood and Timaeus, for example, uses micro-level household data to establish a baseline from which they can examine the impact of HIV on older people in rural KwaZulu-Natal in South Africa, the country in the region with both the highest proportion of old people and one of the severest AIDS epidemics. The authors point out that, partly as a function of a generous social pension program and high rates of rural unemployment and underemployment, older people have maintained their traditional role as a major resource in society, caring for children and maintaining rural households even prior to the HIV epidemic. A recent study of the experiences and needs of older people in Mpumalanga, South Africa, supports this contention. The authors of that study found that almost one in three older people are either now caring for sick adults living in the household or are raising grandchildren whose own parents are either dead or away in the cities on a long-term basis (Makiwane et al., 2004). And 60 percent of all orphans in Mpumalanga are being cared for by their grandparents (Makiwane et al., 2004).

In the absence of detailed longitudinal data, simulation models can be employed to provide critical insights into how the AIDS epidemic may impact certain key demographic variables, such as residential patterns and kinship networks over a protracted period. In their chapters in this volume, Clark and Merli and Palloni use micro- and macromodel-based approaches to examine the likely number of orphans, residential patterns, and kin relations that might result from a severe epidemic.

Formal and Informal Forms of Social Protection[8]

While policy makers in sub-Saharan Africa are becoming increasingly aware of the needs of older people, there is general agreement that the types of social welfare programs in place in other parts of the world are too expensive to replicate in sub-Saharan Africa given the size of their economies (Kalasa, 2001). Thus there is a need to search for alternative approaches that might achieve a similar function but at lower cost.

The concept of social protection is one that is gaining increasing attention in development circles as a useful policy framework for addressing issues of poverty and vulnerability (Garcia and Gruat, 2003). Traditionally in sub-Saharan Africa, social protection for older people is provided by both formal and informal programs and practices that have been developed to reduce poverty and vulnerability in old age. But with per capita income

---

[8]Because no paper on this subject is included in this volume, this section contains an expanded discussion of social protection in sub-Saharan Africa.

TABLE 1-2 Potential Pathways Through Which AIDS Epidemic Can Adversely Affect the Well-Being of Parents of Adult Children with AIDS and Their Possible Specific Consequences

Potential Pathway	Dimension of Well-Being and Possible Specific Consequence (See codes for possible specific consequence below.)			
	Emotional/ Psychological	Economic/ Financial	Physical Health	Social
Caregiving	A, B, C	A	A, B	A, B, C
Coresidence	A, C	—	B	B
Providing financial/material support during illness	C	B, C	C	—
Sponsoring the funeral	C, D	B, C	C	—
Fostering grandchildren	C, D	B, C	C	A, B, C
Loss of child	D, E	D, E	—	—
Negative community reaction	C	F	—	B, D

Possible specific consequences
I. Emotional/psychological
  A. Psychological pain of seeing suffering and decline of health of person who dies of AIDS (PDA)
  B. Feeling overwhelmed by caregiving demands
  C. Psychological pain from anticipated or enacted negative community reaction
  D. Anxiety concerning economic security
  E. Grief from loss of PDA

II. Economic/financial
   A. Opportunity cost of time taken from economic activities
   B. Indebtedness from borrowing money to cover expenses
   C. Depletion of savings or sale of assets to cover expenses
   D. Disruption of PDAs contributions to parents' household
   E. Loss of future support when parents are in old age
   F. Loss of business from former customers out of fear of contagion
III. Physical health
   A. Physical efforts required by caregiving
   B. Risk of exposure to HIV (very low) or opportunistic diseases (especially tuberculosis)
   C. Strain of additional economic activity needed to cover expenses
IV. Social
   A. Time taken away from social activities
   B. Avoidance of social contact by others
   C. Strained intrafamilial relations
   D. Strained social relations

SOURCE: Knodel et al. (2003). Reproduced with permission.

below a few hundred dollars in most sub-Saharan African countries, it is no surprise to find that formal social security systems across the region cover only a small fraction of the population. Except for Mauritius and the Seychelles and a few countries in Southern Africa, including South Africa, Botswana, Lesotho, and Namibia, all of which operate social pension schemes aimed at comprehensive coverage, most countries' formal social security programs never reach the urban or rural poor. Except for these few countries, the extended family unit remains the main source of support for the vast majority of older people in sub-Saharan Africa when they can no longer work.

Social Security Programs

In many Western countries, formal social security is an important policy instrument for governments to redistribute wealth, combat poverty, and reduce inequalities between various segments of society. But in sub-Saharan Africa, current social security schemes are extremely marginal both in terms of percentage of the labor force that is covered and the size of pensions that are received. In most sub-Saharan African settings, national social insurance schemes cover less than 5 percent of the labor force and expend less than 1.5 percent of their gross domestic product on pensions (Fox and Palmer, 2001). Consequently, in the majority of countries in sub-Saharan Africa, social protection programs have a very modest effect on poverty alleviation. The largest social protection programs for older people in sub-Saharan Africa are occupational pension schemes, but these typically cover only people who have worked in the public sector, in state enterprises, or in large private firms in the modern sector. The self-employed, workers in the informal sector, domestic workers, and the vast majority of the population living in rural areas and engaged in subsistence agriculture or other forms of subsistence living, such as nomadic pastoralism, are still excluded from formal social security schemes and must rely on their families for support and protection when they can no longer work.

Bailey (2004) identifies several distinct patterns of social protection schemes that have developed in sub-Saharan Africa. Even though most countries did not introduce programs until after their independence, most schemes have been strongly influenced by their countries' colonial heritage, with the types of programs in Anglophone Africa differing from those in Francophone Africa. At one end of the spectrum are countries, for example South Africa, that have introduced schemes aimed at near universal coverage. Other countries currently provide no form of social security, either because nothing has been set up yet or because previously established schemes have been dismantled or disrupted for various reasons, including, not infrequently, armed conflict. Apart from government schemes, voluntary private pensions can also be found in many countries, although, again, their coverage tends to be restricted to formal sector workers. Most sub-Saharan African pension schemes are financed by contributions made by both employers and employees, with the contribution rate in most cases being higher for the employer. In the case of South Africa's social pension, the scheme is financed through general tax revenue. Given the structure of the schemes and the nature of the labor force in most sub-Saharan African countries, the vast majority of those actually covered by formal social security schemes are neither the poorest of the poor nor women.

In West Africa, several Francophone countries established a voluntary plan during the colonial period for government employees: for example, the West African Retirement Pensions Fund was modeled on a program for French civil servants that linked benefits to length of service and average earnings (Bailey and Turner, 2002). Even today, Senegal has a social security program that determines benefits through a formula that is quite similar to the system used in France (Bailey and Turner, 2002). Cote d'Ivoire, Mali, and other countries in the region have similar defined-benefit programs, with workers contributing between 4 and 9 percent of their earnings to the schemes (Bailey and Turner, 2002).

Social security programs in the countries that were former British colonies are generally more modest than those in Francophone Africa. In several former British colonies, provident funds, such as the Nigerian National Provident Fund, were established. These were seen as relatively easy to operate and amounted to compulsory interest-bearing individual savings accounts for workers that were financed from contributions from both employees and employers (Bailey, 2004). Unlike most social security programs, which typically offer survivor and disability benefits, most provident funds generally provide only a single lump-sum amount at retirement. Generally the level of the lump-sum payment is extremely modest and cannot actually support anyone in retirement. In 1993-1994, for example, retirees enrolled in the Zambian National Provident Fund each received, on average, a lump-sum payment of around US$10 (Mukuka et al., 2002). In a number of countries, for example, Ghana, Nigeria, and Zambia, these early provident funds have now been converted to defined-benefit social security systems.

In some countries, including Sierra Leone, Eritrea, and Somalia, efforts to introduce schemes have been stalled by armed conflicts. In other places, for example Liberia and the Democratic Republic of the Congo, whatever social security programs that once existed have been effectively dismantled and destroyed by armed conflicts.

Finally, a few countries have universal social security programs. Botswana, for example, has a universal flat-rate pension scheme for all residents over the age of 65. South Africa has a means-tested benefit for women age 60 and over and men age 65 and over, and Mauritius offers a basic pension to all residents age 60 or older with supplemented earnings-related benefits (Bailey, 2004). The South African pension scheme was introduced in 1928 as a measure to provide for the poorest retired white workers. The State Pension was extended to all South Africans in 1944, and the value was equalized for all segments of society in 1993 shortly before the first democratic elections in 1994.

In addition to various types of occupational pension schemes that are contributory, some sub-Saharan African countries administer minimal public assistance or social welfare assistance programs to the needy. In Zimbabwe, for example, the government operates a Social Welfare Assistance Scheme that provides assistance to older persons, persons with disabilities, and the chronically ill (Kaseke, 2004). A similar scheme operates in Zambia, the Public Welfare Assistance Scheme, providing benefits to such vulnerable groups as older persons, widows, and the unemployed (Kaseke, 2004). These schemes are far less well documented than contributory pension schemes or provident funds: the amount of assistance provided is typically very small and the coverage of these programs is generally extremely low (Kaseke, 2004).

Problems with Social Security Schemes

Formal social security schemes in sub-Saharan Africa are riddled with a number of well-known problems, including low coverage of the labor force, corruption, and inadequate benefits that are not indexed for inflation. Where occupational pension schemes or provident funds exist, they are only available to a small percentage of workers who have regular paid employment in the formal sector of the economy. In Tanzania, for example, Mchomvu et al. (2002) estimate that formal social security schemes currently cover only 6 percent of the population and about 5 percent of the active labor force, the majority of those covered being men. Schemes are also frequently characterized as suffering from poor and inefficient management and much bureaucracy, leading to high administrative costs, lack of transparency, low or even negative real rates of return on investments, and delays in receiving benefits. In some cases, the number of staff employed to administer the programs is so large that the administrative and management expenses of the fund exceed the investment income. At one point, the Zambian National Provident Fund, the main public scheme in Zambia until January 2000, had more than 1,300 employees. In 1995, administrative expenditures accounted for more than 100 percent of total revenue from contributions (Mukuka et al., 2002). In other cases, the bureaucratic machinery to administer these programs is so unwieldy that it severely hampers the effectiveness of the program. In Uganda and Zimbabwe, for example, the manual processing of claims, combined with the many stages that a claim needs to go through before payment is dispersed, leads to long delays for legitimate recipients waiting to receive their benefits (Dhemba et al., 2002; Kasente et al., 2002). Rates of interest awarded annually to members of provident funds have invariably been negative in real terms, and the lump sums paid out generally represent no more than a few months' earnings (Mchomvu et al., 2002). In addition to these problems, the devaluation of local currencies necessitated by structural adjustment programs has severely eroded the value of benefits in some countries (Kaseke, 2004).

South African Pension Program

No discussion of social protection of older people in sub-Saharan Africa would be complete without a description of the South African social pension program, which is quite unusual in sub-Saharan Africa with respect to its level of coverage and generosity of benefit (Case and Deaton, 1998). South African women age 60 or older and South African men age 65 and older may apply for a state pension irrespective of employment history. In 2006, the state pension was R820 per month (roughly US$115). The pension is means-tested, but the level is set at a point at which 80 percent of all age-eligible Africans may receive the pension (Lam et al., in this volume). Essentially a by-product of the dismantling of the apartheid system, the program, which was originally designed to provide protection for poor whites, is viewed in South Africa today as a way to achieve several broad development goals: providing assistance to households in rural areas, targeting women, and keeping significant numbers of households out of poverty (Ardington and Lund, 1995). It is the sole or major source of income for many poverty-stricken families (van Zyl, 2003).

A considerable body of research has been conducted on the effects of such a large and generous transfer scheme on the welfare of older people and extended family members (Alderman, 1999; Ardington and Lund, 1995; Bertrand, Mullainathan, and Miller, 2003; Case, 2001; Case and Deaton, 1998; Duflo, 2003; Ferreira, 2003; Posel, Fairburn, and Lund, 2004; Lam et al., in this volume). Case and Deaton (1998) argue that the pension program is effective in reaching the poorest households and in fact is a useful tool for reaching the poor in general, not just older people. Because so many older people in South Africa's African population live in multigeneration households, in part because young people tend to join households that receive a pension, the state pension program transfers money into households with children. Roughly one-third of all children age 4 and under live in households in which older people receive pensions, and the percentage of children living with pensioners is even higher among the poorest income quintiles (Alderman, 1999). Case (2001) also found that in the Western Cape, in households that pool income, the state pension appears to protect the health status of all adults and children in the household. Duflo (2003) found that the impact of the program depends on the gender of the recipient: pensions received by men have little effect on children's health status, but pensions received by women have a large impact on the physical stature of girls.

Impact on Older Persons

An important policy question with respect to any social welfare program has to do with the extent to which the program creates dependency and has a negative effect on labor supply. Betrand et al. (2003) found that pensions can have a negative effect on the labor supply of working-age adults residing in pension-receiving households. However, Betrand et al. (2003) investigated only the labor supply of adults resident in the household. Posel et al. (2004) argued that the social pension also affects the propensity of household members to migrate to find work, which acts as a positive supply response to the receipt of a social pension. In their chapter in this volume, Lam et al. contribute to this debate by examining how the social pension affects the decision to withdraw from the labor force by older people. By analyzing census and survey data, the authors found that, although the pension is associated with high rates of withdrawal from the labor force, the rates are somewhat less sharp than those observed for similar programs in Europe.

Another crucial policy question in the region is whether economic growth is needed in order to broaden the social safety net. Kakwani and Subbarao (2005) investigate the likely fiscal implications of providing some sort of social pension to older people in various sub-Saharan African countries and study the impacts on poverty rates. The authors have found that the fiscal cost of providing a universal noncontributory social pension to all of older people in sub-Saharan Africa would be quite high, around 2 to 3 percent of gross domestic product, a level comparable to—or even higher than—the current levels of public spending on health care in some sub-Saharan African nations. The authors argue that the case for universal social pensions also appears to be weak on welfare grounds, inasmuch as there are other groups competing for scarce safety net resources (such as families with many children) whose incidence and prevalence of poverty is much higher than that of older people.

Given that a universal social pension program appears out of reach in most countries and is difficult to defend on purely social welfare grounds, the authors then explore various options for targeted social pensions using a fixed budget constraint of 0.5 percent of gross domestic product and a fixed benefit level of 70 percent or 35 percent of the poverty threshold for older people defined as age 60 or 65 and older. Two household types were considered: households with older people living with children and households with older people only. The authors found that the introduction of social pensions targeted to these groups would yield considerable reductions in the prevalence of household-level poverty, both for the targeted groups and for the national average. Nevertheless, as the authors point out, the operational feasibility of such a program is very weak. The administrative burden of operating such a scheme is enormous and would be likely to lead to dissolution and reformation of certain types of households in order to make them eligible to claim a pension. Bearing this is mind, the authors also investigate the fiscal implications of providing a social pension to only poor older people, regardless of the type of household in which they reside. The authors conclude that the best option is to target the pension only to the poor, keep the benefit level low, and the age of eligibility at 65 and older (Kakwani and Subbarao, 2005).

Informal Schemes

Given the problems and formidable financial and administrative hurdles to expanding formal social security schemes in sub-Saharan Africa, policy makers also need to know whether there are ways to expand and support any of the various forms of informal social protection schemes that exist around the continent as a means to provide a vital safety net for certain vulnerable populations. A wide variety of informal community-based arrangements have been developed in rural areas aimed at spreading risk among friends and extended family members, with neighbors, or with other participants. These can often involve self-help or community based-initiatives that draw on sub-Saharan African traditions of shared support and kinship networks. In parts of Zimbabwe, for example, the government has successfully reintroduced the concept of the *Zunde raMambo* (literally "the Chief's Granary"), which refers to the harvest from a common field that is stored in a common granary and used at the discretion of the chief in order to ensure that the community has sufficient food in the event of a drought or a poor harvest (Dhemba et al., 2002).

There are many other examples of groups that have come together as spontaneous responses to poverty. Rotating savings and credit associations and mutual aid societies, for example, are commonly used throughout sub-Saharan Africa to compensate for failures in existing formal financial markets. In rotating credit and savings associations, participants periodically contribute fixed amounts of money and allocate the fund on a lottery or rotational basis to its members. The scheme encourages small-scale capital accumulation and savings and allows members to meet various welfare objectives, such as to pay school fees, meet medical expenses, or buy food. Funds can also be used to start or promote small businesses and acquire assets, including livestock (Kimuyu, 1999). Burial societies are another form of rotating savings scheme. In burial societies, members pay periodically to the society, and, when the member dies, the family receives money to help offset the funeral expenses. These types of scheme are very popular in sub-Saharan Africa, particularly in urban areas. Much less is known about informal social security systems in sub-Saharan Africa than about formal social security systems, but it is generally believed that informal schemes also suffer from a number of chronic problems and in their current form fail to provide much in the way of long-term protection against various forms of risk (Mchomvu et al., 2002). Nevertheless, there is a need for more detailed country-specific analysis on the nature of both formal and informal schemes, the size and frequency of transfers, and the redistributive effects of those transfer payments on the health and well-being of older people and other household members.

RECOMMENDATIONS

Sub-Saharan African policy makers are increasingly aware of the challenges associated with population aging and with the changing needs and contributions of older people. While aging may not soon have highest priority, such actions as the development and adoption of the African Union Framework and Plan of Action on Ageing, the formulation of the African Common Position on Ageing, and the establishment, for the first time, of national policies on aging in a few sub-Saharan African countries are all indicators of a growing awareness of aging issues across the continent.

Sound understanding of the links between key social and economic trends and the economic security, health and disability, and living conditions of older people in sub-Saharan African contexts is essential if appropriate new policies to enhance their lives are to be established. The recommendations below take into account the research essential to this new understanding, the need to overcome barriers to research, and translation of research findings into programs and policies. The substantive agenda for research was laid out in the previous section on key areas for future research. There are no easy solutions to the problems discussed in this report, but unquestionably understanding of some of the key issues and causal processes we have discussed would be greatly improved if the research community had the resources to use available information and undertake new data collection efforts, particularly those with a repeated sampling or longitudinal design. The consensus of the panel is that this type of longitudinal, multidisciplinary monitoring system would be most useful if implemented in several locations using comparable design. It would not only provide a reliable benchmark on the current socioeconomic situation of older people but would doubtlessly also contribute significantly to scientific knowledge.

In turn, it could inform those charged with the development of new programs and policies for older people. The returns on such an investment may be modest initially but will accumulate over time.

The panel also wishes to emphasize the importance of facilitating research, building local research capacity, and supporting the development of a local research network in sub-Saharan Africa that can support essential studies on the nature and consequences of its population aging and the context in which it is occurring. Top priority for the immediate future should be given to building basic research infrastructure, improving access to data, removing burdensome administrative barriers to carrying out new research, and strengthening international collaboration.[9]

After consideration of the general state of knowledge about aging in sub-Saharan Africa, recent research developments and emerging opportunities, and the strength of local research capacity, the panel arrived at the following recommendations, grouped under research agenda and funding, enhancing research opportunity and implementation, and translation of research findings that they feel could help improve the future development of the field.

Research Agenda

1. Increase Research on Aging in Sub-Saharan Africa

This report provides detail on the substantive agenda of needed research on aging in sub-Saharan Africa. There can be little doubt that, as a function of the emerging fertility transition in sub-Saharan Africa, the changing macroeconomic climate, and the impact of the devastating HIV/AIDS epidemic, researchers are paying increasing attention to the social, economic, and demographic dimensions of aging in sub-Saharan Africa. This attention can be turned into action only with increased funding directed to this arena. Funders should consider mechanisms—existing or new—to enable the research agenda identified in this report to be carried out. These mechanisms should foster international collaborative research in ways that benefit researchers in both the developed and developing worlds.

---

[9]Since the workshop took place, the Oxford Institute of Ageing has established a new network for researchers working on aging in Africa: the African Research on Ageing Network (AFRAN). The network is being coordinated jointly by the Oxford Institute of Ageing and the Council for the Development of Economic and Social Research in Africa (CODESRIA).

2. Explore Ways to Leverage Existing Data Collection Efforts to Learn More About Older People in Sub-Saharan Africa

The ongoing economic and social changes taking place in sub-Saharan Africa as well as the projected changes in both the numbers and proportion of older people in sub-Saharan Africa pose a series of vital policy challenges: How are ongoing economic and demographic changes affecting the family structures, socioeconomic position, and health of older people? How is HIV/AIDS changing the roles and responsibilities of older people? Can some form of social protection scheme be designed and successfully implemented in this part of the world that will partially relieve some of the burden on sub-Saharan African families?

With such vagaries and uncertainties there is a clear need to enhance understanding of the current situation of older people in sub-Saharan Africa as well as to improve understanding of some of the underlying causal processes that relate social and economic change to older people's well-being in the sub-Saharan African context. Given that the proportion of the population that is older is still low, at least relative to other continents, sub-Saharan African policy makers have an important window of opportunity in which to act. Furthermore, as an earlier report of the National Research Council's Committee on Population pointed out, each sub-Saharan African country's response to the challenges of aging is liable to be slightly different. Consequently, a number of natural experiments are either already currently under way, or shortly will be that, provided they are well recorded and documented, could be used to enable countries to learn from each other's experiences (National Research Council, 2001). In order for this to happen, national governments will need both to invest much more in basic research and to develop mechanisms to establish common definitions that will facilitate the harmonization of data collection across countries.

Improving understanding of the situation of older people will also require a better picture of the simultaneous interplay among multiple factors, including health, economic, and social characteristics. Hence, the development and use of multidisciplinary research designs will be essential in the development and production of any new data on aging in sub-Saharan Africa. Furthermore, the very strong a priori assumptions that many researchers and social commentators hold concerning the deteriorating situation of older people over time imply the need for study designs that can trace the experiences of individuals over time. Experience from the United States, Europe, and Asia has shown that data collection efforts that use a multidisciplinary panel approach, involving researchers who are willing to work across traditional domains, can produce significant returns (Börsch-Supan et al., 2005; Hermalin, 2002; National Research Council, 2001). Ideally, data should be reliable, population and community based, and inclusive of all groups, should cover multiple domains of interest, and should be collected both prospectively and continuously.

All of these challenges suggest the need for establishing a foundation of high-quality baseline data and tracking changes in many key variables over time. But collecting high-quality longitudinal data would undoubtedly be an extremely expensive and difficult undertaking. A more feasible first step may be to take advantage of already ongoing data collection efforts. The existing network of community-based population surveillance sites (INDEPTH) offers one likely vehicle for developing such a data collection effort, rather than investing in a completely new sampling framework. Although there are some inherent limitations of site-specific studies, greater investment in a growing number of (predominantly rural) INDEPTH sites around the continent is likely to substantially enrich knowledge of the living arrangements, economic activities, and health status of older people in sub-Saharan Africa if these data are made available and analyzed in a timely fashion. In general with ongoing data collection efforts, it is important to find a balance between protecting confidentiality and increasing access by qualified researchers to these valuable data. Sub-Saharan African researchers are likely to benefit most from greater access to African censuses, surveys, and demographic surveillance site data.

Enhancing Research Opportunity and Implementation

3. Improve Support for Library Infrastructure and Dissemination Tools to Create a More Integrated Body of Knowledge in Sub-Saharan Africa

Researchers and policy makers in sub-Saharan Africa are often poorly informed about previous research that has taken place on their continent or elsewhere. The only sub-Saharan African journal dedicated to publishing the findings of research on various aspects of aging, the *Southern African Journal of Gerontology*, ceased publication in 2000 due to lack of financial support. Furthermore, even when studies are accepted and published in international journals, it is often quite difficult to obtain copies of papers locally. In fact, it is often far easier to obtain copies of research papers outside the country in which they were produced than inside it. In addition, researchers in sub-Saharan Africa are working in three main languages: English, French, and Portuguese, which slows down professional networking and the dissemination of findings. In most sub-Saharan African countries, there is no up-to-date bibliography of research or reports on aging to form a knowledge base, such as was compiled for aging research in Europe in the late 1990s (see Agree and Myers, 1998). Furthermore, there are few opportunities for national and international networking among scholars interested in aging although the recent establishment of the African Research on Ageing Network (AFRAN) may lead to more opportunities in the future. Hence, there is a need for more support for library and information services as well as a need for greater information sharing and professional networking, perhaps through the sponsorship of more local or regional conferences. Given the rapid takeoff of electronic journal retrieval systems, such as JSTOR, increased investment in Internet access—both to high-speed Internet itself and to rights to use resources available on the Internet—may be one of the most effective means of closing the gap between continents in terms of access to existing research.

4. Improve Archiving of Past Censuses and Surveys

Generally speaking, African censuses and surveys have been greatly underutilized and much survey data collected over the past 30 years has deteriorated as a result of poor archiving. Yet even with the limited focus on aging issues in past social surveys, there may be significant potential for furthering knowledge of the social and economic conditions of older people from a more systematic analysis of previously collected data. But that cannot happen without improvements to the ways that data sets are archived and put into the public domain. Data handling and storage technology advance so rapidly that the burden of making data available in a useful format cannot rest with individual researchers. Hence there is a need for a more systematic archiving of sub-Saharan African microdata. The World Bank's web-based African Household Survey database, the Minnesota Integrated Public Use Microdata Series (IPUMS-International), and the University of Pennsylvania's African Census Project are good examples of initiatives designed to save previously collected data from destruction that have eased data constraints and produced new findings about older people (see, for example, Mba, 2002).

5. Improve Access to Ongoing Data Collection Efforts

If investments in new data are to be realized, better mechanisms will need to be put in place to improve storage, retrieval, and access to aging data. The experience of the Health and Retirement Survey and the Asset and Health Dynamics of the Oldest Old Study in the United States has shown that the return on research dollars is highest when the data collected are made available to the broad scientific community in a timely fashion (National Research Council, 2001; Willis, 1999). Yet in the sub-Saharan African context this may be far easier said than done. First, there are a number of ethical issues that need to be explicitly addressed when collecting any individual-level data (Cash and Rabin, 2002). But particularly in the case of such sensitive topics as the HIV status of respondents or their other family members, it is quite easy to see how information collected by researchers could be damaging both to the individual and to others if it were disclosed to a third party. Different countries have different policies in place to protect the privacy and confidentiality of their informants. Issues of confidentiality may require developing complex informed consent procedures that may be difficult to devise and communicate when the concepts are new and foreign and the population being investigated is poorly educated.

Furthermore, much of the best research undertaken to date has been made possible only by the establishment of international research partnerships between researchers in the developed and the developing world. These partnerships are quite complex to establish and maintain, since they involve negotiating such thorny issues as fair allocation of research roles, balance in infrastructure investments, and fairness in ascribing authorship and related credits (Tollman, 2004). At the same time, high functioning North-South institutional partnerships can accomplish a great deal with regard to research training as well as research and may well offer the best prospects for the foreseeable future. Thus, the challenge will be to strengthen these partnerships in ways that both support local institutions and increase timely access to data.

6. Strengthen International Collaboration and Capacity-Building in the Short Term

There is a critical and urgent need to strengthen research capacity in sub-Saharan Africa. More and better research on various dimensions of aging in sub-Saharan Africa cannot happen without an increase in the funding for research, more well-trained local researchers, and improvements in administrative procedures that currently hinder the execution of research projects.

Many sub-Saharan African universities were badly neglected in the 1980s and 1990s. Funding for salaries, maintenance of facilities and equipment, library services, and sometimes even basic office supplies was often entirely inadequate, resulting in the demise of sub-Saharan African universities and the widespread flight of faculty into the private sector (National Research Council, 1996). At the same time, a lack of managerial and administrative capacity can often lead to inefficiencies in the way that available money is allocated.

Although there are signs that African governments are beginning to value the role that science and technology can play in national development, it is unlikely that sub-Saharan African governments are going to increase their level of research funding substantially in the near future. In the short term, foreign financial and technical assistance will remain essential to the development of local universities and the strengthening of local research capacity. Donors should explore funding mechanisms that increase incentives for work in this area, perhaps through the establishment of special funding mechanisms, particularly those that not only advance funding for research on aging in sub-Saharan Africa but also encourage cross-national collaboration and training.

At the same time, African and other governments should do all in their power to facilitate linkages between sub-Saharan African institutions and international research centers in the United States and elsewhere by establishing agreements at the highest levels to expedite local review of projects as expeditiously as possible. Such linkages, especially if built on the basis of a strong mutual interest in collaborative research, can help local universities develop, can assist local researchers by providing funding and in-country technical assistance and training, and can help with the processing of data and the preparation of manuscripts for publication. Experience in a number of sub-Saharan African settings has demonstrated that such collaborations can lead to important scientific advances and be mutually beneficial to all institutions involved (Tollman, 2004).

7. Remove Barriers to Implementation of Research

Collaborative research with sub-Saharan African institutions requires approvals by all collaborating institutions, frequently involving more than one review board for the ethical conduct of research, as well as government offices and officials in the country in which the data collection takes place—whether representatives of the United States or the local government. The panel received informal reports of difficulties and delays in receiving the required approvals even for projects funded by the U.S. National Institutes of Health (NIH) after the usual exacting NIH reviews. One study was delayed for more than a year; another was delayed then finally dropped. If research on these important subjects is to be carried out in a timely fashion, it is essential that institutions, review boards, and government bodies at all relevant levels establish procedures and processes that make speedy review possible, without repetitive reviews of scientific merit.

8. In the Long Term, Sub-Saharan African Governments Must Give Reasonable Priority to Aging Research and Strengthen Local Research Capacity

In the long run, the importance of foreign-supported research in the region must be reduced. It will be up to sub-Saharan African national governments to prioritize aging as a focal area and to find the resources needed to be able to drive the region's aging agenda. Numerous related processes are already under way in Africa aimed at strengthening research institutes and building research capacity, including programs at the Council for the Development of Social Science Research, headquartered in Senegal, and the African Centre for Research and Training in Social Development, headquartered in Ethiopia. Nevertheless, sub-Saharan African governments generally need to place a greater value on the role of higher education and find funding to rebuild and strengthen local universities. In many countries, pay scales will need to be adjusted in order to attract and retain the best researchers.

Translation of Research Findings

9. Improve Dialogue Between Local Researchers and Policy Makers

There is an ongoing need for continued and expanded dialogue between the research and the policy communities. Researchers need to do a better job of drawing out the main policy and programmatic implications of their work, and policy makers need to better articulate what information they most need for more effective planning and program design. At the same time, there is also value in both sides engaging with older people themselves to ensure so that they are not excluded from a dialogue aimed ultimately at enhancing their future well-being. Otherwise, the danger is that local programs and policies will be only marginally based on a solid understanding of local needs and conditions, while research will continue to be undervalued by policy makers and therefore underfunded.

References

Aboderin, I. (2004). Decline in material family support for older people in urban Ghana, Africa: Understanding processes and causes of change. *Journal of Gerontology, 59B(3)*, S128-S137.

Addae-Mensah, I. (2005). Challenges and opportunities of traditional/herbal medicine. Chapter 2 in K. Gyekye, E. Osae, and P. Effah (Eds.), *Harnessing research, science, and technology for sustainable development in Ghana*. Accra, Ghana: National Council for Tertiary Education.

Agesa, R. (2004). One family, two households: Rural to urban migration in Kenya. *Review of Economics of the Household, 2*, 161-178.

Agree, E., and Myers, G. (1998). *Ageing research in Europe: Demographic, social, and behavioural aspects*. Geneva, Switzerland: United Nations Economic Commission for Europe.

Alderman, H. (1999). *Safety nets and income transfers in South Africa*. (Discussion Paper No. 19335). Washington, DC: World Bank.

Apt, N.A. (1996). *Coping with old age in a changing Africa: Social change and the elderly Ghanaian*. Aldershot, England: Ashgate.

Ardington, E., and Lund, F. (1995). Pensions and development: Social security as complementary to programmes of reconstruction and development. *Development Southern Africa, 12(4)*, 557-577.

Asamoah-Odei, E., Garcia Calleia, J.M., and Boerma, J.T. (2004, July). HIV prevalence and trends in sub-Saharan Africa: No decline and large subregional differences. *Lancet, 364*, 35-40.

Bailey, C. (2004). *Extending social security coverage in Africa*. (Working Paper, ESS No. 20). Geneva, Switzerland: International Labour Office.

Bailey, C., and Turner, C. (2002). Social security in Africa: A brief review. *Journal of Aging and Social Policy, 14(1)*, 105-114.

Barrientos, A., Gorman, M., and Heslop, A. (2003). Old age poverty in developing countries: Contributions and dependence in later life. *World Development, 31(3)*, 555-570.

Becker, C.M., and Grewe, C.D. (1996). Cohort-specific rural-urban migration in Africa. *Journal of African Economics, 5(2)*, 228-270.

Behrman, J.R. (1997). Intrahousehold distribution and the family. In M.R. Rosenzweig and O. Stark (Eds.), *Handbook of population and family economics* (vol. 1A, pp. 125-187). Amsterdam, The Netherlands: Elsevier Science.

Bertrand, M., Mullainathan, S., and Miller, D. (2003). Public policy and extended families: Evidence from pensions in South Africa. *World Bank Economic Review, 17*(1), 27-50.

Börsch-Supan, A., Brugiavini, A., Jürges, H., Mackenbach, J., Siegrist, J., and Weber, G. (Eds.). (2005). *Health, ageing and retirement in Europe: First results from the survey of health, ageing, and retirement in Europe.* Mannheim, Germany: Mannheim Research Institute for the Economics of Aging.

Case, A. (2001). *Does money protect health status? Evidence from South African pensions.* (NBER Working Paper No. 8495). Cambridge, MA: National Bureau of Economic Research.

Case, A., and Deaton, A. (1998). Large cash transfers to the elderly in South Africa. *The Economic Journal, 108,* 1330-1361.

Cash, R.A., and Rabin, T.L. (2002). Overview of ethical issues in collecting data in developing countries with special reference to longitudinal designs. In National Research Council, *Leveraging longitudinal data in developing countries: Report of a workshop* (pp. 75-94). Committee on Population, V.L. Durrant and J. Menken (Eds.). Division of Behavioral and Social Sciences and Education. Washington, DC: National Academy Press.

Chayanov, A.V. (1925). *Peasant farm organization.* Moscow: The Co-operative Publishing House. (Reprinted in D. Thorner, B. Kerblay, and R.E.F. Smith (Eds.). (1986). *A.V. Chayanov on the theory of peasant economy.* Madison: University of Wisconsin Press.)

Commission for Africa. (2005). *Our common interest. Report of the Commission for Africa.* London, England: Author.

Cooper, R.S., Osotimehin, B., Kaufman, J.S., and Forrester, T. (1998). Disease burden in sub-Saharan Africa: What should we conclude in the absence of data? *The Lancet, 351,* 208-210.

Dayton, J., and Ainsworth, M. (2004). The elderly and AIDS: Coping with the impact of adult death in Tanzania. *Social Science and Medicine, 59,* 2161-2172.

de Savigny, D., Debpuur, C., Mwageni, E., Nathan R., Razzaque A., and Setel, P. (Eds.). (2005). *Measuring health equity in small areas: Findings from demographic surveillance sites.* Aldershot, England: Ashgate.

Deaton, A., and Paxson, C.H. (1992). Patterns of aging in Thailand and Côte d'Ivoire. In D.A. Wise (Ed.), *Topics in the economics of aging* (pp. 163-206). Chicago, IL: University of Chicago Press.

Deng, F.M. (1984). *The Dinka of the Sudan.* Long Grove, IL: Waveland Press.

Dhemba, J., Gumbo, P., and Nyamusara, J. (2002). Social security in Zimbabwe. *Journal of Social Development in Africa, 17*(2), 111-156.

Duflo, E. (2003). Grandmothers and granddaughters: Old-age pensions and intrahousehold allocation in South Africa. *World Bank Economic Review, 17*(1), 1-25.

Feachem, R.G.A., Kjellstrom, T., Murray, C.J.L., Over, M., and Phillips, M.A. (Eds.). (1992). *The health of adults in the developing world.* New York: Oxford University Press.

Ferreira, M. (1999). Building and advancing African gerontology. *Southern African Journal of Gerontology, 8*(1), 1-3.

Ferreira, M. (2003). The impact of South Africa's social security system on traditional support systems: More generally, should we be looking backwards or forwards in Africa? In I.H. Goldenberg (Ed.), *Sustainable structures in a society far all ages* (pp. 22-23). New York: United Nations.

Fox, L., and Palmer, E. (2001). New approaches to multipillar pension systems: What in the world is going on? Chapter 3 in R. Holzmann and J.E. Stiglitz (Eds.), *New ideas about old age security: Towards sustainable pension systems in the 21st century.* Washington, DC: World Bank.

Garcia, A.B., and Gruat, J.V. (2003). *Social protection: A life cycle continuum investment for social justice, poverty reduction, and sustainable development.* (Working Paper). Geneva, Switzerland: International Labour Office.

Gillian, C., Turner, J., Bailey, C., and Latulippe, D. (2000). *Social security pensions: Development and reform.* Geneva, Switzerland: International Labour Office.

Gwatkin, D.R., Guillot, M., and Heuveline, P. (1999). The burden of disease among the global poor. *The Lancet, 354*(9188), 1477.

Hermalin, A.I. (Ed.). (2002). *The well-being of the elderly in Asia: A four-country comparative study.* Ann Arbor: University of Michigan Press.

House, W.J. (1991). The nature and determinants of socioeconomic inequality among peasant households in southern Sudan. *World Development, 19*(7), 867-884.

House, W.J., and Phillips-Howard, K. (1990). Socio-economic differentiation among African peasants: Evidence from Acholi, Southern Sudan. *Journal of International Development, 2*(1), 77-109.

Internal Displacement Monitoring Center. (2006). *Internal displacement: Global overview of trends and developments in 2005.* Geneva, Switzerland: Norwegian Refugee Council.

Joint United Nations Programme on HIV/AIDS. (2006). *Report on the global AIDS epidemic: Executive summary.* Geneva, Switzerland: Author.

Kakwani, N., and Subbarao, K. (2005). *Ageing and poverty in Africa and the role of social pensions.* (International Poverty Centre, Working Paper No. 8). New York: United Nations Development Programme.

Kalasa, B. (2001). *Population and ageing in Africa: A policy dilemma?* Paper presented at the International Union for the Scientific Study of Population's XXIV General Population Conference, August 18-24, Salvador de Bahia, Brazil.

Kaseke, E. (2004). *An overview of formal and informal social security systems in Africa.* Paper presented at the National Academy of Sciences and University of the Witwatersrand Workshop on Aging in Africa, July 27-29, Johannesburg, South Africa.

Kasente, D., Asingwire, N., Banugire, F., and Kyomuhenda, S. (2002). Social security in Uganda. *Journal of Social Development in Africa, 17*(2), 157-184.

Kimuyu, P.K. (1999). Rotating saving and credit associations in rural East Africa. *World Development, 27*(7), 1299-1308.

Knight, J.B., and Sabot, R.H. (1990). *Education, productivity, and inequality: The East African natural experiment.* Washington, DC: Oxford University Press for the World Bank.

Knodel, J. (2005). Researching the impact of the AIDS epidemic on older-age parents in Africa: Lessons from studies in Thailand. *Generations Review: Journal of the British Society of Gerontology, 15*(2), 16-22.

Knodel, J., Watkins, S., and VanLandingham, M. (2003). AIDS and older persons: An international perspective. *Journal of Acquired Immune Deficiency Syndrome, 33*, S153-S165.

Laxminarayan, R., Chow, J., and Shahid-Salles, S.A. (2006). Intervention cost-effectiveness: Overview of main messages. In D.T. Jamison, J.G. Breman, A.R. Measham, G. Alleyne, M. Claeson, D.B. Evans, P. Jha, A. Mills, and P. Musgrove (Eds.), *Disease control priorities in developing countries* (pp. 35-86). New York: Oxford University Press for the World Bank.

Lopez, A.D., Mathers, C.D., Ezzati, M., Jamison, D.T., and Murray, C.J.L. (Eds.). (2006). *Global burden of disease and risk factors.* New York: Oxford University Press for the World Bank.

Lucas, R.E.B., and Stark, O. (1985). Motivations to remit: Evidence from Botswana. *Journal of Political Economy, 93*(5), 910-918.

Makiwane, M., Schneider, M., and Gopane, M. (2004). *Experiences and needs of older persons in Mpumalanga.* Report written for Human Science Research Council and Department of Health and Social Services, Mpumalanga, South Africa.

Makoni, S., and Stroeken, K. (2002). *Ageing in Africa: Sociologinguistic and anthropological approaches.* Aldershot, England: Ashgate.

Marshall, M.G., and Gurr, T.R. (2005). *Peace and conflict 2005: A global survey of armed conflicts, self-determination movements, and democracy.* College Park, MD: Center for International Development and Conflict Management.

Mathers, C.D., Salomon, J.A., Ezzati, M., Begg, S., Vander Hoom, S., and Lopez, A.D. (2006). Sensitivity and uncertainty analyses for burden of disease and risk factor estimates. In A.D. Lopez, C.D. Mathers, M. Ezzati, D.T. Jamison, and C.J.L. Murray (Eds.), *Global burden of disease and risk factors* (pp. 399-426). New York: Oxford University Press for the World Bank.

Mba, C. (2002). Determinants of living arrangements of Lesotho's elderly female population. *Journal of International Women's Studies, 3*(2), 1-22.

McCabe, J.T. (2004). *Cattle bring us to our enemies. Turkana ecology, politics, and raiding in a disequilibrium system.* Ann Arbor: University of Michigan Press.

Mchomvu, A.S.T., Tungaraza, F., and Maghimbi, S. (2002). Social security systems in Tanzania. *Journal of Social Development in Africa, 17*(2), 11-63.

Montgomery, M.R., Gragnolati, M., Burke, K.A., and Paredes, E. (2000). Measuring living standards with proxy variables. *Demography, 37*(2), 155-174.

Mukuka, L., Kalikiti, W., and Musenge, D. (2002). Social security systems in Zambia. *Journal of Social Development in Africa, 17*(2), 65-110.

Murray, C.J.L., and Evans, D.B. (Eds.). (2003). *Health systems performance assessment: Debates, methods, and empiricism.* Geneva, Switzerland: World Health Organization.

Murray, C.J.L., and Lopez, A.D. (Eds.). (1996). *The global burden of disease.* Cambridge, MA: Harvard University Press.

Murray, C.J.L., Tandon, A., Salomon, J.A., Mathers, C.D., and Sadana, R. (2002). New approaches to enhance cross-population comparability of survey results. In C.J.L. Murray, J.A. Salomon, C.D. Mathers, and A.D. Lopez (Eds.), *Summary measures of population health: Concepts, ethics, measurement, and applications* (pp. 421-431). Geneva, Switzerland: World Health Organization.

Murray, C.J.L., Özaltin, E., Tandon, A., Salomon, J.A., Sadana, R., and Chatterji, S. (2003). Empirical evaluation of the anchoring vignette approach in health systems. In C.L.J. Murray and D.R. Evans (Eds.), *Health systems performance assessment: Debates, methods, and empiricism* (pp. 369-399). Geneva, Switzerland: World Health Organization.

National Bureau of Statistics (Tanzania). (2002). *Household budget survey, 2000/2001.* Dares Salaam, Tanzania: Author.

National Research Council. (1996). *Preventing and mitigating AIDS in Sub-Saharan Africa: Research and data priorities for the social and behavioral sciences.* Panel on Data and Research Priorities for Arresting AIDS in Sub-Saharan Africa. B. Cohen and J. Trussell (Eds.). Washington, DC: National Academy Press.

National Research Council. (2001). *Preparing for an aging world: The case for cross-national research.* Panel on a Research Agenda and New Data for an Aging World. Washington, DC: National Academy Press.

National Research Council and Institute of Medicine. (2005). *Growing up global: The changing transitions to adulthood in developing countries.* Panel on Transitions to Adulthood in Developing Countries. C.B. Lloyd (Ed.). Committee on Population and Board on Children, Youth, and Families. Division of Behavioral and Social Sciences and Education. Washington, DC: The National Academies Press.

National Statistics Office (Malawi). (2005). *Malawi second integrated household survey (HIS-2), 2004-2005*. Zomba, Malawi: Author.

Nyambedha, E.O., Wandibba, S., and Aagaard-Hansen, L. (2003). Changing patterns of orphan care due to the HIV epidemic in western Kenya. *Social Science and Medicine, 57,* 301-311.

Omram, A.R. (1971). The epidemiological transition: A theory of the epidemiology of population change. *Milbank Memorial Fund Quarterly, 49,* 509-538.

Peachey, K., and Nhongo, T. (2004). *From piecemeal action to integrated solutions: The need for policies on ageing and older people in Africa*. Paper presented at the National Academy of Sciences and University of the Witwatersrand Workshop on Aging in Africa, July 27-29, Johannesburg, South Africa.

Porter, E., Robinson, G., Smyth, M., Schnabel, A., and Osaghae, E. (2005). *Researching conflict in Africa: Insights and experiences*. Tokyo, Japan: United Nations University Press.

Posel, D., Fairburn, J.A., and Lund, F. (2004). *Labour migration and households: A reconsideration of the effects of the social pension on labour supply in South Africa*. Paper presented at the National Academy of Sciences and University of the Witwatersrand Workshop on Aging in Africa, July 27-29, Johannesburg, South Africa.

Poullier, J.P., Hernandez, P., and Kawabata, K. (2003). National health accounts: Concepts, data sources, and methodology. In C.J.L. Murray and D.R. Evans (Eds.), *Health systems performance assessment: Debates, methods, and empiricism* (pp. 185-193). Geneva, Switzerland: World Health Organization.

Poullier, J.P., Hernandez, P., Kawabata, K., and Savedoff, W.D. (2003). Patterns of global health expenditures: Results for 191 countries. In C.J.L. Murray and D.R. Evans (Eds.), *Health systems performance assessment: Debates, methods, and empiricism* (pp. 195-203). Geneva, Switzerland: World Health Organization.

Rapoport, B. (2004). Why do African households give hospitality to relatives? *Review of Economics of the Household, 2,* 179-202.

Rowntree, B.S. (1901). *Poverty: A study of town life*. London, England: Macmillan.

Salomon, J.A., Tandon, A., and Murray, C.J.L. (2003). Unpacking health perceptions using anchoring vignettes. In C.L.J. Murray and D.R. Evans (Eds.), *Health systems performance assessment: Debates, methods, and empiricism* (pp. 401-407). Geneva, Switzerland: World Health Organization.

SASPI Team. (2004). The social diagnostics of stroke-like symptoms: Healers, doctors, and prophets in Agincourt, Limpopo Province, South Africa. *Journal of Biomedical Science, 36,* 433-443.

Stark, O. (1991). *The migration of labor*. Cambridge, MA: Blackwell.

Stark, O. (1995). *Altruism and beyond: An economic analysis of transfers and exchanges within families and groups*. Cambridge, England: Cambridge University Press.

Thomas, D., and Frankenberg, E. (2002). The measurement and interpretation of health in social surveys. In C.J.L. Murray, J.A. Salomon, C.D. Mathers, and A.D. Lopez (Eds.), *Summary measures of population health: Concepts, ethics, measurement, and applications* (pp. 387-420). Geneva, Switzerland: World Health Organization.

Todaro, M.P. (1969). A model of labor migration and urban unemployment in less developed countries. *American Economic Review, 49,* 138-148.

Tollman, S. (2004). Establishing long-term research partnerships: Aligning rhetoric and reality. *Scandinavian Journal of Public Health, 32,* 1-3.

Tollman, S., Doherty, J., and Mulligan, J.A. (2006). General primary care. In D.T. Jamison, J.G. Breman, A.R. Measham, G. Alleyne, M. Claeson, D.B. Evans, P. Jha, A. Mills, and P. Musgrove (Eds.), *Disease control priorities in developing countries* (pp. 1193-1209). Washington, DC: International Bank for Reconstruction and Development and the World Bank.

Toulmin, C. (2006). *Securing land rights for the poor in Africa: Key to growth, peace, and sustainable development.* Paper prepared for the High Level Commission on the Legal Empowerment of the Poor. New York: United Nations.

United Nations. (2005). *World population prospects: The 2004 revision highlights.* New York: United Nations Department of Economic and Social Affairs, Population Division.

United Nations. (2006). *List of least developed countries.* New York: Author. Available: http://www.un.org/special-rep/ohrlls/ldc/list.htm [accessed April 25, 2006].

United Nations High Commission for Refugees. (2006). *The state of the world's refugees: Human displacement in the new millennium.* Oxford, England: Oxford University Press.

Üstün, T.B., Chatterji, S., Mechbal, A., Murray, C.J.L., and WHS Collaborating Groups. (2003). The world health surveys. In C.J.L. Murray and D.R. Evans (Eds.), *Health systems performance assessment: Debates, methods, and empiricism* (pp. 797-808). Geneva, Switzerland: World Health Organization.

van de Walle, E. (Ed.). (2006). *African households: Censuses and surveys.* London, England: M.E. Sharpe.

van Zyl, E. (2003). Old age pensions in South Africa. *International Social Security Review, 56,* 3-4.

Williams, A. (2003). *Ageing and poverty in Africa: Ugandan livelihoods in a time of HIV/AIDS.* Aldershot, England: Ashgate.

Williams, A., and Tumwekwase, G. (2001). Multiple impacts of the HIV/AIDS epidemic on the aged in rural Uganda. *Journal of Cross-Cultural Gerontology, 16,* 221-236.

Willis, R.J. (1999). Theory confronts data: How the HRS is shaped by the economics of aging and how the economics of aging will be shaped by the HRS. *Labour Economics, 6*(2), 119-145.

World Bank. (2005). *World development indicators 2005.* Washington, DC: Author.

World Bank. (2006a). *Global monitoring report 2006.* Washington, DC: Author.

World Bank. (2006b). *Global economic prospects 2006: Economic implications of remittances and migration.* Washington, DC: Author.

World Health Organization. (2002). *Impact of AIDS on older people in Africa: Zimbabwe case study.* Geneva, Switzerland: World Health Organization.

Zimmer, Z., and Dayton, J. (2005). Older adults in sub-Saharan Africa living with children and grandchildren. *Population Studies, 59*(3), 295-312.

Part II

Papers

2

Aging in Sub-Saharan Africa: The Changing Demography of the Region

Victoria A. Velkoff and Paul R. Kowal

INTRODUCTION

Population aging will become perhaps the most important demographic dynamic affecting families and societies throughout the world in the coming decades. Nearly 63 percent of the population age 60 and older currently resides in developing countries, and this percentage will increase to nearly 73 percent over the next 25 years. Yet the limited understanding of the demographics of aging in most developing countries stands in stark contrast to the comparatively well-documented course and implications of aging in developed countries.

A combination of factors contributes to the limited understanding of the situation of older people in Africa: they constitute a smaller proportion of the population and their proportions are projected to grow fairly slowly relative to other areas in the world.[1] In addition, other more pressing political, demographic, and health issues have confronted the subcontinent over the past two decades, and the systems to collect data essential for

---

[1]While we recognize the limitations of using a chronological age to define older persons in sub-Saharan Africa, most comparisons in this paper will focus on the population age 60 and over. Largely derived from the creation of a state social welfare system for older workers in developed countries, the use of the age group 60 and over or 65 and over has evolved to become a relatively standard definition of old age worldwide. Age 60 and over was adopted by the United Nations as the standard definition. This standard is not able to fully account for the cultural and societal differences in the definition of "old" between and within countries; however, using this chronological age to define "old" is practical and commonly used for official purposes.

accurate demographic estimates and projections are largely lacking. Resources available for addressing demographic changes and health problems in Africa have focused on issues of more immediate concern to the great majority of people who are not yet old: infant, child, and maternal health; nutrition; and HIV/AIDS. However, the consequences of recent social and political upheavals—HIV/AIDS, poverty, and violent conflicts—have shaken the core of societies and thrust older people into new roles in families and communities.

Despite the fact that the older population makes up a small proportion of the population in most sub-Saharan African countries, the number of older people is growing. In 2005, there were 34 million people age 60 and over in sub-Saharan Africa, and this number is projected to increase to over 67 million by 2030. In fact, the number of older people is growing more rapidly in sub-Saharan Africa than in the developed world. This increase in the number of older people will occur despite the excess mortality due to AIDS that many countries are currently experiencing.

This paper is divided into two sections. The first section focuses primarily on the demographic aspects of aging in sub-Saharan African countries with a special subsection examining the impact of AIDS on population aging. The demographic data in this first section are from the U.S. Census Bureau's International Programs Center's International Data Base. The second section compares and contrasts the estimates and projections from the U.S. Census Bureau with those of the United Nations (UN) Population Division. This section presents, compares, and contrasts these two sources of demographic estimates and projections, focusing on populations age 60 and older. The underlying models and assumptions, input data, and the resulting output data are examined to describe the demographic aspects of aging in sub-Saharan African countries. The concluding section provides suggestions for future work in the area.

DEMOGRAPHIC DIMENSIONS

The world is aging at an unprecedented rate. The numbers of older persons and pace of aging vary widely between and within regions, and typically more developed regions have higher proportions of their populations in older age groups than do developing regions (Figure 2-1). For example, nearly 21 percent of Europe's population was age 60 and over in 2005. In contrast, less than 5 percent of sub-Saharan Africa's population was age 60 and over. In other developing regions, those aged 60 and over make up between 7 and 9 percent of the population. In all regions of the world, the proportion age 60 and over is projected to increase in the future.

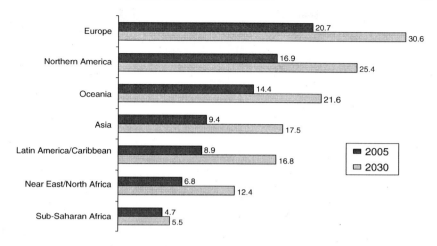

FIGURE 2-1 Percentage age 60 and over by region of the world: 2005 and 2030. SOURCE: U.S. Census Bureau (2005).

By 2030, over 30 percent of Europeans are projected to be age 60 and over. In Asia and Latin America and the Caribbean, the proportions age 60 and over are projected to nearly double in less than 25 years. Again, sub-Saharan Africa stands in contrast to the other regions of the world with the proportion age 60 and over projected to grow only slightly, from 4.7 percent in 2005 to 5.5 percent in 2030.

The Misconception of "No Older People" in Africa

The small increase in the *proportion* age 60 and over in sub-Saharan Africa masks a large increase in the *number* of people in this age group. The number of people age 60 and over in sub-Saharan Africa will nearly double from over 34 million in 2005 to over 67 million in 2030. The number of older people is growing more rapidly in sub-Saharan Africa than in the developed world and will continue to do so in the future (Figure 2-2). The average annual growth rate of the population age 60 and over in sub-Saharan Africa is over 2 percent and will increase over the next 50 years to nearly 4 percent. In contrast, the average annual growth rate of this population in developed countries is less than 2 percent and is projected to decline to less than 1 percent over the next several decades.

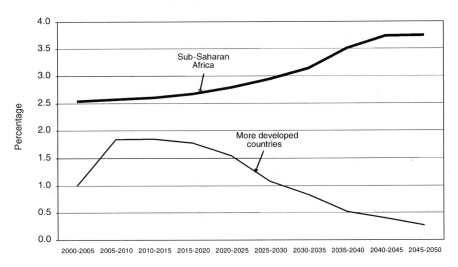

FIGURE 2-2 Average annual growth rates of the age 60 and over population in sub-Saharan Africa versus more developed countries: 2000 to 2050.
SOURCE: U.S. Census Bureau (2005).

Country Comparisons

Population aging in sub-Saharan Africa is not uniform. Both the size of the 60 and over population and the proportion of the population they account for varies among the countries of the region.[2]

Eight Countries Have at Least 1 Million People Age 60 and Over

In 2005, Nigeria ranked among the top 30 countries in the world on the basis of the size of its population age 60 and over. Nigeria had the largest older population in sub-Saharan Africa, with over 6 million people age 60 and over; South Africa had just over 3.4 million (Figure 2-3). Six additional sub-Saharan African countries had over 1 million people age 60 and over in 2005.

---

[2]There are 50-53 countries in sub-Saharan Africa. The UN Population Division includes 50 countries and the U.S. Census Bureau, 51. This paper focuses on 42 countries that had total populations of at least 1 million in 2005. The countries not included in tables and figures are Cape Verde, Comoros, Djibouti, Equatorial Guinea, Mayotte, Reunion, Saint Helena, Sao Tome and Principe, and Seychelles.

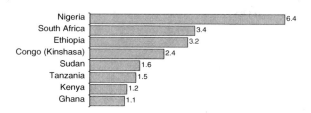

FIGURE 2-3 Sub-Saharan African countries with at least 1 million people age 60 and over: 2005 (number of people age 60 and over in millions). SOURCE: U.S. Census Bureau (2005).

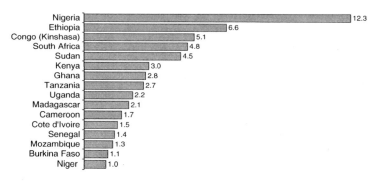

FIGURE 2-4 Sub-Saharan African countries with at least 1 million people age 60 and over: 2030 (number of people age 60 and over in millions). SOURCE: U.S. Census Bureau (2005).

The size of older populations in many sub-Saharan African countries is roughly equivalent to certain developed countries. For instance, Nigeria's older population is roughly the same size as those in South Korea and Canada.

The list of countries with at least 1 million people age 60 and over is projected to increase to 16 by the year 2030 (Figure 2-4). Again, Nigeria will have the largest older population, with over 12 million people age 60 and over, and Ethiopia will rank second, with over 6 million people. Congo (Kinshasa) and South Africa are projected to have nearly 5 million older people in 2030. Burkina Faso, Cameroon, Cote d'Ivoire, Madagascar, Mozambique, Niger, Senegal, and Uganda are all projected to have their older populations grow to over 1 million people by 2030.

Mauritius Is the Oldest Country in Sub-Saharan Africa

Although the proportion age 60 and over is just under 5 percent for sub-Saharan Africa as a whole, a number of countries have much higher proportions in this age group (Figure 2-5). Over 9 percent of Mauritius's population was age 60 and over in 2005, making it the oldest country in sub-Saharan Africa. South Africa had 7.8 percent of its population age 60 and over in 2005 and nearly 7 percent of Lesotho's population was in this age group. At the other end of the spectrum are such countries as Benin, Burundi, Kenya, Mauritania, Rwanda, Uganda, and Zambia, where the older population accounted for less than 4 percent of the total population.

By 2030, nearly 22 percent of the population of Mauritius is projected to be age 60 and over. In South Africa over 12 percent of the population is projected to be 60 and over (Figure 2-6). While the proportion of this population group is projected to increase in some countries (for example, Congo [Brazzaville], Ghana, Mauritius, and South Africa), the proportion age 60 and over is projected to remain fairly stable in many sub-Saharan African countries. For instance, 4 percent of Burundi's population in 2005 was age 60 and over, and this proportion is projected to stay the same in 2030. In other countries, the proportion is projected to decrease slightly. In Malawi, the percentage is projected to decrease from 4.2 percent in 2005 to 3.7 percent in 2030.

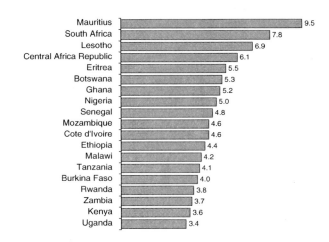

FIGURE 2-5 Percentage age 60 and over in selected sub-Saharan African countries: 2005.
SOURCE: U.S. Census Bureau (2005).

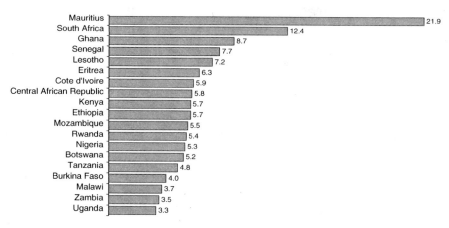

FIGURE 2-6 Percentage age 60 and over in selected sub-Saharan African countries: 2030.
SOURCE: U.S. Census Bureau (2005).

Although the proportion age 60 and over is on average projected to remain stable or decrease slightly in many countries, the absolute number of people in this age group is projected to grow in most countries. For example, the decrease in the proportion age 60 and over in Malawi between 2003 and 2030 masks an increase in the absolute number of people in this age group of around 280,000.

Older Populations Projected to Grow in Sub-Saharan African Countries

The change in the proportion of the population age 60 and over in most sub-Saharan African countries does not indicate the magnitude of change. The absolute number of people age 60 and over is projected to increase over the next three decades. However, there are exceptions, such as Botswana, Lesotho, and Swaziland. These three countries are severely affected by the AIDS epidemic, and their populations age 60 and over are projected to decrease between 2005 and 2030. Conversely, the number of older people in some countries is projected to more than double by 2030. In Sudan, for example, the number is expected to nearly triple (Figure 2-7).

Composition of Older Age Groups

In many countries in the world, the oldest old (those age 80 and over) is the fastest growing segment of the population. This is true for a majority of

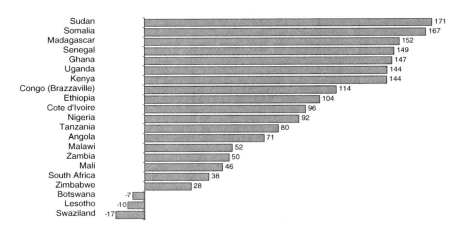

FIGURE 2-7 Percentage increase in the population age 60 and over in selected sub-Saharan African countries: 2005 to 2030.
SOURCE: U.S. Census Bureau (2005).

sub-Saharan African countries as well. In sub-Saharan Africa there were around 2.4 million people age 80 and over in 2005, and this number is projected to nearly triple to 6.1 million by 2030. Despite the rapid growth in the number of people age 80 and over, the oldest-old population accounted for less than 1 percent of the total population of sub-Saharan Africa in the years 2005 and 2030.

While the oldest old account for a very small proportion of the total population, they accounted for 7.1 percent of the 2005 population age 60 and over in sub-Saharan Africa. By 2030, the proportion will increase to 9.1 percent. In the more developed region, the oldest old will account for 22.6 percent of the population age 60 and over in 2030 and 12 percent in countries in the less developed regions.

Factors Affecting Population Structure

Impact of AIDS Seen in Population Pyramids

The extensive spread of HIV started in sub-Saharan Africa in the late 1970s, but it was not until the late 1980s that the epidemic exploded in Southern Africa (Joint United Nations Programme on HIV/AIDS and World Health Organization, 2003). Whereas the HIV/AIDS pandemic has consisted of various distinct epidemics, with geographic and population differences, almost all countries in sub-Saharan Africa have generalized epidemics. At the end of 2004, about 25.4 million of the estimated 39.4 million people worldwide living with HIV/AIDS were in this region, accounting for approximately two-thirds of the global burden (Joint United Nations Programme on HIV/AIDS, 2004). South Africa has the largest number of people living with HIV/AIDS in the world, 5.3 million. Botswana and Swaziland have the highest prevalence levels, both approaching 40 percent with no signs of leveling off. West Africa has been relatively less affected by HIV infection than other regions of sub-Saharan Africa, but the spread of HIV from forced migration in this subregion is a significant cause for concern.

In those countries most affected by HIV/AIDS, the age-specific impact on mortality is reshaping population structures. The death of adults in their prime reproductive and economically productive years has changed age pyramids, through declining fertility and increasing mortality, resulting in very atypical age distributions both now and for the next few decades.

Specific details of the impact are provided in the next section, but a good illustration of the impact is evident on examination of the population pyramids for Botswana and Zimbabwe. Comparisons of the age and sex structures over time for each country reveal the magnitude of the devastation. Figures 2-8 through 2-11 show the age and sex structure of the populations of Botswana and Zimbabwe for 2005 and 2030. These pyramids show the population estimates and projections with AIDS mortality incorporated into the projections and what the population structures would have looked like without AIDS mortality.

The 2005 population of Botswana is somewhat smaller than it would have been if there was no AIDS mortality (Figure 2-8). By 2030, Botswana's population age and sex structure is projected to be dramatically different from what it would have been without AIDS mortality (Figure 2-9). Botswana's total population in all age groups is projected to decrease slightly between 2005 and 2030, dropping from about 1.6 million in 2005 to 1.5 million in 2030. The population age 60 and over is also projected to decrease slightly over the same time period. In 2005, there were 86,000 people age 60 and over, and by 2030 this population is projected to be 80,000.

The age and sex structures for Zimbabwe also show the impact of AIDS mortality; however, the impact is slightly less severe than that on Botswana. Zimbabwe's population in 2005 is somewhat smaller than it would have been without AIDS mortality (Figure 2-10). By 2030, the impact of AIDS can clearly be seen in the age and sex structure of the population (Figure 2-11). Unlike Botswana, the total population in Zimbabwe will be larger in 2030 than it was in 2005, despite the impact of AIDS. The older population will also continue to grow in Zimbabwe. In 2005, there were 614,000 people age 60 and over, and this number is projected to grow to 783,000 by

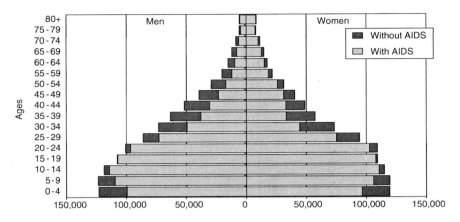

FIGURE 2-8 Population by age and sex in Botswana, with and without AIDS mortality incorporated into the estimate: 2005.
SOURCE: U.S. Census Bureau (2005).

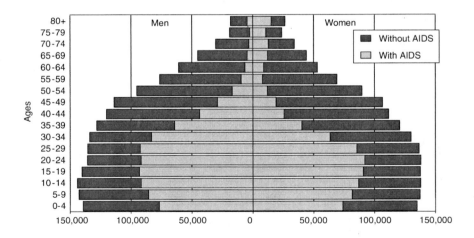

FIGURE 2-9 Population by age and sex in Botswana, with and without AIDS mortality incorporated into the projection: 2030.
SOURCE: U.S. Census Bureau (2005).

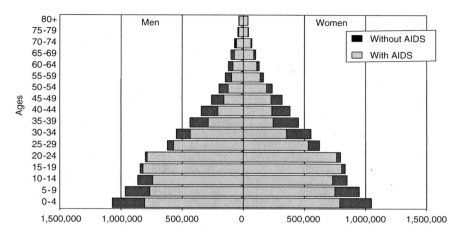

FIGURE 2-10 Population by age and sex in Zimbabwe, with and without AIDS mortality incorporated into the estimate: 2005.
SOURCE: U.S. Census Bureau (2005).

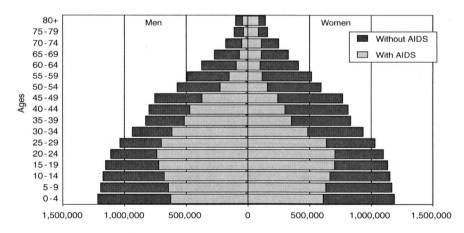

FIGURE 2-11 Population by age and sex in Zimbabwe, with and without AIDS mortality incorporated into the projection: 2030.
SOURCE: U.S. Census Bureau (2005).

2030. So even though AIDS is having a severe impact on Zimbabwe's population, the older population will continue to grow.

Impact of AIDS on Life Expectancy

Perhaps a more intuitive understanding of mortality is obtained by considering the life expectancy at birth, the number of years a newborn child is expected to live given the existing health and other environmental conditions of the country. Projection models have usually indicated a steady increase in life expectancy under the assumption that improvements in public health and health care, particularly child immunizations, would decrease mortality.

Life expectancy in sub-Saharan African countries ranges from a high of 72.4 in Mauritius to a low of 33.2 in Swaziland (Figure 2-12). Life expectancy at birth is below 50 years in 28 sub-Saharan African countries. Eight countries have life expectancy less than 40 years. These low levels of life expectancy at birth are related to many factors, including poor access to health care, low living standards and economic oppression, and civil unrest and violent conflict. However, in most countries, the main reason for these low levels is the AIDS pandemic.

Figures 2-13 and 2-14 show trends in life expectancy by sex for

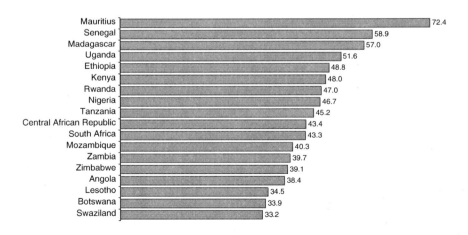

FIGURE 2-12 Life expectancy at birth for selected sub-Saharan African countries: 2005.
SOURCE: U.S. Census Bureau (2005).

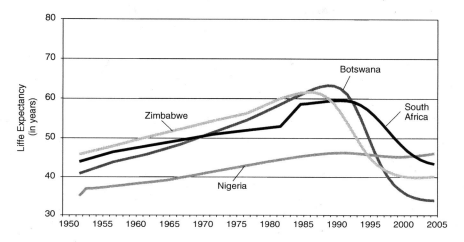

FIGURE 2-13 Male life expectancy at birth in four countries: 1950 to 2005.
SOURCES: United Nations (2001) and U.S. Census Bureau (2005).

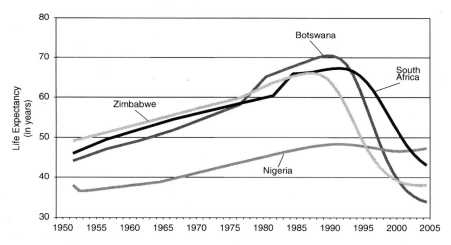

FIGURE 2-14 Female life expectancy at birth in four countries: 1950 to 2005.
SOURCES: United Nations (2001) and U.S. Census Bureau (2005).

Botswana and three other countries affected by AIDS. Life expectancy at birth increased steadily in all four countries for both men and women during the 1950s, 1960s, and 1970s. In the mid-1980s, there was a dramatic downturn in the trajectory of life expectancy at birth, mainly related to the increased mortality due to AIDS.

The trend in life expectancy at birth in Botswana is a good illustration of the devastation of AIDS on populations in Africa. In Botswana, male life expectancy at birth fell from 63.3 years the late 1980s to just 33.9 years in 2005, a decrease of 29.4 years (Figure 2-13). The loss for women is even larger: life expectancy dropped by 36.7 years over the same time period. Zimbabwe also experienced large decreases in life expectancy at birth, a drop of 21.4 years for men and 28.0 years for women. The AIDS pandemic has had, and will continue to have, an enormous impact on mortality in Africa.

Life Expectancy With and Without AIDS

Another way to illustrate the impact of AIDS on life expectancy at birth is to calculate life expectancies with and without AIDS mortality for one point in time. Taking the example of Botswana again, in 2005 life expectancy at birth for men was 40 years lower than it would have been if there was no mortality due to AIDS. AIDS mortality has had an even larger impact on female life expectancy. Life expectancy at birth for women in Botswana in 2005 was estimated at 33.8 years, 44.6 years lower than it would have been without the excess mortality due to AIDS. The net impact of AIDS on life expectancy at birth in Lesotho, Swaziland, and Zimbabwe is also large—with net differences of over 25 years in male life expectancy and 30 years in female life expectancy (see Table 2-1). That is, life expectancies at birth in these three countries are over 30 years lower for women than they would have been without AIDS mortality.

COMPARISON OF U.S. CENSUS BUREAU AND UN POPULATION DIVISION ESTIMATES AND PROJECTIONS

The U.S. Census Bureau and the UN Population Division both produce population estimates and projections for all countries of the world.[3] They share data sets but use different modeling techniques and assumptions to produce their demographic estimates and projections. In this section we compare the population estimates and projections from the two organizations. We also examine the input data used for the two sets of projections and compare the assumptions that are made about fertility, mortality (particularly about the impact of the HIV epidemic), and migration.

---

[3]For comparison purposes we use the UN's medium variant.

TABLE 2-1 Life Expectancy at Birth, With and Without AIDS, by Sex for Selected Sub-Saharan African Countries: 2005 (countries with a difference of 5 or more years in life expectancy for at least one sex)

Country	Men			Women		
	With AIDS	Without AIDS	Difference	With AIDS	Without AIDS	Difference
Botswana	33.9	73.9	−40.0	33.8	78.4	−44.6
Burkina Faso	47.0	51.4	−4.4	50.0	55.6	−5.6
Burundi	49.6	56.7	−7.1	51.0	60.1	−9.1
Cameroon	50.7	58.6	−7.9	51.1	61.3	−10.2
Central African Republic	43.3	56.6	−13.3	43.5	60.8	−17.2
Cote d'Ivoire	46.1	52.0	−6.0	51.3	60.4	−9.1
Ethiopia	47.7	51.7	−4.0	50.0	55.3	−5.3
Gabon	53.6	62.2	−8.6	56.5	67.4	−10.9
Kenya	48.9	57.3	−8.4	47.1	57.7	−10.7
Lesotho	35.5	62.8	−27.3	33.4	68.2	−34.8
Malawi	41.7	55.9	−14.2	41.2	59.0	−17.8
Mozambique	39.9	49.6	−9.7	40.8	52.3	−11.5
Namibia	44.7	68.2	−23.5	43.1	72.6	−29.5
Nigeria	46.2	51.4	−5.2	47.3	54.5	−7.2
Rwanda	45.9	51.0	−5.1	48.0	54.5	−6.5
South Africa	43.5	63.5	−20.0	43.1	70.6	−27.5
Swaziland	32.5	70.8	−38.3	34.0	76.0	−42.0
Tanzania	44.6	53.4	−8.9	45.9	57.6	−11.7
Togo	55.0	60.8	−5.8	59.1	66.7	−7.6
Uganda	50.7	56.8	−6.1	52.5	60.6	−8.1
Zambia	39.4	54.5	−15.0	40.0	58.9	−18.9
Zimbabwe	40.2	69.2	−29.0	38.0	73.5	−35.5

SOURCE: U.S. Census Bureau (2005).

Population

Table 2-2 compares the U.S. Census Bureau and the UN estimates and projections of the proportion of the population age 50 and over, age 60 and over, and age 80 and over for the world, the developed regions, the developing regions, and sub-Saharan Africa for 2005 and 2030. In 2005, the percentage of older persons in sub-Saharan Africa was low compared with other regions, and these percentages will increase at a slower rate than in other regions. The proportion age 60 and over is remarkably similar in the two data sets. The Census Bureau estimates that 4.7 percent of the population in sub-Saharan Africa was age 60 and over in 2005, and the UN estimates 4.9 percent. By 2030, both organizations project that the proportion in the older ages will increase but the increase is fairly small, less than 1 percentage point for both data sets. The differences in percentages, when comparing Census Bureau with UN data, are surprisingly small (see Table 2-2).

If we examine the absolute numbers of older people by regions, we see more of a difference between the two data sets, particularly for certain regions (e.g., Asia and North Africa); however, the difference is still small. For sub-Saharan Africa, the Census Bureau estimates 34.1 million people age 60 and over and the UN estimates 36.6 million, a difference of about 2.5 million. By 2030, the projected difference in the number of older people in sub-Saharan Africa is larger, 3.7 million people. Both organizations project that the number of people age 60 and over in sub-Saharan Africa will roughly double in size between 2005 and 2030 (see Table 2-3).

Country-level comparisons of these two data sets provide an illustration of the results of applying different assumptions to the input data. Figure 2-15 presents the differences between the two data sets in the estimates for the number of people age 60 and over in 2005. The UN estimates for Ethiopia, Sudan, and Tanzania are much larger in 2005 than are the Census Bureau's, while the estimates for Nigeria and South Africa are larger from the Census Bureau (see Figure 2-15).

Comparing the Census Bureau and UN projections for 2030, one sees that the magnitude of the difference increases substantially, especially in Ethiopia, Nigeria, South Africa, and Tanzania (see Figure 2-16). The UN projects that in Ethiopia there will be around 7.5 million people age 60 and over and the Census Bureau projects that there it will be around 6.6 million, a difference of nearly 1 million people. For other countries, not only the magnitude but also the sign of the difference changes. For example, in 2005 the Census Bureau's estimate for South Africa was larger than the UN estimate by around 236,000 people. In 2030, the Census Bureau's projection for the number of older people in South Africa is smaller than that of the UN's projection by over 1 million people. Similarly, the Census Bureau

TABLE 2-2 Percentage of the Population Age 50 and Over, 60 and Over, and 80 and Over: 2005 and 2030

Region[a]	Year	Percentage Age 50 and Over		Percentage Age 60 and Over		Percentage Age 80 and Over	
		Census	UN	Census	UN	Census	UN
World	2005	19.2	19.3	10.4	10.4	1.4	1.3
	2030	27.8	27.6	16.8	16.7	2.5	2.4
More Developed	2005	33.3	33.2	20.2	20.2	3.7	3.7
	2030	42.5	42.0	29.3	28.9	6.6	6.3
Less Developed	2005	16.0	16.1	8.1	8.2	0.8	0.8
	2030	25.1	24.9	14.6	14.5	1.7	1.7
Sub-Saharan Africa	2005	9.6	9.9	4.7	4.9	0.3	0.3
	2030	11.2	11.2	5.5	5.7	0.5	0.5

[a]More developed region = all countries of Europe, plus North America, Australia, New Zealand, and Japan. Less developed region = all countries in Africa, Asia (excluding Japan), Latin America and the Caribbean, Micronesia and Polynesia. For UN region definition, see http://esa.un.org/unpp/definition.html.

SOURCES: U.S. Census Bureau (2005) and United Nations (2005).

TABLE 2-3 Number of Older People by Age and Region of the World: 2005 and 2030

Region[a]	Year	Age 50 and Over		Age 60 and Over		Age 80 and Over	
		Census	UN	Census	UN	Census	UN
Europe	2005	245,614,448	245,015,520	151,291,593	150,591,254	26,169,672	25,725,770
	2030	312,561,235	304,613,381	214,331,028	207,605,773	45,929,877	41,947,901
North America	2005	97,313,814	97,343,151	55,589,473	49,339,590	11,903,309	6,700,336
	2030	147,652,565	145,846,216	102,554,119	100,570,697	21,936,520	19,998,266
Oceania	2005	8,246,024	8,194,953	4,700,674	4,594,260	874,076	846,739
	2030	13,693,849	13,838,186	8,857,103	9,103,985	1,793,838	1,793,470
Asia	2005	691,162,428	706,996,181	355,182,191	364,860,938	38,087,333	38,103,899
	2030	1,390,710,312	1,404,019,914	824,256,449	833,038,827	1,793,838	102,982,325
Latin America/Caribbean	2005	93,146,632	93,344,375	49,256,543	49,339,590	6,314,087	6,700,336
	2030	200,780,113	199,873,771	117,985,102	117,900,557	17,350,971	18,277,533
North Africa	2005	25,672,557	25,888,659	12,765,209	12,868,919	1,059,691	1,058,834
	2030	63,948,861	59,986,758	34,179,192	32,047,078	106,120,112	3,079,500
Sub-Saharan Africa	2005	70,591,644	74,237,838	34,110,260	36,594,051	2,427,129	2,626,207
	2030	137,419,008	140,021,970	67,335,106	71,033,103	6,097,609	6,549,537

[a]In this table, regions follow the practice of the United Nations. For region definitions, see http://esa.un.org/unpp/definition.html.
SOURCES: U.S. Census Bureau (2005) and United Nations (2005).

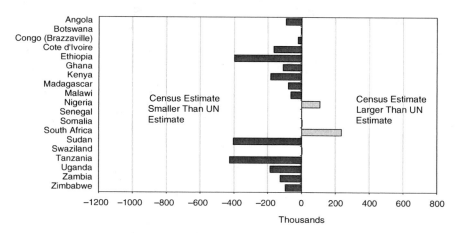

FIGURE 2-15 Difference between U.S. Census Bureau and UN estimates of the population age 60 and over in selected sub-Saharan African countries: 2005. SOURCES: U.S. Census Bureau (2005) and United Nations (2005).

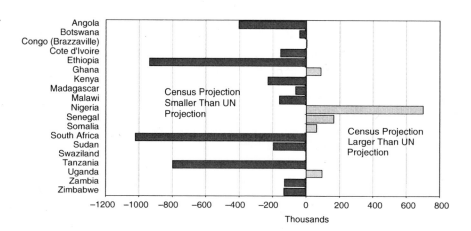

FIGURE 2-16 Difference between U.S. Census Bureau and UN estimates of the population age 60 and over in selected sub-Saharan African countries: 2030. SOURCES: U.S. Census Bureau (2005) and United Nations (2005).

estimates for Swaziland were larger than the UN estimates in 2005. However, by 2030 the Census Bureau projections of the older population for this country are smaller than the UN's. The opposite is true for Congo (Brazzaville), Ghana, Senegal, and Uganda, in that the Census Bureau's estimate in 2005 was smaller than the UN's, but by 2030, the Census Bureau's projection of the population age 60 and over is larger than the UN's.

A closer inspection of country-specific data reveals some unique differences between the two data sources. A number of patterns emerge when the numbers and percentages of older persons are examined from 1990 to 2030. The Census Bureau's figures are often lower than the UN data, a situation that is probably due to the differences in assumptions about the future path of the AIDS epidemic (discussed below). The impact of violent conflict in a number of countries in sub-Saharan Africa resembles an epidemic, but, again, reliable data on the effect of these conflicts on population size are not available (see Table 2-4 for estimates of war deaths). Countries with a large impact from the HIV epidemic and countries affected by violent conflict over the past decades show the greatest differences.

Examination of population estimates and projections for Botswana demonstrate the extent to which the Census Bureau and the UN data sets differ. Both organizations project that the total population of Botswana will decrease slightly between 2005 and 2030, but the magnitude of the decrease differs. The Census Bureau projects the total population of Botswana will decline from 1.6 million in 2005 to 1.5 million by 2030, a decrease of just over 100,000 people. The UN also projects a decline, but it is slightly larger, just over 120,000 people. For the older population, the two data sources also differ. The Census Bureau projects that the 2030 older population will be about 6,000 people *smaller* than the 2005 older population. The UN projects that the older population in 2030 will be around 30,000 people *larger* than the 2005 older population.

Factors Affecting Population Projections

Comparison of input data and assumptions used in the Census Bureau and UN estimates and projections help explain the differences between the two data sets. The main differences are linked to the different assumptions about AIDS mortality.

Input Data

The four main sources of input data are censuses, vital registration, national household surveys, and demographic surveillance sites. Census data are the most often used source for the baseline population data in population projections. Figure 2-17 indicates the most recent rounds of census

TABLE 2-4 U.S. Census Bureau and the United Nations Population Division Estimates and Projections of Numbers and Percentages of Older People for Selected Countries in Sub-Saharan Africa: 1990, 2005, 2015, and 2030

Country	Total Population	Population Age 50 and Over		Population Age 60 and Over		Population Age 80 and Over	
		Number	Percentage	Number	Percentage	Number	Percentage
Countries affected by HIV/AIDS (epidemic characteristics in parentheses)							
Botswana (AIDS—late start, explosive growth, very high prevalence)							
Census							
1990	1,263,643	128,233	10.1	70,170	5.6	9,991	0.8
2005	1,640,115	159,976	9.8	86,480	5.3	13,296	0.8
2015	1,634,216	150,760	9.2	86,008	5.3	16,342	1.0
2030	1,537,295	126,666	8.2	80,348	5.2	19,638	1.3
UN							
1990	1,428,510	112,310	7.9	55,405	3.9	4,344	0.3
2005	1,764,926	191,667	10.9	90,829	5.1	7,923	0.4
2015	1,690,491	213,034	12.6	124,154	7.3	10,539	0.6
2030	1,642,498	165,469	10.1	120,744	7.4	19,305	1.2
Kenya (AIDS—mid-start, steady growth, moderate prevalence)							
Census							
1990	23,358,413	1,836,738	7.9	918,152	3.9	90,394	0.4
2005	33,829,590	2,652,930	7.8	1,223,610	3.6	97,231	0.3
2015	42,702,635	3,615,823	8.5	1,632,772	3.8	117,860	0.3
2030	52,472,826	6,808,107	13.0	2,987,402	5.7	214,778	0.4
UN							
1990	23,430,275	1,901,586	8.1	969,845	4.1	78,372	0.3
2005	34,255,722	2,929,834	8.6	1,406,063	4.1	130,706	0.4
2015	44,194,402	3,963,630	9.0	1,971,956	4.5	186,585	0.4
2030	60,605,792	6,791,920	11.2	3,217,455	5.3	286,887	0.5

continued

TABLE 2-4 Continued

Country	Total Population	Population Age 50 and Over		Population Age 60 and Over		Population Age 80 and Over	
		Number	Percentage	Number	Percentage	Number	Percentage
Malawi (AIDS—mid-start, steady growth, high prevalence)							
Census							
1990	9,286,655	857,924	9.2	408,213	4.4	27,867	0.3
2005	12,707,464	1,082,383	8.5	535,960	4.2	34,683	0.3
2015	16,074,826	1,237,020	7.7	646,935	4.0	48,633	0.3
2030	22,030,253	1,677,073	7.6	815,850	3.7	81,753	0.4
UN							
1990	9,459,434	821,864	8.7	393,630	4.2	16,041	0.2
2005	12,883,935	1,190,090	9.2	599,583	4.7	40,825	0.3
2015	15,997,810	1,402,139	8.8	760,846	4.8	55,848	0.3
2030	21,686,512	1,823,220	8.4	976,112	4.5	97,728	0.5
Senegal (AIDS—early start, no growth, low prevalence)							
Census							
1990	7,844,199	706,826	9.0	331,655	4.2	21,438	0.3
2005	11,706,498	1,176,631	10.1	566,950	4.8	42,071	0.4
2015	14,488,615	1,658,431	11.4	812,355	5.6	66,623	0.5
2030	18,292,033	2,837,929	15.5	1,409,079	7.7	133,766	0.7
UN							
1990	7,977,487	776,870	9.7	388,355	4.9	31,543	0.4
2005	11,658,172	1,124,724	9.6	567,479	4.9	43,394	0.4
2015	14,538,255	1,511,727	10.4	744,539	5.1	62,697	0.4
2030	18,677,539	2,563,428	13.7	1,243,949	6.7	105,774	0.6

Uganda (AIDS—early start, now falling, moderate prevalence)

Census

Year						
1990	17,074,034	1,361,305	8.0	637,004	3.7	23,301	0.1
2005	27,269,482	1,794,941	6.6	917,712	3.4	70,907	0.3
2015	39,142,167	2,573,062	6.6	1,177,362	3.0	110,004	0.3
2030	67,604,495	4,921,994	7.3	2,242,143	3.3	185,678	0.3

UN

Year						
1990	17,757,955	1,476,737	8.3	727,634	4.1	42,637	0.2
2005	28,816,229	2,161,017	7.5	1,102,864	3.8	88,130	0.3
2015	41,918,305	2,648,080	6.3	1,413,514	3.4	127,436	0.3
2030	72,077,803	5,052,488	7.0	2,146,531	3.0	213,187	0.3

Zimbabwe (AIDS—early start, rapid growth, very high prevalence)

Census

Year						
1990	10,152,933	907,069	8.9	454,203	4.5	43,323	0.4
2005	12,160,782	1,159,985	9.5	613,557	5.0	70,709	0.6
2015	12,772,015	1,243,544	9.7	689,141	5.4	92,825	0.7
2030	12,842,466	1,433,303	11.2	782,899	6.1	132,727	1.0

UN

Year						
1990	10,564,857	925,692	8.8	474,510	4.5	35,717	0.3
2005	13,009,534	1,318,238	10.1	708,585	5.4	69,789	0.5
2015	13,804,252	1,443,927	10.5	846,788	6.1	94,154	0.7
2030	14,699,962	1,559,117	10.6	915,002	6.2	132,787	0.9

Countries affected by violent conflict (approximate start-end dates, estimated number of deaths where available)

Angola (conflict—1980-2002, 1.1 million)

Census

Year						
1990	8,290,856	863,766	10.4	348,563	4.2	14,854	0.2
2005	11,827,315	1,123,136	9.5	535,548	4.5	21,680	0.2
2015	14,655,105	1,400,587	9.6	614,873	4.2	33,557	0.2
2030	19,375,631	1,976,052	10.2	915,775	4.7	47,282	0.2

continued

TABLE 2-4 Continued

Country	Total Population	Population Age 50 and Over		Population Age 60 and Over		Population Age 80 and Over	
		Number	Percentage	Number	Percentage	Number	Percentage
UN							
1990	10,532,123	934,779	8.9	440,043	4.2	20,766	0.2
2005	15,941,392	1,332,437	8.4	628,394	3.9	36,601	0.2
2015	20,946,513	1,783,002	8.5	831,941	4.0	53,078	0.3
2030	30,049,775	2,752,104	9.2	1,318,818	4.4	87,641	0.3
Congo (Kinshasa) (conflict—1996-2003, 2.5 million)							
Census							
1990	39,064,041	3,536,186	9.1	1,652,198	4.2	101,560	0.3
2005	60,764,490	5,061,774	8.3	2,435,275	4.0	169,009	0.3
2015	82,030,429	6,551,088	8.0	3,219,551	3.9	250,680	0.3
2030	122,223,300	10,750,219	8.8	5,072,914	4.2	461,695	0.4
UN							
1990	37,764,442	3,519,601	9.3	1,673,012	4.4	97,789	0.3
2005	57,548,744	4,985,882	8.7	2,453,022	4.3	158,931	0.3
2015	78,016,089	6,275,692	8.0	3,125,250	4.0	222,217	0.3
2030	117,493,959	9,786,515	8.3	4,616,225	3.9	372,096	0.3
Mozambique (conflict—1976-1992, 1 million)							
Census							
1990	12,655,732	1,153,393	9.1	494,735	3.9	22,496	0.2
2005	19,406,703	1,927,506	9.9	884,866	4.6	49,334	0.3
2015	21,731,142	2,237,793	10.3	1,089,297	5.0	73,623	0.3
2030	24,322,705	2,557,453	10.5	1,328,732	5.5	119,627	0.5

continued

UN

Year						
1990	13,429,408	1,438,878	10.7	703,162	5.2	36,550	0.3
2005	19,792,295	2,020,773	10.2	1,026,078	5.2	73,491	0.4
2015	23,512,692	2,427,029	10.3	1,287,419	5.5	109,552	0.5
2030	29,603,641	3,138,367	10.6	1,703,205	5.8	178,798	0.6

Rwanda (conflict—1990-1994, 1 million)

Census

Year						
1990	6,923,738	596,714	8.6	304,205	4.4	17,831	0.3
2005	8,440,820	705,435	8.4	319,140	3.8	27,462	0.3
2015	10,687,704	994,796	9.3	446,765	4.2	36,168	0.3
2030	14,441,869	1,653,133	11.4	778,778	5.4	55,589	0.4

UN

Year						
1990	7,096,089	556,337	7.8	258,594	3.6	14,669	0.2
2005	9,037,690	737,815	8.2	356,014	3.9	23,354	0.3
2015	11,261,747	980,829	8.7	464,783	4.1	32,979	0.3
2030	14,367,933	1,542,229	10.7	733,961	5.1	56,673	0.4

Sierra Leone (conflict—1991-2002, 50,000)

Census

Year						
1990	4,220,883	471,635	11.2	214,460	5.1	17,430	0.4
2005	5,867,426	609,524	10.4	303,234	5.2	17,371	0.3
2015	7,367,438	676,494	9.2	355,074	4.8	23,563	0.3
2030	10,094,211	980,562	9.7	465,791	4.6	37,164	0.4

UN

Year						
1990	4,078,436	487,974	12.0	231,798	5.7	8,434	0.2
2005	5,525,478	626,839	11.3	303,550	5.5	13,463	0.2
2015	6,897,404	760,093	11.0	367,546	5.3	17,825	0.3
2030	9,649,911	1,062,311	11.0	528,521	5.5	28,856	0.3

TABLE 2-4 Continued

Country	Total Population	Population Age 50 and Over		Population Age 60 and Over		Population Age 80 and Over	
		Number	Percentage	Number	Percentage	Number	Percentage
Sudan (conflict—1983-2004, 2 million)							
Census							
1990	26,627,366	2,235,135	8.4	966,290	3.6	86,478	0.3
2005	40,187,486	3,677,107	9.1	1,643,233	4.1	81,263	0.2
2015	50,848,938	5,155,041	10.1	2,479,011	4.9	136,234	0.3
2030	66,346,176	9,302,769	14.0	4,454,353	6.7	361,476	0.5
UN							
1990	26,066,123	2,659,892	10.2	1,270,552	4.9	74,536	0.3
2005	36,232,945	4,127,418	11.4	2,047,024	5.6	153,513	0.4
2015	44,035,008	5,665,452	12.9	2,870,760	6.5	240,413	0.5
2030	54,511,049	9,007,892	16.5	4,650,247	8.5	451,380	0.8

SOURCES: U.S. Census Bureau (2005); United Nations (2005); Zaba, Marston, and Floyd (2003); Smith (2003); U.S. Central Intelligence Agency (2004); Leitenberg (2003).

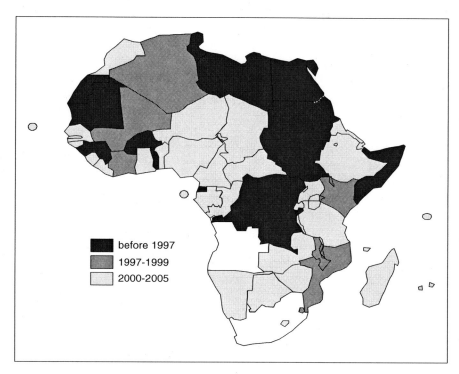

FIGURE 2-17 Most recent census dates.
SOURCE: U.S. Census Bureau (2005).

data collection for each country. While censuses provide invaluable data, they have the disadvantage of long time periods between rounds and time lags (sometimes significant) between data collection and data availability. Some sub-Saharan countries have data from a recent census (taken less than five years ago). However, others have postponed censuses from 2000 out to 2005 or later. Although certain countries took censuses near 2000, the data are not always available for use until much later (e.g., Senegal took their census in 2002 but the data have not yet been released).

Other data sources, such as vital registration data, demographic surveillance sites, and national surveys are also used as input data. However, many of these other sources have limitations, particularly for the countries of sub-Saharan Africa. Vital registration systems with high coverage are uncommon in most countries in sub-Saharan Africa. Where they do exist, coverage is variable (the World Health Organization has data from only nine countries in sub-Saharan Africa, with coverage rates ranging from 5 percent in Mozambique to 99 percent in the Seychelles) (Kowal, Rao, and Mathers, 2003). Thus, vital registration data that can be used as input data for projections are not available for use in most projections of sub-Saharan populations.

Another source of input data is national demographic surveys, such as the Demographic and Health Surveys (DHS). These surveys are often conducted more frequently than censuses and produce high-quality data for estimations of fertility and infant and child mortality, but they do not provide adult mortality estimates. Typically, infant and child mortality estimates derived from DHS data are matched to model life tables to produce estimates of adult mortality patterns. However, given that the model life tables available were developed before the onset of the HIV/AIDS epidemic, they cannot be used without major adjustments to take into account the impact of AIDS deaths.

Demographic surveillance field sites, such as those in INDEPTH, potentially provide high-quality data; however, the data are not typically nationally representative.[4] Data from demographic surveillance sites have not been used by the Census Bureau or the UN in the estimates and projections discussed in this paper.

Migration data are derived from various sources, including the UN (the United Nations High Commission for Refugees, the United Nations Statistics Division, and the United Nations Economic Commission for Europe Statistics Division) and the International Organization for Migration. Migration data are notoriously difficult to obtain and available data are generally considered to be unreliable. The political will throughout Africa to address migration policies and to obtain these data is improving, yet the realities of current data collection systems suggest that improvements will take time (African Union Commission, 2004). Data on forced, internal, and international migration are fraught with problems. Cross-border migration and internal displacement continue to create migration flows that remain difficult to track as the frequency, timing, and duration of migration patterns are subject to rapidly changing factors, such as household disintegration due to HIV/AIDS, economic forces driven by globalization, and natural and manmade disasters, many of which disproportionately affect countries in this region.

In addition, new migration patterns have developed as a result of AIDS, countering the urbanization trends: adult children "going home to die," moving from urban areas to rural homes, to be cared for by their parents

---

[4]INDEPTH is an international network of field sites with continuous demographic evaluation of populations and their health in developing countries.

and families (Foster, 1995). AIDS deaths are contributing to the disintegration of households, resulting in orphaned children being forced to relocate, and usually to poor areas (Richter, 2004).

Both the Census Bureau and the UN use data on HIV/AIDS prevalence rates provided by the Joint United Nations Programme on HIV/AIDS (UNAIDS) and World Health Organization (WHO) Epidemiology Reference Group (Joint United Nations Programme on HIV/AIDS and World Health Organization, 2004a). These prevalence rates are based on the best available data from different national sources, including antenatal clinic surveillance sites and national surveys. Both organizations used the UNAIDS 2004 release of HIV prevalence rates in their projections. The prevalence rates that underlie the mortality assumptions for both the Census Bureau and the UN projections are presented in Table 2-5. The characteristics and impact of HIV/AIDS vary throughout the subcontinent, which affects the magnitude and timing of their effects on demographic estimates and projections.

In general, UNAIDS divides the magnitude of the infection into three states: (1) *generalized,* defined as HIV prevalence consistently over 1 percent in pregnant women; (2) *concentrated*, defined as HIV prevalence consistently over 5 percent in at least one subpopulation at highest risk and prevalence below 1 percent in the general adult population ages 15 to 49 in urban areas; and (3) *low,* defined as HIV prevalence has not consistently exceeded 5 percent in any defined subpopulation (Joint United Nations Programme on HIV/AIDS and World Health Organization, 2003).

Fertility Assumptions

Historically, declines in fertility have been the main determinant of population aging in developing countries. Countries that have experienced rapid declines in fertility have also experienced rapid increases in aging (for example, South Korea and Thailand). Fertility rates for most countries in sub-Saharan Africa are still high. In many, fertility is declining slowly, which contributes to the relatively slow rate of population aging in the region (United Nations, 2003a). Future trends in fertility will affect the way that countries in the region will age.

According to Census Bureau estimates, sub-Saharan African countries accounted for 8 of the top 10 highest fertility rates in the world in 2005. Niger and Mali had the two highest total fertility rates in the world, at more than 7 births per woman, and Somalia's estimated total fertility rate was 6.8. Only three countries in the subregion (Botswana, Mauritius, and South Africa) had total fertility rates below 3.0 children per women, and only Mauritius had a total fertility rate below the replacement level fertility of 2.1.

TABLE 2-5 Prevalence Rates for Sub-Saharan Africa HIV Adults Ages 15 to 49 from the Joint United Nations Programme on HIV/AIDS: End of 2003

	Adult Prevalence (%)	(Low Estimate and High Estimate)
Sub-Saharan Africa	7.5	[6.9 - 8.3]
Angola	3.9	[1.6 - 9.4]
Benin	1.9	[1.1 - 3.3]
Botswana	37.3	[35.5 - 39.1]
Burkina Faso	4.2	[2.7 - 6.5]
Burundi	6.0	[4.1 - 8.8]
Cameroon	6.9	[4.8 - 9.8]
Central African Republic	13.5	[8.3 - 21.2]
Chad	4.8	[3.1 - 7.2]
Congo (Brazzaville)	4.9	[2.1 - 11.0]
Congo (Kinshasa)	4.2	[1.7 - 9.9]
Côte d'Ivoire	7.0	[4.9 - 10.0]
Djibouti	2.9	[0.7 - 7.5]
Eritrea	2.7	[0.9 - 7.3]
Ethiopia	4.4	[2.8 - 6.7]
Gabon	8.1	[4.1 - 15.3]
Gambia	1.2	[0.3 - 4.2]
Ghana	3.1	[1.9 - 5.0]
Guinea	3.2	[1.2 - 8.2]
Kenya	6.7	[4.7 - 9.6]
Lesotho	28.9	[26.3 - 31.7]
Liberia	5.9	[2.7 - 12.4]
Madagascar	1.7	[0.8 - 2.7]
Malawi	14.2	[11.3 - 17.7]
Mali	1.9	[0.6 - 5.9]
Mauritania	0.6	[0.3 - 1.1]
Mozambique	12.2	[9.4 - 15.7]
Namibia	21.3	[18.2 - 24.7]
Niger	1.2	[0.7 - 2.3]
Nigeria	5.4	[3.6 - 8.0]
Rwanda	5.1	[3.4 - 7.6]
Senegal	0.8	[0.4 - 1.7]
South Africa	21.5	[18.5 - 24.9]
Swaziland	38.8	[37.2 - 40.4]
Togo	4.1	[2.7 - 6.4]
Uganda	4.1	[2.8 - 6.6]
Tanzania	8.8	[6.4 - 11.9]
Zambia	16.5	[13.5 - 20.0]
Zimbabwe	24.6	[21.7 - 27.8]

SOURCES: Joint United Nations Programme on HIV/AIDS and World Health Organization (2004b).

Fertility rates used in the estimates are derived from census and national household survey data. For its projections, the Census Bureau takes trends in observed fertility rates for a country and calculates the decline in the future based on a logistic function. The UN assumes that fertility decline follows a path derived from models of fertility decline that it has established on the basis of the past experiences of countries with declining fertility during the period 1950 to 2000 (United Nations, 2005). Projected fertility is compared with recent fertility trends in each country and adjusted so that the projected fertility is consistent with the most recent fertility trends. Projected fertility rates for a number of sub-Saharan countries are shown in Figures 2-18a (Census Bureau) and 2-18b (UN). Both the Census Bureau and the UN project fertility to decrease in all of the countries of sub-Saharan Africa between 2005 and 2030; however, the size of the decrease differs. The Census Bureau projects that fertility will be at or below replacement level in only five countries in sub-Saharan Africa by 2030, and the UN projects that two countries will be at or below replacement by this date. The total fertility rate in 2030 is projected to remain above 4 children per woman in 15 of the 42 countries, according to the Census Bureau. These relatively high fertility rates ensure that the proportion in the older ages will remain fairly low in many sub-Saharan African countries well into the future.

It is unclear how fertility rates will be affected by HIV/AIDS, but at the individual level, as the time infected increases, pregnancy rates drop. Overall, the most likely result is that an HIV epidemic will slightly reduce fertility, but at this point the data are not available to make reasonable assumptions about the impact (Stover and Stanecki, 2003).

Mortality Assumptions

Although declines in fertility have historically been the driving force behind population aging in the countries of sub-Saharan Africa, mortality contributes to population aging, especially in countries highly affected by AIDS. The impact of AIDS has been so large in many of these sub-Saharan countries that it will significantly affect how their populations age.

In countries with AIDS mortality, the impact is seen clearly in mortality rates for the adult age groups. These groups are projected to have high mortality rates when AIDS mortality is incorporated into the projections.

The mortality rates are adjusted on the basis of HIV prevalence rates. The adult HIV prevalence rate for the countries in sub-Saharan Africa ranges from 0.6 in Mauritania to 38.8 in Swaziland (see Table 2-5) (Joint United Nations Programme on HIV/AIDS and World Health Organization,

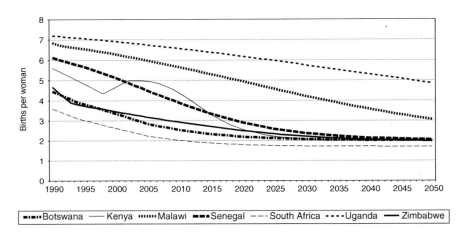

FIGURE 2-18a Total fertility rates for selected sub-Saharan African countries: 1990 to 2050 (U.S. Census Bureau data).
SOURCE: U.S. Census Bureau (2005).

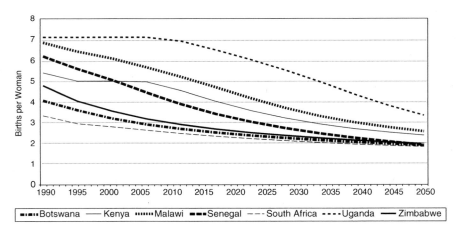

FIGURE 2-18b Total fertility rates for selected sub-Saharan African countries: 1990 to 2050 (UN data).
SOURCE: United Nations (2005).

2004a).[5] These figures are based on HIV prevalence in women attending antenatal clinics, from which assumptions about infection rates are applied to derive rates for the general population (Joint United Nations Programme on HIV/AIDS, 2004). Despite the limitations and without a functioning vital registration system or representative national-level surveys, prevalence rates derived from antenatal clinic data provide the best source of routinely collected information currently available.[6]

The Census Bureau incorporated AIDS mortality in 54 countries into their 2005 International Data Base. Of these 54 countries, 39 were in sub-Saharan Africa. The Census Bureau obtained estimates of AIDS-related mortality using a new application that incorporates estimates of HIV prevalence from the Estimation and Projection Package (EPP)—an epidemiologically realistic model developed and used by the WHO and UNAIDS. EPP produces a national "best fit" curve of adult HIV prevalence using sentinel surveillance data pertaining to pregnant women. The Census Bureau used country-specific adult HIV prevalence estimates from EPP for years from the beginning of the epidemic to 2010. The Census Bureau applied assumptions from the WHO/UNAIDS Epidemiological Reference Group about the age and sex distribution of HIV incidence, sex ratios of new infections, mother-to-child transmission rate, and disease progression. The model allows for competing risk of death and projects HIV incidence implied by the EPP estimates of HIV prevalence through 2010, assuming a decline in HIV incidence of 50 percent by 2050. The model can include the impact of antiretroviral therapy, but the current projections assume no one will receive treatment (U.S. Census Bureau, 2005).

In its 2004 revision, the UN Population Division increased the total number of countries with substantial excess deaths caused by HIV/AIDS to 60; of these 60 countries, 40 are located in sub-Saharan Africa (United Nations, 2005). A slow pace of mortality decline in countries highly affected by the AIDS epidemic was used for mortality risk not related to HIV/AIDS. For countries not considered "most affected" by HIV/AIDS, mortality is projected based on models of changing life expectancy produced by the UN.

Infection prevalence data from models created by UNAIDS were used

---

[5]The proportion of adults ages 15 to 49 living with HIV/AIDS at the end of 2003.

[6]There is recent evidence that using data from antenatal clinics to estimate prevalence rates for the entire population may not be appropriate. A recent national survey in Kenya, which tested respondents for HIV infection, found that only 7 percent of the adult population was HIV positive. This contrasts with the estimate of 15 percent prevalence estimated using antenatal clinic data. In other words, the antenatal clinic overestimated the prevalence rate by 100 percent.

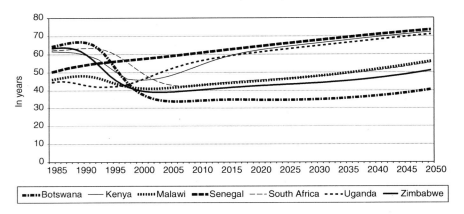

FIGURE 2-19a Life expectancy at birth in selected sub-Saharan African countries: 1990 to 2050 (U.S. Census Bureau data). SOURCE: U.S. Census Bureau (2005).

to estimate past dynamics and create projections for annual incidences of HIV infection. The 2004 UN revision projects the impact of HIV/AIDS to be less severe than was previously forecast in the 2002 revision. This difference is due to the revised and lower estimates of HIV prevalence in several countries (based on UNAIDS data for 2003) (United Nations, 2005; Joint United Nations Programme on HIV/AIDS, 2004). Also in the 2004 revision, the UN has assumed that beginning in 2005 changes in behavior and treatment will reduce the chances of infection in the future.

Both the Census Bureau and the UN project that life expectancy at birth will continue to decline for countries in which AIDS mortality is present (see Figures 2-19a and 2-19b). However, life expectancy at birth is projected to increase in most countries beginning some time after 2010.

CONCLUSION

Accurate statistics on basic demographic events are the foundation of rational health and public policy, yet many countries lack sound demographic information. In particular, data on both the number and causes of death in sub-Saharan African countries are virtually nonexistent. Reliable adult mortality data on levels, let alone causes, simply do not exist for the majority of the countries in sub-Saharan Africa. Mortality estimates are modeled from limited sources of data, such as surveys, censuses, and demographic surveillance sites (in the small number of countries where they exist). Currently there is a paucity of high-quality country-level data on mor-

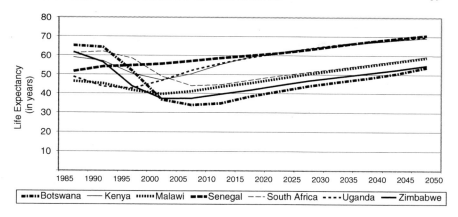

FIGURE 2-19b Life expectancy at birth in selected sub-Saharan African countries: 1990 to 2050 (UN data).
SOURCE: United Nations (2005).

tality for the sub-Saharan countries, and this has an impact on population estimates and projections. Efforts are currently under way to improve the collection of demographic data in many sub-Saharan countries, which will improve the future projections and assist in elucidating how these countries will age in the future.

The impact of HIV/AIDS on adult mortality rates in sub-Saharan Africa has reshaped the population structure and age distribution in most countries. Approximately 2.3 million people died of AIDS in 2004 (Joint United Nations Programme on HIV/AIDS, 2004). By the year 2020, it is projected that a total of 75 million Africans will have lost their lives to AIDS since the beginning of the epidemic. The impact of AIDS dramatically affects how countries in sub-Saharan Africa will age over the next several decades. Despite the huge impact of AIDS, sub-Saharan Africa is aging and will continue to age. The number of older people is projected to nearly double in less than 30 years. These growing numbers of older people will age in countries that are ill equipped to deal with the challenges that aging populations pose.

Explanation of Acronyms/Abbreviations

AIDS   Acquired Immunodeficiency Syndrome
HIV   Human Immunodeficiency Virus
HMN   Health Metrics Network

INDEPTH	An international network of field sites with continuous demographic evaluation of populations and their health in developing countries
IOM	International Organization of Migration
SAVVY	Sample Vital Registration and Verbal Autopsy
UN	United Nations Population Division
UNECE	United Nations Economic Commission for Europe Statistics Division
UNHCR	United Nations High Commission for Refugees
UNSD	United Nations Statistics Division
UNAIDS	Joint United Nations Programme on HIV/AIDS
USCB	U.S. Census Bureau
WHO	World Health Organization

REFERENCES

African Union Commission. (2004, March). Experts Group Meeting on the Policy Framework on Migration in Africa, Addis Ababa, Ethiopia. Opening speech by Adv. Bience Gawanas, African Union Commissioner for Social Affairs.

Foster, S.A. (1995). *A study of adult diseases in Zambia: Final report.* London, England: Overseas Development Agency.

Joint United Nations Programme on HIV/AIDS. (2004). *2004 report on the global AIDS epidemic.* Executive Summary. Geneva, Switzerland: Author.

Joint United Nations Programme on HIV/AIDS and World Health Organization. (2003, September). *A history of the HIV/AIDS epidemic with emphasis on Africa.* Training Workshop on HIV/AIDS and Adult Mortality in Developing Countries. New York: United Nations.

Joint United Nations Programme on HIV/AIDS and World Health Organization. (2004a, December). *AIDS epidemic update.* UNAIDS/04.45E.

Joint United Nations Programme on HIV/AIDS and World Health Organization. (2004b, December). *Technical report on improving estimates and projections of HIV/AIDS.* Based on a meeting of the UNAIDS/WHO Reference Group for Estimates, Modelling, and Projections, Sintra, Portugal. Geneva, Switzerland: Author.

Kowal, P.R., Rao, P.V.C., and Mathers, C. (2003). *Report on a WHO workshop: Minimum data set on ageing and adult mortality data in Sub-Saharan Africa.* Geneva, Switzerland: World Health Organization.

Leitenberg, M. (2003). *Death in wars and conflicts between 1945-2000.* New York: Cornell University. Peace Studies Program.

Richter, L.M. (2004, May). *The impact of HIV/AIDS on the development of children.* Presented at the Seminar on HIV/AIDS, Vulnerability, and Children: Dynamics and Long-term Implications for Southern Africa's Security, 4 April, 2003, Pretoria. Institute for Security Studies monograph no. 109.

Smith D. (2003). *The atlas of war and peace.* New York: Penguin Putnam.

Stover, J., and Stanecki, K.A. (2003). *Estimating and projecting the size and impact of the HIV/AIDS epidemic in generalized epidemics: The UNAIDS Reference Group approach.* Geneva, Switzerland: Joint United Nations Programme on HIV/AIDS.

United Nations. (2001). *World population prospects: The 2000 revision.* New York: Author.

United Nations. (2003a). *The impact of HIV/AIDS on mortality.* (Workshop on HIV/AIDS and Adult Mortality in Developing Countries. UN/POP/MORT/2003/14). New York: Author.

United Nations. (2003b). *World population prospects: The 2002 revision.* New York: Author.

United Nations. (2005). *World population prospects: The 2004 revision.* (ESA/P/WP.193). New York: Author.

U.S. Census Bureau. (2004). *The AIDS pandemic in the 21st century.* (International Population Reports No. WP/02-2, available from the U.S. Government Printing Office). Washington, DC: U.S. Department of Commerce.

U.S. Census Bureau. (2005). *International programs center, international database.* Available: http://www.cia.gov/cia/publications/factbook/ [accessed August 2006].

U.S. Central Intelligence Agency. (2004). *The world fact book.* Available: http://www.census.gov/ipc/wwf [accessed Sept. 2006].

Zaba, B., Marston, M., and Floyd S. (2003). *The effect of HIV on child mortality trends in sub-Saharan Africa.* Presented at the Training Workshop on HIV/AIDS and Adult Mortality in Developing Countries, Population Division, Department of Economic and Social Affairs, United Nations Secretariat, September 8-13, New York.

3

Demographic Impacts of the HIV Epidemic and Consequences of Population-Wide Treatment of HIV for the Elderly: Results from Microsimulation

Samuel J. Clark

INTRODUCTION

The high levels and continued increase in HIV prevalence in parts of sub-Saharan Africa are bringing with them substantial increases in adult mortality (Dorrington, Bourne, Bradshaw, Laubsher, and Timaeus, 2001; Timaeus, 1998; Joint United Nations Programme on HIV/AIDS, 2002) and decreases in fertility (Gregson, 1994; Gregson, Zaba, and Garnett, 1999; Zaba, 1998). Together these change the composition of infected populations significantly with important consequences for the elderly. Added to this is the potential for widespread prevention and treatment programs that will have substantial impacts of their own.

One of the most important and widely recognized consequences for the elderly is the creation of a large number of "AIDS orphans"—children who lose one or both of their parents as a result of HIV-related mortality. The report *Children on the Brink: 2002* indicates that there were 38 million orphans in Africa in 2001, 11 million of whom were attributable to AIDS mortality (Joint United Nations Programme on HIV/AIDS, UNICEF, and U.S. Agency for International Development, 2002). The same report predicts it is likely that there will be 42 million orphans in Africa in 2010, 20 million of whom are the result of AIDS mortality; others make even larger estimates of the number of orphans by 2010 (Monk, 2002). Bicego, Rutstein, and Johnson (2003) observed a strong correlation between the percentage of children who are orphans and national HIV prevalence for several African countries during the 1990s, lending weight to the conclusion that HIV is related to the rise in the number of orphans.

The sheer number of orphans being created is unusual in human history, as is the fact that many are *dual* orphans, children who have lost both parents and must be cared for by someone else. Compounding the problem for the elderly is the fact that their own numbers and the proportion of the population they constitute are also being affected by the epidemic, and all of the changes wrought by an HIV epidemic evolve as the epidemic grows and stabilizes. Accordingly, to adequately understand the total impact of the epidemic on the number and proportion of children who are orphans and on the number of grandparents and other family members who will be alive to care for them, one must employ a "whole population" model. Such a model takes into account all of the major avenues through which HIV impacts a population and how these interact with one another. Gregson, Garnett, and Anderson (1994) constructed one such model in the mid-1990s and used it to predict the major increase in the number and proportion of children who are orphaned as a result of HIV. Many of their theoretical findings are being validated now, as the epidemic unfolds and large numbers of orphans begin to appear in the worst affected African countries (Joint United Nations Programme on HIV/AIDS, UNICEF, and U.S. Agency for International Development, 2002).

Gregson and colleagues (1994) also examined more general demographic impacts of an HIV epidemic and demonstrate significant changes in the age-specific sex ratio, population age structure, and overall growth rates—all of which affect the elderly as the underlying structure and size of the population changes. Results presented here largely corroborate their findings while adding some additional nuances.

The work presented here employs a different modeling strategy from that used by Gregson and colleagues (1994) to explore many of the same questions. The individual-level microsimulator used here is capable of modeling marriage, sex, and the biological and behavioral impacts of HIV. The individual-level nature of the model allows it to track the *links* between parents and children and grandparents and grandchildren. In comparison to the deterministic, compartmental model used by Gregson and colleagues, this model provides a direct means through which to measure the number of orphans and the number of grandparents who could be living with orphaned grandchildren. In addition, it is able to realistically model two different types of intervention: a preventive, largely behaviorally mediated intervention and an antiretroviral treatment program, which reduces viral load and increases the time between infection and death without having other specific preventive effects. Treatment programs of these two types are simulated in the late phase of an HIV epidemic to ascertain their overall effects and how these affect the situation of the elderly. It is important to keep in mind that the microsimulator used here is a *heuristic* tool that allows us to explore the intricate, interrelated processes operating to create an HIV epidemic. A heuristic tool of this kind is not designed to faithfully reproduce a specific population, but rather to represent a generalized population of a given type, sub-Saharan African in this case, and to provide a virtual sandbox in which to manipulate that population in order to gain better understandings of the inner workings of a system of that type.

Below we discuss the specific questions to which the model is addressed and provide some context for each. Following that is a brief discussion of the simulator itself. A full description of the model and its calibration is outside the scope of this work but can be found in detail elsewhere (Clark, 2001a). Finally there is a detailed presentation of the results from 15 40-year simulations, three in each of five scenarios: (1) a stable population with no HIV, (2) a population with untreated HIV, (3) a population with HIV treated with a preventive program, (4) a population with HIV treated with antiretrovirals, and (5) a population with HIV treated with both preventive and antiretroviral treatment programs.

QUESTIONS

Orphans can be created either through the loss of one or both of a child's parents or through abandonment by one or both parents. Orphans of the first type are genealogical or demographic orphans, while those of the second type are social orphans. HIV-related mortality in Africa is primarily creating orphans of the first, genealogical, type. The strong household and extended family structure in many African settings is absorbing the vast number of orphans created by HIV-related morbidity and is thereby preventing the creation of a large number of social orphans. In addition to other related adults, elderly people play a critical role in this extended family.

This work addresses the demographic and structural consequences of heterosexually spread HIV epidemics and the impacts of different treatment strategies on elderly people. Consequently, the following investigations address structural questions relating to genealogical or demographic orphanhood. This in and of itself is a surprisingly complicated set of issues, which must be well understood in order to begin studying the very urgent and important social problems wrought by the creation of so many genealogical orphans. Future work will add household and extended family structures to the existing modeling framework in order to begin addressing questions relating to the impact of orphanhood on a more broadly defined set of older kin.

As a heterosexually transmitted HIV epidemic grows and a substantial fraction of the general adult population is infected, the structure of the population gradually changes as a result of the influences of HIV—often mediated through behavioral mechanisms—on mortality, and perhaps more important, on fertility. These structural changes have significant implications for older people, and it is specifically these impacts that are the focus of the questions posed here.

In addition to the structural changes resulting from the disease directly, prevention and treatment programs have significantly different structural effects that arise from their varied effects on the transmission and progression of HIV infections. Taking this into account, the two primary questions posed below are examined in five different treatment scenarios to ascertain the impacts of both the HIV epidemic itself and various treatment programs.

Number of Orphans

One of the most discussed impacts of heterosexually transmitted HIV epidemics is the excess number of orphans they can generate, and the potential for those orphans to place additional burdens on the elderly. Throughout the remainder of this work I use the word "orphan" to indicate genealogical or demographic orphans—children who have lost one or both of their biological parents. Establishing the relationship between the population prevalence of HIV and the number of additional orphans generated is complicated by the facts that (1) the HIV-related mortality of women and their children is strongly correlated, leading to significant excess HIV-related mortality of orphans who result from women's HIV-related mortality and (2) the magnitude of non-HIV-related excess mortality suffered by orphans as a result of simply being orphans is poorly measured. This is mainly because orphans have historically been relatively rare, are often difficult to identify if they have been fostered, are less likely than nonorphans to be covered by many data collection systems, and finally because the excess mortality seems to persist for only a short period immediately after the death of the parent(s), making it less likely that dead children who have very recently been orphaned are properly categorized as orphans at the time of their deaths.

Given that accurate reliable empirical data describing orphans are unusual, one must turn to modeling to gain a better understanding of the relationship between overall indicators of an HIV epidemic and the number and sex and age distribution of orphans. To accurately model the creation of orphans, the link between *individual* parents and their *individual* children must be represented—something that is possible only in an individual-level modeling framework like the one employed here. In the context of an HIV epidemic, maternal, paternal, and dual orphans are of interest, which requires the model to represent and account for marriage so that children who lose their father can be identified. However, simply accounting for the links between parents and children is insufficient because the overall number of orphans of a given age is a function of fertility, adult mortality, child mortality rates, and the size of the base population of adults and orphans to which those rates are applied. Consequently, to realistically model orphanhood, it is necessary to accurately model an entire two-sex population at the individual level with realistic pairing dynamics.

The model utilized for this work is of this type and is suitable to accurately model orphanhood dynamics in the context of a whole population. Because mother-to-child transmission of HIV is modeled and infection with the virus has realistic duration-since-infection impacts on the mortality of both adults and children, the correlation between the mortality of mothers and children resulting from HIV infection is correctly modeled. However, the model does not account for the additional non-HIV-related excess mortality associated with being an orphan; empirical work in progress by the author suggests that there is substantial excess mortality associated with becoming an orphan—during the first year after losing their mother for young children (Clark, 2004). Taking this into account, the mortality of orphans is underrepresented in the model and consequently the model produces a conservative (slight over-) estimate of the number of orphans.

A number of specific questions relate to the number and fraction of all children who are maternal, paternal, and dual orphans as an HIV epidemic grows and stabilizes:

1. How many and what percentage of children are maternal, paternal, and dual orphans in a rapidly growing population with relatively high mortality but no HIV?

2. How many and what percentage of children are maternal, paternal, and dual orphans in the same population infected with HIV, and how do these indicators change as the HIV epidemic grows and stabilizes?

3. What impact do preventive (behavioral) and antiretroviral treatment programs have on the number and percentage of children who are maternal, paternal, and dual orphans after an HIV epidemic has stabilized?

Numbers of Children and Grandchildren

The important intergenerational consequence (alluded to above) of a significant increase in the number of orphans is that after children lose both parents, other members of the extended family, including grandparents, often must take responsibility for them. If large numbers of maternal and dual orphans are produced, these orphaned children will become a significant challenge for the extended family, the social services that may be available to assist them, and, particularly in the case of dual orphans, for grandparents who must care for them. Recognizing that a variety of related adults will contribute to the care of orphans, the specific aim of this work is to examine the impacts of HIV and its treatments on the elderly, and consequently the focus is on genealogically related grandparents who are likely to be the elderly people most closely related to the orphans.

To adequately describe and investigate this issue, all links between parents and children must be known so that links between grandparents and grandchildren can be reconstructed. Empirical studies of this issue must both record these links and have good data to describe orphans—something that very few empirical studies have. This strongly motivates a modeling approach to gain insight into these issues. The model employed here produces a realistic base population affected by HIV, including the number and age distribution of children, orphans, adults, and adults age 50 and over. Combined with the links between parents and children, it is possible to examine changes in the average number of orphaned grandchildren per grandparent age 50 and over, taking into account sex differentials brought about by the sex differentials in HIV-related mortality and consequent distortions in the age-specific sex ratio.

A number of specific questions relate to the number of orphaned grandchildren per grandparent age 50 and older as an HIV epidemic grows and stabilizes:

1. How many and what percentage of adults age 50 and older have surviving orphaned grandchildren but no surviving children in a rapidly growing population with relatively high mortality but no HIV?

2. How many and what percentage of adults age 50 and older have surviving orphaned grandchildren but no surviving children in the same population infected with HIV, and how do these indicators change as the HIV epidemic grows and stabilizes?

3. Are there different numbers and percentages of elderly women and men age 50 and older who have surviving grandchildren but no surviving children as an HIV epidemic grows? How much of a difference is there?

4. As an HIV epidemic grows and stabilizes, how are the different numbers and percentages of elderly women and men age 50 and older with surviving grandchildren but no surviving children related to the prevalence of HIV in the population as a whole and the prevalence of HIV among those age 50 and older?

5. What impact do preventive (behavioral) and antiretroviral treatment programs have on the number and percentage of adults age 50 and older who have surviving orphaned grandchildren but no surviving children after an HIV epidemic has stabilized?

METHODS

The questions posed above are generally not amenable to empirical investigation *in their entirety* because that would require observation of whole populations over the entire period during which HIV epidemics subjected to various forms of treatment grow and stabilize. In addition, the level of detailed information necessary to investigate the intergenerational questions is typically not available from empirical studies. And finally, ethical concerns relating to measuring the incidence and prevalence of HIV would make empirical studies of this type prohibitively expensive and in most cases impossible—through the influence of the investigation on the process.

In contrast, modeling is comparatively very cheap, flexible, fast, and ethically neutral. The primary disadvantage is that models are not the real thing, nor will they even reflect the real thing very well; so whatever insights are gained through modeling are transmitted through a comparatively blurry, low-resolution lens. In addition, the closer a model is to representing the complexity of reality, the more difficult it is to parameterize with empirically observed parameters. So, one lives with relatively simple models that average the internal complexity of reality and reflect the aggregate reality well, or more complex models that begin to adequately reflect the internal complexity of reality but do not reflect aggregate reality well because complete sets of empirically observed parameter values are not available. Vast quantities of accurate, detailed, individual-level data are required to adequately parameterize models of the second type, and this heavy data requirement often limits the application of such models. Models in the first group are useful to project or predict into the future with reasonable accuracy, while models in the second group are useful to probe the inner workings of a system and understand how the components of a system are related to each other in a dynamic sense over time and as the system is perturbed.

To understand how heterosexually transmitted HIV affects populations, one needs to understand how it affects various components of a population and how these effects in turn affect other components of the population and interact synergistically to produce the population-level impacts observed. Investigations of this type are best pursued by using the second type of model that offers an ability to manipulate and observe the inner workings of a process in detail.

The questions posed here are investigated using a two-sex, individual-level stochastic microsimulator (Clark, 2001d) parameterized with empirically observed mortality, fertility, and nuptiality parameters describing a rural population living in southern Zambia[1] between 1950 and 1995

---

[1]The choice of the population from southern Zambia is arbitrary and simply reflects the

(Clark, 2001c). The populations it simulates closely resemble rapidly growing, high-fertility, high-mortality, polygynous populations similar to those now living in parts of Southern Africa. The simulator models polygynous marital and both polygynous and polyandrous nonmarital pairings[2] of men and women, and, within all these types of union, individual sexual intercourse events. The sexual intercourse events lead to both conceptions and the transmission of the human immunodeficiency virus, thereby tightly and accurately coupling reproduction of the population and transmission of the virus. Once infected with the virus, an individual gradually develops AIDS and eventually dies. During this progression, the disease impacts both their behavior and biology, causing them to be, among many things, less likely to enter into unions of all types, less likely to have sex, more likely to be divorced, increasingly more likely to die and, if female, less likely to conceive and more likely to miscarry.

Simulator

In this section is a very brief description of the simulator, containing just enough detail to understand what it is, how it works, and what it produces. For a detailed description of the simulator, see Clark (2001d), and for a complete exposition of the large set of demographic parameters and how they were calculated, see Clark (2001c).[3] Both these references can be downloaded from Clark (2001b).

The simulator contains entities corresponding to *individual people, individual unions* (both marital and extramarital) between men and women, *fertility histories* for women, and *pregnancies* for women. Together with the union-mediated *links* between spouses or partners and between parents and children, this is sufficient to model all the important dynamics of a whole population. Planned additions to the simulator include modeling households, but this requires a significant amount of so far unavailable quantitative data describing the detailed dynamics of households.

---

availability of a rich and unique source of longitudinal data describing this population over 40 years, 30 of which occurred before HIV began to have an impact. Data of this sort that describe all important demographic aspects of a relatively large African population before HIV are essentially unavailable in Africa leaving very little choice in the selection of an empirically based parameter set for a model of this type.

[2]The parameters governing the formation and dissolution of nonmarital pairings are not empirically based because these processes are not yet well understood in Africa and there is insufficient quantitative data to adequately describe them. The quantity of nonmarital sexual activity is calibrated to reproduce observed fertility rates when added to the sexual activity that occurs within unions.

[3]Due to stringent length restrictions of this paper, the approximately 250 pages of references that completely describe the simulator are only briefly summarized here.

Simulated time is incremented in units of one month, and during each month every entity is exposed to the risk of the events for which it is eligible. Event hazards governing the monthly probability of occurrence of each event are compared with random numbers to decide which events occur during a given month. These occurrences and their repercussions are recorded—often changing the eligibility of the affected entities for future events—and the process is repeated until the desired number of months has been simulated.

The simulator utilizes a relational database to store the long event histories generated by this process. The Structured Query Language (SQL) is used to manipulate the database—both to conduct the simulation and to extract data for analysis. The additional logic necessary to run the simulator is written in Visual Basic for Applications® (a standard programming language) that makes changes to the database by executing SQL. A significant benefit of this architecture is that the entire history of every modeled entity is recorded permanently, a situation that allows unlimited ad hoc analysis of the resulting simulated population using the same tools one would employ to analyze similar data describing a real population. Another benefit is that any simulation can be stopped and restarted without having to employ any special logic or procedures. Additional benefits include the ability to easily utilize both time-invariant and time-varying parameters, and through the straightforward use of SQL, to employ dynamically scaled parameters that are functions of aggregate indicators that are calculated on the fly as the simulation progresses.

Simulator Components

The simulator is organized around modules that manage events relating to (1) mortality, (2) fertility, (3) nuptiality, (4) extramarital unions, or affairs, and (5) sexual intercourse—which occurs with differing frequency in the context of the two types of unions. An additional module manages the effects of infection with HIV on the event probabilities that are managed by the other five modules. See Clark (2001d) for a detailed description of these components and how they interact.

The set of parameters used to parameterize the simulator is too large to describe here; see Clark (2001d) for details. The parameter values are derived from 40 years of observation of a population living in southern Zambia. Those data are unique for Africa and make it possible to calculate a complete, internally consistent set of parameters describing the dynamics of an African population. With very few exceptions, such data are unavailable for other parts of Africa, and it is primarily for this reason that they were chosen to parameterize the simulator. Stable populations unaffected by HIV that result from running the simulator for many years with the parameter set used for this work have (1) mortality levels associated with expectations of life at birth of about 50 years for men and about 52 years for women, (2) fertility levels associated with a total fertility rate of about 6.2, and (3) annual proportionate growth rates of about 4 percent. These and more specific indicator values closely match the empirical values describing the population of Gwembe Tonga (in southern Zambia), from which the parameter values are taken (see Clark, 2001d).

Effects of HIV

An HIV disease progression (DP) indicator is used to govern the progress of an infected individual's HIV infection. The DP indicator consists of a time series of values that correspond loosely to an infected individual's viral load as the disease progresses. The shape of this indicator with time is different for children and adults, reflecting the different pace of the disease in children and adults. The shape of the DP indicator with time is that of a lop-sided U with the initial value being small but rapidly decreasing to a very small value that persists for some time and very slowly increases. For children the rapid increase begins at about 18 months after infection, and for adults the DP begins to increase steadily from about 80 months, reaching substantial levels at about 120 months.

HIV treatment programs that utilize antiretroviral pharmaceuticals to suppress viral load and extend the life of infected individuals are modeled by changing the shape and time scale of the DP indicator. For adults, the whole curve is stretched by about 10 years and the intermediate values are diminished to approximately zero—mimicking the effects of properly administered antiretroviral drugs. For children, the curve is stretched by about three years.

The DP indictors translate into average times between death and infection of about 10 years for adults and 2 years for children with no antiretroviral treatment, and 20 years for adults and 5 years for children with antiretroviral treatment.

Transmission of HIV between adults occurs only through heterosexual sexual intercourse from an infected individual to their partner, with an average per intercourse probability of transmission of roughly 10^{-3} over the course of an HIV infected individual's disease. Individuals can be infected more than once, but their DP indicator starts at the date of their first infection. The actual transmission probability applied to each intercourse event is scaled by the DP indicator of the infected individual, allowing the transmission probability to change as the disease progresses and roughly reflect the infected individual's viral load and hence their potential to transmit.

Infected mothers transmit the virus to their newborns at birth, with an average transmission probability of about .3 over the course of an infected woman's disease. Again, the specific transmission probability applied to a given birth is scaled by the mother's DP indicator, allowing her transmission probability to track the progress of her disease and accurately reflect her viral load and hence her potential to transmit at each time following her own infection.

The transmission probability utilized in both the horizontal and vertical modes of transmission is governed by the infected individual's DP indicator, allowing changes in the DP indicator—such as those that implement the virtual antiretroviral treatment program—to be reflected in the transmission probabilities.

Infection with HIV has a number of other effects whose details are not discussed here beyond mentioning that they are implemented; see Clark (2001d) for details on these effects. Being HIV positive affects

- the probability that a conception will lead to a miscarriage,
- the fecundity of an infected woman,
- the daily hazard of intercourse between a man and a woman if one or both are infected,
- the probability of transmitting the virus from an infected to an uninfected individual through sexual intercourse,
- the probability of transmitting the virus from an infected woman to her newborn child through the birth process,
- the probability that a possible couple with one or both possible partners infected will form a marital union,
- the probability that a marital union will dissolve if one or both of the partners are infected, and
- the probability that an infected individual will die.

Indicators

Indicators presented to explore the questions posed above include measures of the composition of the population through time and the prevalence of HIV in various sex and age groups. The majority of these are familiar, are calculated in the standard way, and should be self-explanatory in terms of definitions and calculation methods (see Preston, Heuveline, and Guillot, 2001).

The orphanhood indicators relate to maternal (mother dead), paternal (father dead), and dual (both parents dead) orphans age 15 and younger. The percentage of children who are orphans of each type are presented as a function of time. The percentage of children who are orphans is calculated as the ratio of the number of children who are orphaned (by type) to the total number of children, including the orphans.

The grandchildren indicators relate the total number of adults age 50 and over (by sex) to the number of their surviving children and grandchildren over time. The indicators presented here are the sex-specific: (1) total number of adults age 50 and older, (2) the total number of adults age 50 and older who have *no* surviving children but at least one surviving grandchild under the age of 15, and (3) the percentage of total adults age 50 and older who have *no* surviving children but at least one surviving grandchild under the age of 15.

HIV Prevalence

Sex- and age-specific HIV prevalence is calculated as the ratio of the number of person-years lived infected with HIV to the total number of person-years lived. Age-specific HIV prevalence values are weighted by the age structure of wider age groups to aggregate HIV prevalence across those wider age groups (i.e., 15-64).

Running the Simulator: Five Scenarios

To start the analysis presented here, a stable population consisting of 1,271 women and 1,230 men was created by letting the simulator run for 150 years from an initial population consisting of 15 women and 15 men of young reproductive age. This stable population served as the starting point for all of the simulations presented here and is referred to as P0 below.

The choice was made to begin "treatment" in the treated simulations in year 31 of the 40 years that are simulated for each of the scenarios described below. This is to roughly mimic the sequence of events in the HIV epidemics in Southern Africa. HIV has been affecting Central Africa for 30 to 40 years and Southern Africa for 15 to 30 years. Widespread treatment programs are in the near future for South Africa and perhaps for other nations in the region, so it seems appropriate to let the HIV epidemics grow for three decades before instituting treatment programs in order to roughly mirror the time scale of the real epidemics and their potential treatment in Southern Africa. Future work will address the impact of treatment programs earlier and later in the life of the epidemic.

Population Without HIV

Three simulations were run from P0 for 40 years without any HIV infection, resulting in final population sizes of roughly 12,000 individuals. These three simulations serve as the healthy "control" to which the HIV-affected simulations can be compared. They also provide some feel for the level of stochastic variability that one may expect to see in the various indicators unaffected by HIV. Averages of these three simulations are presented as the "No HIV" results below.

Population with Untreated HIV

Three simulations were run from P0 for 40 years with HIV. Throughout these simulations there was a very low hazard of "external" infection (equal to 15 per 100,000 per month) for adults ages 15 to 49. Because the simulated population is a closed one, the epidemic has to be seeded in some reasonably realistic way, and without modeling special high-risk groups and their subdynamics within the population, this seems like the most reasonable approach. Over the course of a typical 40-year HIV simulation, about 2 to 3 percent of all adult infections ages 15 to 49 resulted from "random external" transmission—a value that does not seem unreasonable. Averages of these three are presented as the "HIV" results below.

Population with HIV Treated with Behavioral Preventative Programs

A behaviorally mediated HIV prevention program was simulated using the three HIV simulations. Starting in year 31 and running for 10 years through year 40, each of the three HIV populations was subjected to a complete cessation of the formation of extramarital relationships. This had the immediate effect of reducing women's exposure to intercourse and completely curtailed the high levels of sexual mixing across age groups that results from formation and dissolution of extramarital relationships. The immediate consequences are a sharp reduction in fertility and a concurrent sharp reduction in the transmission (incidence) of HIV. Although this is a drastic and ultimately "unreal" treatment strategy, in keeping with the heuristic nature of this work the results clearly demonstrate what the *total* overall effect of such a program could be and clearly illuminate the important dynamic and structural characteristics of such a treatment strategy. Realistic implementations could attain at best substantially less impact than that demonstrated here, and it is important to keep in mind that the results of this simulated treatment are exaggerated. Averages of these three simulations are presented as the "HIV with 'Behavioral' Treatment Starting in Year 31" results below.

Population with HIV Treated with Pharmacological Antiretroviral Programs

A pharmacologically mediated HIV treatment program was simulated using the three HIV simulations. Starting in year 31 and running for 10 years through year 40, in each of the three HIV populations the untreated

DP indicator was removed and replaced with the lengthened and reduced DP indicator described above in "Effects of HIV" that reflects the impact of antiretroviral drugs on the progression of HIV disease and a treated infected individual's viral load. This had the effect of substantially reducing the transmission of HIV from mothers to children and between adults and of dramatically reducing the other impacts of HIV, including its fertility-reducing and mortality-elevating effects. This virtual treatment was applied to *all* HIV-infected individuals and so, like its behavioral corollary, does not reflect a real-world treatment program that would undoubtedly reach only a limited fraction of HIV-infected individuals. That understood, it reveals the maximum effect that such a treatment program could have and a typical time course over which that effect might be observed. Averages of these three simulations are presented as the "HIV with Antiretroviral Treatment Starting in Year 31" results below.

Population with HIV Treated with Both Preventative and Antiretroviral Programs

The last set of three simulations applies both types of treatment using the three HIV simulations starting in year 31. Averages of these three simulations are presented as the "HIV with Both 'Behavioral' and Antiretroviral Treatment Starting in Year 31" results below.

FINDINGS

In the course of conducting this work, a number of other questions were investigated to fully understand the results relating to orphans. To keep the page count reasonable, in-depth discussion of these investigations is not possible, and consequently they are summarized briefly. After 40 years of an untreated HIV epidemic, the annual proportionate growth rate of the population is reduced to zero or below; the age structure converges on a younger, two-tiered shape with fewer young children and adults; the age-specific sex ratio attains a high of roughly 1.5 men per woman in the 45-49 age range and a low of 0.5 men per woman at ages older than 70; and the dependency ratio falls substantially. While discussing the results related to orphans, it is useful to keep these general findings in mind.

Number of Orphans

Panel A of Figure 3-1 demonstrates that the percentage of children under the age of 15 who are maternal, paternal, and dual orphans remains constant in the population unaffected by HIV and, importantly, that the percentage of children who are dual orphans is literally negligible in the

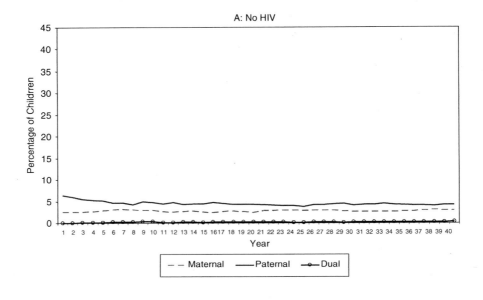

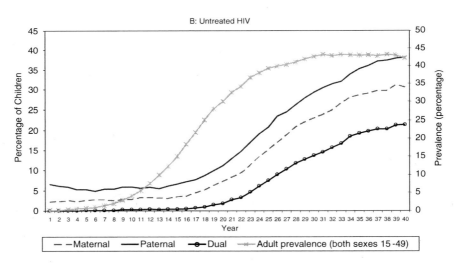

FIGURE 3-1 Trends in the percentage of all children age 15 and younger who are orphans and adult prevalence.

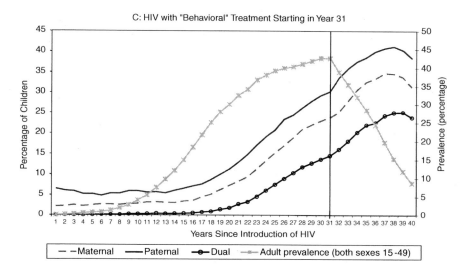

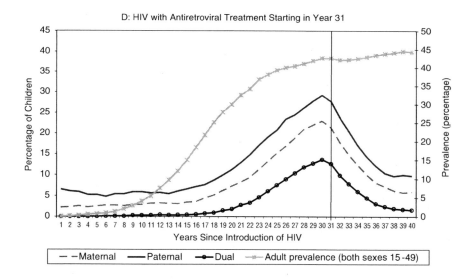

FIGURE 3-1 Continued.

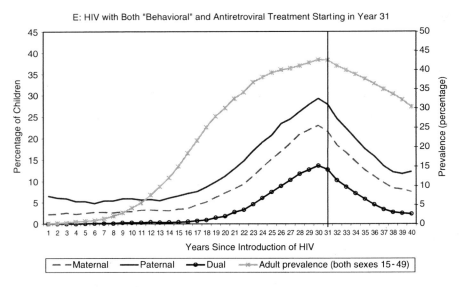

FIGURE 3-1 Continued.

HIV-free population. There are always a few more paternal orphans resulting from the slightly higher adult mortality of men.

Panel B in Figure 3-1 displays the same numbers for the untreated population with HIV. Added to this plot is the trend in the adult (both sexes ages
15 to 49) prevalence of HIV. About 20 years after HIV is introduced, the
number of orphans begins to rise significantly. Interestingly the number of
orphans begins to increase about 10 to 15 years after the adult prevalence
begins its rise, and the number of orphans does not reach significant levels
until HIV has been affecting the population for at least 20 years—a significant lag associated with the average time between infection and death of
roughly 10 years for adults. Given that most HIV epidemics in sub-Saharan
Africa are less than 20 years old, big increases in the numbers of orphans
may yet be coming. Looking at panel B of Figure 3-1 reveals the stunning
fact that 37 percent of all children under age 15 are maternal orphans by
year 40, 30 percent are paternal orphans, and 22 percent are dual orphans.
Compare this number to the figure just above 0 percent in panel A of Figure
3-1. The 15-year (or so) lag is very apparent in this plot when comparing
the trends in the percentage of children who are orphans and adult prevalence. The dramatic increase in the percentage of children who are orphans
is driven both by the falling number of children (denominator) and by the

rising number of those who are orphans (numerator); working together, these two movements create a large fraction of children who are orphaned.

Examining the impacts of the behavioral preventive treatment program in panel C of Figure 3-1 reveals the familiar sharp drop in adult prevalence induced by the treatment, accompanied by a strong reduction in the total number of children ages 0 to 15 but no big drop in the number of orphans until the latest years of the simulation, 38 through 40. This results from the fact that adult HIV-related mortality is unaffected by this treatment, and hence the parents of existing children keep dying as they did until near the end of the 10-year period of the treatment, when the reservoir of HIV-infected adults begins to thin and the number of HIV-related deaths among adults begins to abate. Panel C makes clear that there is a sharp downturn in the percentage of children who are orphans toward the end of the treatment period. Keep in mind that the behavioral treatment implemented here is extreme, in that all extramarital sexual activity is eliminated; this clearly shows the type and direction of the effects of such a treatment but overestimates the magnitudes of both positive and negative consequences.

The antiretroviral treatment program has the opposite effect on orphanhood. Immediately after the treatment begins, the total number of children begins to climb again as the HIV-mediated reduction in fertility is ameliorated, and concurrently the number of orphans begins to decline because the treatment defers HIV-related adult mortality to older adult ages that are attained after the children have lived to age 15, and existing orphans age out of the 0 to 15 age range. These changes translate into a very sharp decline in the percentage of children who are orphans, panel D of Figure 3-1, that softens and flattens out toward the end of the treatment period as the system begins to stabilize.

Combining the two treatment programs produces a result similar to the antiretroviral treatment program, except accompanied by a clear decrease in the total number of children and in adult HIV prevalence (panel E).

Clearly, HIV-induced changes in the numbers and percentage of children who are orphaned are very significant and will produce substantial intergenerational tensions in the population, as well as the necessity to reallocate resources to the caregivers of these orphans. Now we examine this same question from the point of view of those caregivers—in this case, adults age 50 and over.

Numbers of Children and Grandchildren

Figure 3-2 describes the number and percentage of adults age 50 and older who have surviving grandchildren less than 15 years of age but no surviving children. Panel A indicates that in a population unaffected by HIV, the number of adults age 50 and older rises at a constant proportion-

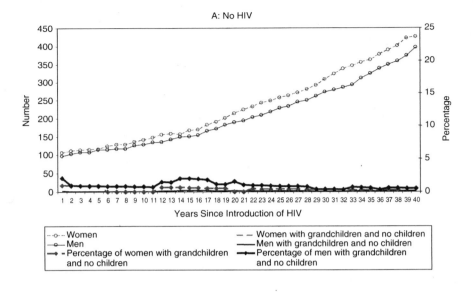

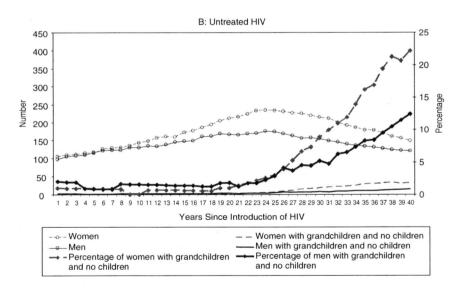

FIGURE 3-2 Trends in the number and percentage of adults age 50 and over with surviving grandchildren but no surviving children.

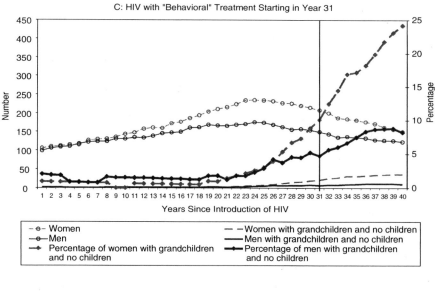

C: HIV with "Behavioral" Treatment Starting in Year 31

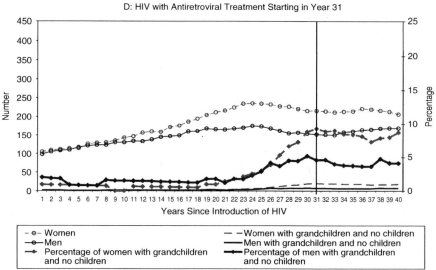

D: HIV with Antiretroviral Treatment Starting in Year 31

FIGURE 3-2 Continued.

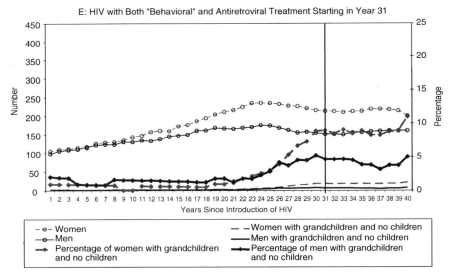

FIGURE 3-2 Continued.

ate rate with slightly fewer men than women—a natural result of the mortality of adult men exceeding that of adult women. The number and percentage of older people of either sex who have surviving grandchildren without surviving children are negligible and constant.

When HIV is introduced to the population in panel B the situation changes; about 20 to 25 years into the epidemic—10 years or so after prevalence begins rising—the number of adults age 50 and older plateaus and immediately starts declining. At the same time, the number and percentage of adults age 50 and older with surviving grandchildren but no surviving children begins to rise. Because the total number of adults age 50 and older is declining while the number with surviving grandchildren but no surviving children is rising, the percentage with surviving grandchildren but no surviving children rises very quickly. Roughly 22 percent of women age 50 and older and roughly 12 percent of men are in this category by year 40. The discrepancy between the female and male percentages probably results from the fact that women can have children only during the years when they are fertile, whereas men can have children over a wider (and older) range of ages. This results in an oldest age at which women as a population reproduce, and as a consequence they cannot replenish their pool of children as they age and therefore more quickly lose *all* of their children, compared with men, who always have the potential to have another child. In this way, men are able to maintain their pool of children longer than women.

Introducing the behavioral preventive treatment program in panel C of Figure 3-2 has little impact because most of the transmission is happening at much younger ages, which do not impact the total number of adults age 50 and older during the comparatively short period of 10 years over which the treatment is applied. The existing HIV-positive population at the time the treatment started continues to die as it did over the 10 years of the treatment, thereby continuing to create the orphans that contribute to the percentage of adults age 50 and over who have surviving grandchildren but no surviving children.

In contrast, the antiretroviral treatment program has an immediate and very positive impact on this indicator, panel D of Figure 3-2. The number of adults age 50 and older stabilizes because HIV-related adult mortality is deferred, and the number of adults age 50 and older with surviving grandchildren but no surviving children also stabilizes for the same reason. The net result is a stabilization of the percentage of adults age 50 and older with surviving grandchildren but no surviving children at a level of about 9 percent for women and 4 percent for men.

The combined treatment program (panel E) produces a result almost identical to the antiretroviral program—as expected given the fact that the behavioral preventive program had little effect.

HIV-mediated changes in the number and percentage of adults age 50 and older who are in a position to be required to care for young children are very significant and display a strong sex differential. By the time a vigorous HIV epidemic stabilizes, up to one-quarter of women age 50 and older may have surviving orphaned grandchildren for whom they must care, while up to 15 percent of older men may be in the same position. The 40 years simulated here are not sufficient to see these indices stabilize; they are still rising steadily in year 40. Given the 20- to 25-year lag between the time HIV is introduced to the population and the beginning of the rise in this indicator, the future is ominous for those who will be age 50 and older in sub-Saharan Africa over the next 10 to 15 years.

CONCLUSION

Taken as a whole, the findings presented here paint a nuanced picture of the impact of HIV on a population, and in particular of the consequences for older people. Results obtained in the course of this work but not presented here indicate that through subtle changes in the age structure, driven by changes in both fertility and mortality, the dependency ratio is likely to fall and that furthermore the decline is largely driven by changes in the male age structure. Additional big changes are wrought on the age structure, resulting in a stable age structure with a "stepped" shape after the epidemic has stabilized that is likely to be younger than the pre-HIV age structure.

Because of the sex differentials in age-specific incidence and prevalence, women die of HIV-related causes at younger ages than men, leading to severe distortions in the age-specific sex ratio that result in a substantial predominance of women living at older ages in HIV-infected populations. And overall the population growth rate is likely to fall substantially, to the vicinity of 0 percent per annum. The average time from infection to death of roughly 10 years appears in many guises—mainly the typical duration of the lag between the initial rise in prevalence and the appearance of some other effect, such as the creation of excess numbers of orphans.

Perhaps the most salient results with respect to the older segment of an HIV-infected population have to do with the creation of a large number of orphans of all three types—maternal, paternal, and dual. The situation grows even grimmer when viewed from the point of view of the elderly themselves, with the result that nearly 25 percent of women older than age 50 potentially live with surviving grandchildren but no surviving children after 40 years of an HIV epidemic. Taken together with the impact of HIV on the age-specific sex ratio, which after 40 years of an epidemic results in two-thirds of the population age 50 and older being female, the final result is that fully one-fifth of the total population over 50 years of age will potentially be in a position of some obligation to care for grandchildren. Acknowledging that each grandchild has two grandmothers, two grandfathers, a number of aunts and uncles on both sides of the family, and in some cases social services designed to help them, the entire burden will be diluted. Despite this, the fact remains that a substantial fraction of older people, who will be largely women under any circumstances, will be caring for young children.

The impacts of the behavioral preventive and antiretroviral treatment programs are varied and often work in opposite directions. The most important impacts of the prevention program have to do with its effect on fertility, the fact that it can, depending on the scope and success of the intervention, substantially reduce fertility. This feeds back through the age structure to affect other processes in the population and the indicators used to measure the impact of HIV, such as the dependency ratio. The fertility impacts of the preventive programs are felt immediately, whereas the drop in incidence does not work through to have an impact on HIV-related mortality for about 10 years, which produces a lag in the mortality impact; because the treatment programs were simulated for only 10 years, these mortality impacts were largely not yet evident.

In comparison, the antiretroviral programs have little effect on fertility, and what little they do increases rather than decreases fertility. In contrast, they have an immediate impact on mortality by deferring it for an average of 10 years or so in adults. These mortality reduction/deferment impacts were evident immediately and often led to positive changes in the trend of the epidemic. It is critical to note that these changes are temporary and result only from the immediate deferment of mortality. Again, because the simulated treatment lasted only 10 years, there was not sufficient time to see the rebound of HIV-related mortality as the deferment expired and HIV-related mortality began to reassert itself at a new level slightly lower than what it had been before the treatment began—because of the reduction in incidence brought about by the suppression of viral load and lowered transmission probability.

In general it appears that some mixture of the two types of treatment program is best; the combined approach often leads to a smoother result with less dramatic short-term changes, and often the two complement each other. It is clear that treatment alone does not solve all, or even most, of the problems associated with an HIV epidemic.

An important next step in this investigation is to restart all of the 15 simulations whose results are presented here and simulate another 40 years. This will provide ample time for the perturbations wrought by the treatment programs to stabilize and for the epidemics to reach new equilibria. In general there appear to be two important time scales in the temporal evolution of all of these epidemics. The first has to do with the latency between infection and death—about 10 years for adults. The second has to do with fertility, the latency between a change in fertility and the time when the children who were born at the time of that change reach reproductive ages themselves, or about one generation. This is the period over which the perturbations in fertility reverberate through the age structure. After about one generation, the fluctuations in the age structure are significantly reduced in magnitude, but at least one to two more generations are required for the echoes of a fertility perturbation to completely disappear.

Extending the investigation still further, work needs to be done to incorporate the household and larger extended social structures into the model so that their interactions with HIV-positive adults, the children of those adults, and eventually orphans can be properly studied. In a similar vein, the investigation also needs to widen to take into account the effects of HIV-related adult morbidity and the burden that this places on children and other adults in the social networks that support the HIV-positive adults. Challenging these expansions of the model is the need for reasonably accurate empirical data describing these structures and their dynamics; data that are so far very difficult to find.

The most important impression provided by the findings presented here is that the impacts of HIV on a population are subtle and multifaceted and must be understood together in the context of their joint impact on a whole population. Ignoring one or more of the major impacts results in a distorted view of the other impacts. It is also clear that the time scales over which an epidemic grows and treatments have their impacts are on the order of decades or quarter-centuries, and that many will echo through the age structure for on the order of 50 to 100 years. These long time scales are important in motivating urgency in treatment but also cautioning patience after a program is instituted, because it may take some time for the effects to be strongly felt and even longer for a new equilibrium to be reached.

REFERENCES

Bicego, G., Rutstein, S., and Johnson, K. (2003). Dimensions of the emerging orphan crisis in sub-Saharan Africa. *Social Science and Medicine, 56*(6), 1235-1247.

Clark, S.J. (2001a). *An investigation into the impact of HIV on population dynamics in Africa.* (Ph.D. dissertation in demography). Philadelphia: University of Pennsylvania.

Clark, S.J. (2001b). *An investigation into the impact of HIV on population dynamics in Africa.* Available: http://www.samclark.net/ [accessed Oct. 2, 2006].

Clark, S.J. (2001c). Part 2: The demography of the Gwembe Tonga. In *An investigation into the impact of HIV on population dynamics in Africa* (pp. 55-195). (Ph.D. dissertation in demography). Philadelphia: University of Pennsylvania.

Clark, S.J. (2001d). Part 3: A two-sex stochastic microsimulation of a population with HIV. In *An investigation into the impact of HIV on population dynamics in Africa* (pp. 196-355). (Ph.D. dissertation in demography). Philadelphia: University of Pennsylvania.

Clark, S.J. (2004, April). *Survival of orphans: Examples from southern Zambia and South Africa.* Presentation at the annual meeting of the Population Association of America, Boston, MA.

Dorrington, R., Bourne, D., Bradshaw, D., Laubsher, R., and Timaeus, I.M. (2001). *The impact of HIV/AIDS on adult mortality in South Africa.* (Report). Cape Town: South African Medical Research Council.

Gregson, S. (1994). Will HIV become a major determinant of fertility in sub-Saharan Africa? *Journal of Development Studies, 30*(3), 650-679.

Gregson, S., Garnett, G.P., and Anderson, R.M. (1994). Assessing the potential impact of the HIV-1 epidemic on orphanhood and the demographic structure of populations in sub-Saharan Africa. *Population Studies, 48*(3), 435-458.

Gregson, S., Zaba, B., and Garnett, G.P. (1999). Low fertility in women with HIV and the impact of the epidemic on orphanhood and early childhood mortality in sub-Saharan Africa. *Aids, 13*(Suppl. A), S249-257.

Joint United Nations Programme on HIV/AIDS. (2002, July). *Report on the global HIV/AIDS pandemic.* Geneva, Switzerland: Author.

Joint United Nations Programme on HIV/AIDS, UNICEF, and U.S. Agency for International Development. (2002). *Children on the brink 2002: A joint report on orphan estimates and program strategies.* Washington, DC: Author.

Monk, N.O. (2002). Enumerating children orphaned by HIV/AIDS: Counting a human cost. Available: http://www.albinasactionfororphans.org/learn/OVCstats.pdf [accessed September 24, 2003].

Preston, S.H., Heuveline, P., and Guillot, M. (2001). *Demography: Measuring and modeling population processes.* Oxford, England: Blackwell.

Timaeus, I.M. (1998). Impact of the HIV epidemic on mortality in sub-Saharan Africa: Evidence from national surveys and censuses. *Aids, 12*(Suppl. 1), S15-S27.

Zaba, B. (1998). Evidence of the impact of HIV on fertility in Africa. (International conference). *AIDS, 12*(abstract no. 24196), 479.

4

The HIV/AIDS Epidemic, Kin Relations, Living Arrangements, and the African Elderly in South Africa

M. Giovanna Merli and Alberto Palloni

INTRODUCTION

Although the effects of HIV/AIDS on individuals who contract it have been relatively well known for sometime (Quinn, Mann, Curran, and Piot, 1986), the understanding of the plethora of indirect effects and their pervasiveness in many realms of individual and social life is much less complete. Age selectivity, together with the disease's relatively long periods of incubation and the associated morbidity and lethality, may affect a number of social relations and social organizations that are either unique or distinctly more powerful than those observed for other diseases in Africa or anywhere else. In particular, the levels and age patterns of the incidence of HIV and future increases in prevalence are likely to have a large impact on kin relations, residential patterns, household organization, and the well-being of family members. Faced with the escalating burden of excess morbidity leading to the disruption of normal activities and functions, families and households are likely to adopt coping strategies to contain the damaging effects of the epidemics. An interesting issue is the magnitude and nature of the costs borne by individuals and families as a consequence of the adoption of these strategies and whether or not they will be put into place without threatening the very fabric of family relations as they are known today.

Ten years ago, Palloni and Lee (1992) reviewed the potential effects of the HIV/AIDS epidemic on mortality levels at various ages that would affect household and family organization. The main idea is that when levels of widowhood and orphanhood rise as much as they could due to the HIV/AIDS effects on mortality alone (excluding effects on fertility and migration), the material basis of traditional kin relations (kin availability) and of

117

household organization (residential patterns) will weaken or cease to operate. In their place, one could expect to see the emergence of new forms of social relations. In addition to projecting high levels of widowhood and orphanhood, the authors anticipated the collapse of traditional family organization, kin networks, and the erosion of the foundations of typical household arrangements. They also predicted increasing prevalence of households in which children live with grandparents in the absence of their parents.

In this paper, we update the work of Palloni and Lee and use a modified version of their model to calculate the demographic impact of HIV/AIDS on the elderly. Our evaluation rests on newly available data for South Africa.

The AIDS epidemic is far worse in Southern Africa than it is in Central and Eastern Africa, where it first began. With its 5.3 million cases (Department of Health, 2003), South Africa is the country with the largest number of people infected with HIV. The rapidity with which HIV has spread is exceptional. In less than a decade, adult HIV prevalence from antenatal surveys increased from 1 percent in 1990, to 7.6 percent in 1994, to 27.9 in 2003 (Department of Health, 2003). On the basis of a combination of vital registration data and estimates derived from AIDS modeling, Dorrington, Bourne, Bradshaw, Laubscher, and Timaeus (2001) attributed to AIDS a significant increase in mortality at young and middle adult ages since the late 1980s, estimating that 40 percent of the deaths of adults ages 15-49 in 2000 were from AIDS. A more recent study estimates the increases in mortality related to HIV between 1996 and 2000-2001 at 7 per 1,000 among children, 2.7 per 1,000 among women ages 30-34, and 2.6 per 1,000 among men ages 35-39 (Groenewald, Nannan, Bourne, Laubscher, and Bradshaw, 2005). This age-specific increase is consistent with an AIDS-related acceleration of mortality in the latter part of the 1990s, estimated from demographic surveillance system data in KwaZulu-Natal (Hosegood, Vanneste, and Timaeus, 2004). Without treatment to prevent the progression from HIV to AIDS, Dorrington et al. (2001) estimate that the cumulative number of AIDS deaths is expected to reach between 5 and 7 million by 2010.

Furthermore, in South Africa, as in much of the rest of Africa, the African elderly have been until very recently primarily supported by intra- and intergenerational familial networks. In particular, coresidence with an adult child is a common form of living arrangement and a form of exchange (Møller and Devey, 1995). Thus what we observe among the African population of South Africa may be replicated in other countries with similar patterns of intergenerational relations.[1]

---

[1]The advent of a pension system in South Africa may be changing some of these patterns of generational transfers and may be consequential for the coresidence of the elderly and some or all of their adult children.

Strategies adopted by households and families to cope with the depletion of human and material resources induced by HIV/AIDS may range from changes in household structure, to reorganization of the division of labor in the domestic domain, to shifts in norms regarding female, child, and elderly labor force participation, and depletion of assets and cash reserves. The particular menu of strategies chosen will depend on the social group, and some, though not all, of the changes in household structure introduced by HIV/AIDS will be reflected in observable shifts in the living arrangements of the elderly. Increases in AIDS morbidity and mortality will reduce the availability of members of the young adult generation. Adult children will be sick or disabled for long periods of time and later die. They may lose the capacity to earn the income that would have been otherwise transferred to their aging parents. They may also require additional resources for their own support and medical care. Thus the elderly suffer a double burden with likely implications for their own health status and well-being: they become caregivers of the younger generations, first of their adult children and then of the AIDS orphans, and they may find themselves without the income transfers from the middle generations, so that net resource flows may be *from* rather than *to* aging parents.

Moreover, the physical and psychological well-being of older persons will be affected not only by the death of adult children and foregone transfers of income, goods, and services, but also by the need to raise additional cash by diluting assets or deploying more hours of work to satisfy the increased burden entailed by the protracted nature of the illness. With its implied long-lasting health impairments on adult individuals, the disease jeopardizes households' ability to generate resources for the care of their most vulnerable members, namely, children and the elderly, and thus aggravates the social and psychic costs of the illness (Ainsworth and Dayton, 2001).

This damaging consequence of the disease will start long before the time of death of those already infected. This phenomenon is what was referred to early on as the "bottom of the iceberg" (Palloni and Lee, 1992:82). The effects of deterioration of the health status of adults on the well-being of children and the elderly is in all likelihood much larger than those implied by the direct effect via excess mortality.

Our central objective in this paper is rather modest, since we only estimate the effects of HIV/AIDS on residential patterns of the South African elderly and evaluate observable changes in their living arrangements over a decade. We eschew assessment of other effects of the epidemic on the elderly but argue that these may be reflected, at least in part, in changes in residential arrangements. We use information from three data sources collected before and after the onset of the HIV/AIDS epidemic in South Africa: the 1991 census of the Republic of South Africa, the 10 percent sample of

South Africa's first postapartheid census conducted in 1996, and the 10 percent sample of the 2001 census.

We proceed in two steps. First, we evaluate macromodels of the epidemic through backward and forward projections of HIV incidence and related mortality. The models are based on a backward projection of a current population of elderly people who are then projected forward, subjecting their children to an estimated HIV/AIDS regime. These models yield estimates of the expected availability of adult children for the elderly, lower bounds for the prevalence of sickness among the children born to elderly people, and 10- to 15-year projections of changes in the availability of adult children and the prevalence of sickness. Second, we use the macromodel to contrast some of the epidemic's expected outcomes derived from the model with observed changes in living arrangements of the elderly over time and across provinces. These contrasts depend on descriptions of observable patterns. We focus on the impact of AIDS mortality as well as the burden of illness associated with the presence of sick adult children. A significant difficulty made evident by these comparisons is that of identifying the direction and magnitude of changes in the living arrangements of the elderly that can be unequivocally associated with the impact of HIV/AIDS.

PREVIOUS RESEARCH ON THE IMPACT OF EPIDEMICS ON FAMILIES AND HOUSEHOLDS

Demographically speaking, the HIV/AIDS epidemic is not far removed from the large shocks suffered by preindustrial populations. In fact, all evidence available to us seems to point to a catastrophe of much larger proportions. Although the parallel suggests that we could learn from the past by examining studies of the population impact of epidemics, famines, and wars, this literature is in general devoid of systematic analysis of the complex effects on family and household organization. Attempts to assess the relation between past crisis mortality and the day-to-day operation of households, families, and social relations are scarce. The effects most successfully examined are those directly related to global excess mortality, deficits in fertility, and increased regional displacement of individuals.[2]

Only rarely have extant studies of past population crises attempted to identify mechanisms translating raised levels of individual mortality or morbidity into shifts of the size distribution of households and the likelihood of fusion, fission, or outright disappearance of family units. An important exception is Livi-Bacci's (1978) assessment of the demographic effects of epi-

---

[2]For a summary of this literature, see Palloni (1990).

demics suffered by preindustrial populations on the distribution of families by size.[3] We attempt to follow this lead to understand the effects of HIV/AIDS on the living arrangements of the African elderly in South Africa, but we adopt completely different assumptions to reflect the operation of a unique epidemic, with a distinct age pattern of incidence, a protracted period of incubation and infectiousness, and singular lethality.

With the exception of a few studies on the direct economic costs for individuals and households (Ainsworth and Over, 1999), most research on the effects of the African epidemic focus on particular members of families, such as mothers or children, and on the impact of adult male deaths that raise widowhood and orphanhood. Studies of the impact of HIV/AIDS on widowhood have focused on traditional behaviors, such as the role of widow inheritance, where a widow is inherited by one of her husband's brothers or other male relatives, in exposing women to HIV infection, and the changes in such traditional arrangements due to the epidemics in Uganda (Mukiza-Gapere and Ntozi, 1995). Ntozi, Ahimbisibwe, Ayiga, Odwee, and Okurut (1999a) found that the stigmatization of AIDS widows upon the loss of their spouse in Uganda influenced their movements. Less healthy widows were more likely to leave their late husbands' homes and seek care in their natal villages, while healthier AIDS widows were more likely to remarry or form new sexual partnerships.

A review of a series of case studies on the impact of HIV/AIDS on orphanhood by Zaba and Gregson (1998) reveals that in areas with high HIV/AIDS prevalence, the prevalence of paternal orphanhood was higher than that of maternal orphanhood. It was attributed to polygynous unions whereby, at the father's death, all children born to his widows become orphans. In Tanzania, Urassa and colleagues (1997) found that 8 percent of children under age 15 and 9 percent of children under age 18 had lost one or both parents. In the region of Manicaland in Zimbabwe, the rapid increase in the number of parental deaths posed demands that exceed the capacity of relatives to fulfill their traditional role of caring for orphans and triggered the emergence of child-headed households (Foster, Makufa, Drew, and Kralovec, 1997). In the Kagera region of Tanzania, excess adult deaths not only implied higher levels of orphanhood but severely affected the nutritional status of orphaned children (Ainsworth and Semali, 1998).

Community studies provide evidence for the effects of the epidemic on household organization (Barnett and Blaikie, 1992; Boerma, Urassa,

---

[3]Livi-Bacci's original idea (1978), in his work on demographic crises, was to use this technique to retrieve a measure of the intensity of the mortality crisis from observed statistics on the size distribution of families during the period following the crisis.

Senkoro, Klokke, and Ng'weshemi, 1999; Ntozi and Zirimenya, 1999; Urassa et al., 1997). In Uganda's Rakai district, two or three generations with at least one orphan and individuals living alone were more common in AIDS-affected households than unaffected ones, and in a significant fraction of households containing AIDS victims, grandparents cared for orphans (Barnett and Blaikie, 1992). The burden of AIDS mortality and morbidity for households is shared by their members in a strict hierarchy. In Uganda, care of AIDS orphans was left to the surviving parent, then to grandparents, followed by older orphans, stepparents, and members of the extended family, such as uncles. Paternal orphans were more likely to be fostered by uncles than cared for by their mothers, because children belong to their father's lineage (Ntozi, Ahimbisibwe, Odwee, Ayiga, and Okurut, 1999b). In a study in Zimbabwe, grandparents were the main care providers to AIDS orphans (Foster et al., 1995). Data from the Kisesa community study show that terminally ill people travel back to rural homes in search of care by the extended family (Urassa et al., 2001). Elderly parents are the most likely caregivers of their infected children, because parents are the most sympathetic and are likely to be informed of their children's AIDS diagnosis first (Ntozi, 1997). Strikingly, similar patterns of caregiving were found in Thailand (Knodel, VanLandingham, Saengtienchai, and Im-em, 2001), where 27 percent of adults with "symptomatic" AIDS were cared for by a parent. Two-thirds of the adults who died of an AIDS-related disease had lived with or next to a parent by the terminal stage of illness, and a parent, usually the mother, had acted as a main caregiver for about half. For 70 percent, either a parent or other older-generation relative had provided at least some care. The vast majority of parents were age 50 or more and many were 60 or older.

The foregoing summary identifies two important albeit weak regularities. First, most studies underscore transformations of living arrangements to accommodate AIDS orphans and widows, with an increased prevalence of households composed of the elderly with their widowed children and grandchildren, as well as households with grandparents and grandchildren but no member of the intermediate generation. Second, there is a rearrangement of the household to adjust to the needs of caring for sick adult children. These changes may lead to increases in headship among the elderly and to a more influential presence of households composed of elderly parents, their adult children, and grandchildren.

Besides the somewhat elusive evidence connecting HIV/AIDS and concomitant changes in families and households, demographic models that attempt to identify the population-level effects of HIV/AIDS have not succeeded in providing a benchmark against which to evaluate empirical evidence (Zaba and Gregson, 1998). For example, although orphanhood is the most amenable outcome to modeling because it requires assumptions only about mortality and fertility, modeling the impact of HIV/AIDS on orphanhood is complicated by time lags between the onset of HIV and orphanhood and the difficulties of quantifying pre-HIV/AIDS levels and patterns of orphanhood. Models predicting the impact of HIV on widowhood require additional conjectures about nuptiality and are more complicated to implement, especially in sub-Saharan Africa, where polygyny and remarriage are frequent.[4]

Changes in household organization in general and in the living arrangements of the elderly in particular have proven to be even less amenable to modeling than orphanhood or widowhood. This is because, in addition to information on demographic determinants, one needs to assess the influence of propensities to coreside and of internal migration flows, both of which may mimic the effects of HIV/AIDS on the availability of kin and confound the epidemic's independent effect. Efforts to isolate the contribution of each of these factors are rare, as they generally require the combined use of simulation and empirical observations. One study uses microsimulation, in combination with aggregate demographic analysis, to estimate how patterns of coresidence of elderly parents in Thailand would adjust in response to the HIV/AIDS epidemic (Wachter, Knodel, and VanLandingham, 2002). The authors project that 11.9 percent of the present generation of Thai elderly (age 50 and over) will lose one or more children to AIDS, and 13 percent of those who lose at least one child will lose two or more before death. They also estimate that, of the cohort of Thai men and women age 55 in 1995, 1 in 9 could expect to experience the loss of at least one child to AIDS, while 1 in 14 could expect to have lived with a child during illness and have provided care.

The most important lesson emerging from this brief review of previous studies is that even the most direct effects—those working through augmented levels of orphanhood and widowhood—present themselves in a veiled form or not at all in aggregate data. Problems with identification of the proper time lags, imperfect knowledge of relations prevailing in the period preceding the epidemic, and the widespread use of norms typical of most African societies, such as those regulating fosterage and remarriage, tend to mask or dampen the observed effects of the epidemic.

---

[4]The practice of levirate, or remarriage to members of the widow's former husband's family, is common in parts of Africa (Potash, 1986). To the extent that it takes place rapidly after widowhood, levirate will conceal the impact of excess adult mortality. Similarly, child fosterage accompanied by a blurring of the distinction between biological and foster parents will lead to underestimates of the impact of adult mortality.

THE IDENTIFICATION PROBLEM

Minimum Identification Conditions

Efforts to estimate empirically the impact of HIV/AIDS on the residential arrangements of the elderly can be successful only if a set of minimum identification conditions are satisfied at the outset. These conditions are associated with processes that either uniquely determine or loosely bound the observable patterns of the elderly's living arrangements.

Living arrangements of the elderly are determined by two factors. The first is a function of purely demographic forces and influences the availability of kin. Preexisting levels and patterns of mortality, fertility, and migration limit the supply of kin that could reside with older people and therefore affect the ability to observe certain types of living arrangements. The second factor is the set of individual propensities to live with blood kin and other relatives. Residential propensities are a function of culturally bounded patterns of preferences and are likely to vary greatly across social classes and ethnic groups in the same society.

Thus the prevalence of living alone or with a spouse but no children among the elderly age x at time t, $P(x,t)$, is simply the product of $D(x,t)$, a measure of the supply of children available to the elderly age x—the proportion of elderly who have surviving children to live with—and $p(x,t)$, a measure of the conditional probability of residing with one of the surviving children.[5] Since excess mortality associated with HIV/AIDS affects $D(x,t)$, one could argue that the difference between estimates of demographic availability in contexts with and without HIV/AIDS is sufficient to identify the effects of HIV/AIDS on living arrangements of the elderly. But this line of thought ignores a number of difficulties.

First, when examining changes in the living arrangements of the elderly, both $D(x,t)$ and $p(x,t)$ need to be identified simultaneously. While changes in $D(x,t)$ can be assessed through a variety of procedures, including micro- and macrosimulations, estimation of $p(x,t)$ is almost always problematic. This difficulty has already confronted scholars who have worked on microsimulation of households and families (Ruggles, 1987; Wachter, Hammel, and Laslett, 1978), but it has been met with no straightforward solution. Furthermore, the relationship among the observed distribution of living arrangements of the elderly, the demographic availability of kin, and individual propensities involves sources of misidentification that, if not properly neutralized, will bias inferences regarding the effects

---

[5]To simplify, we ignore the possibility of age variation (across children and elderly) in $p(x,t)$.

of HIV/AIDS on the living arrangements of the elderly. While some of these sources of misidentification are unique to South Africa, others apply to broader contexts.

In the foregoing formulation, we assumed that the estimation of past levels and patterns of vital events (including nuptiality and migration) is unproblematic. Although this may be so for fertility, mortality, and nuptiality, it is not so for migration. Migration exerts a severe drag on the supply of adult children. In the absence of proper controls for out-migration flows, one can mistake a decline in $P(x,t)$ for changes in other demographic determinants, particularly mortality. In the absence of direct estimates of the tug of migration, *a minimum first condition for the identification of the effects of HIV/AIDS is a comparison of measured effects across areas exposed to similar incidence of HIV/AIDS but experiencing different levels of migration.*

The second source of misidentification is peculiar to the nature of HIV/AIDS. Because the median duration from infection to full-blown AIDS and mortality in sub-Saharan Africa is about 7.5 years (Boerma, Nunn, and Whitworth, 1998), one cannot expect to see large changes in patterns of living arrangements until some time after the onset of the epidemic. In South Africa, the first AIDS cases were reported in 1984-1985 (Sher, 1986), but the full force of the epidemics could not have been felt before 1995. Using a data source for a year before 1995 is tantamount to choosing a baseline against which changes induced by the epidemic can be measured. The selection of a target date is also problematic, for it should be sufficiently distanced from the benchmark to allow time for the effects to accumulate. *Thus, a second minimum identifying condition is to examine information on residential arrangements after 1995 relative to those prevailing some time before this benchmark date.*

Third, the above formulation rests on a "whopper" assumption—to paraphrase Ruggles's terminology (Ruggles, 1987)—namely, that changes in demographic forces do not significantly alter individual residential preferences. However, sudden changes in mortality levels could simultaneously shift preferences among kin by decreasing the propensity of the elderly to live with a surviving adult child. If one is unaware of this, one will attribute a larger fraction of changes in $P(x,t)$ to observed changes in mortality levels than one ought to, with an ensuing exaggeration of the effects of exogenous changes in mortality due to HIV/AIDS. Conversely, a sudden rise in adult morbidity may increase the propensity to live with a surviving (and possibly ill) adult child. The resulting increase in $p(x,t)$ will offset the mortality-induced decrease in $D(x,t)$ and yield an error in the opposite direction, namely, an underestimation of the demographic effects of excess mortality. These examples ignore time lags and the precise mechanisms through which demographic availability influences residential preferences, but the main idea should be transparent: if our mission is to assess the impact of an external event on $P(x,t)$ and to determine how much of this change occurs via changes in $D(x,t)$ alone, identification will be problematic insofar as we do not account for the impact of changes in $D(x,t)$ on $p(x,t)$. It follows that *a third minimum condition for the identification of HIV/AIDS effects is the assessment of changes during a period of time short enough to support the assumption that endogenous effects have not significantly altered residential preferences prevailing prior to the onset of HIV/AIDS.*

It should be noted, however, that if one is interested in the total effect of HIV/AIDS, the third identification condition is superfluous. Indeed, in this case all we need is a rough measure of change in $P(x,t)$—whether reflecting changes in $D(x,t)$ or in $p(x,t)$ induced by the epidemic itself. The only caveat is that inconsistent estimates of the effects of the epidemic will obtain if any of the changes in $p(x,t)$ are exogenous to the event of interest. Furthermore, if changes in $D(x,t)$ and $p(x,t)$ offset each other perfectly, no changes in $P(x,t)$ will be observed, leading one to conclude that the HIV/AIDS epidemic is inconsequential for living arrangements.

Identification Conditions in South Africa

In South Africa, identification problems are exacerbated by the fact that the period of fastest growth of the incidence rates in HIV/AIDS coincided with a period of tumultuous social and demographic transformations that occurred just before and after the collapse of apartheid.

Apartheid and its associated system of separate development imposed restrictions on spatial mobility, education, and employment of black South Africans, by forcibly resettling them to the homelands, four of which were made "independent states" in the 1960s and 1970s (Transkei, Bophuthatswana, Venda, and Ciskei, or the TBVC states). This regime supported a migrant labor system, of circular character, which affected almost every African household. Through the enforcement of influx control laws, African men working in the mining industries, on white farms, and in towns and cities were systematically denied the right to settle there with their families. Single sex hostels were built in all major cities to host rural African laborers. This system encouraged male out-migration but kept families divided by forcing heavy restrictions on residential changes by migrants' wives, children, and elderly relatives (Murray, 1980, 1987; Russell, 1998). What were once undivided rural households became "stretched households," that is, spatially divided units connected by kinship and remittances (Spiegel, Watson, and Wilkinson, 1996). After the collapse of apartheid, migration involved broader age groups as well as women (Collinson, Tollman, Kahn, and Clark, 2003; Posel and Casale, 2002). The intensification of migration resulted in the rapid periurbanization of formerly rural areas bordering large metropolitan areas and the swelling of the population of black townships living in backyard shacks (Kinsella and Ferreira, 1997; Percival and Homer-Dixon, 1995; Spiegel et al., 1996).

If death were the only reason for children to be cared for by grandparents, we would expect a higher proportion of the elderly living in skipped-generation households—which are households composed by grandparents and grandchildren without members of the middle generation, in areas where the prevalence of HIV/AIDS is high. But in South Africa, children may lose a parent to migration as well as death (Bray, 2003), and migration provides a condition for grandparents to take in and support their grandchildren (Smit, 2001). Thus, an increase in the prevalence of grandparents living with their grandchildren without the presence of an adult child may not be due to HIV/AIDS but to high rates of population mobility.

Apartheid and its forced labor migration system also changed the economic function of black South African households, from agricultural production to labor in South Africa's gold mines and industrial development (Martin and Beitel, 1987; Marwick, 1978). Theories of modernization hold that economic transformations, brought about by industrialization and the establishment of wage labor, have decoupled production from the family division of labor characteristic of traditional agricultural societies. In line with these theories, the changes brought about by apartheid might have led to an erosion of social control over family members and a weakening of emotional ties that sustain traditional adherence to the family and its patriarch. Disintegration of the traditional intergenerational relationships has implications for the living arrangements of the elderly, for whom modernization assumes a shift from a preference for coresidence with adult children and grandchildren to a preference for solitary living. Thus, an observed increase in the prevalence of solitary living among the elderly may be due to forces of modernization rather than the outcome of demographic constraints imposed by HIV/AIDS.

Moreover, in South Africa, there is a distinctive reason for alterations in the living arrangements of the elderly: a pension system that was extended to all South African elderly in 1993, mostly by increasing the benefits received by Africans. With rising rates of unemployment, pension sharing with an elderly relative has become a reason for adult children to join their elderly parents' households (Burman, 1996; Møller and Sotshongaye, 1996). Nearly 80 percent of age-qualified Africans reported receiving a social pension in 1996 (Case and Deaton, 1998). Similar to the effects of HIV/AIDS, which may draw adult children back to their elderly parents' homes, the elderly pension system may affect the propensities of adult children to coreside with the elderly, thus introducing another source of misidentification.

Operationalization of Minimum Conditions

In order to partially satisfy the identification conditions, we utilize three different strategies. The first strategy is model-based and consists of estimating expected demographic impacts, that is, changes in $D(x,t)$ associated with mortality increases due to HIV/AIDS. These estimates are obtained through the application of simple multistate models relying on estimated patterns of age-specific HIV incidence, incubation periods, and HIV/AIDS-related mortality. They provide us with a benchmark for the magnitude and direction of expected changes in living arrangements of the elderly $(P(x,t))$ due to changes in the availability of adult children $(D(x,t))$ in the absence of changes in $p(x,t)$. They also provide a baseline to evaluate the burden of disease borne by their adult children. Observed data derived from data sources for the period 1991-2001 are then compared with expected (model-based) values. This first strategy contributes to the first and second identification conditions, since it provides us with a sense of the magnitude of the expected changes in availability due to changes in demographic forces in the absence of endogenous or exogenous changes in residential propensities.

Second, for the comparison of model outcomes with empirical data, we choose the period 1991-2001, which brackets the sharp increase in the incidence of HIV/AIDS. Differences in the patterns of living arrangements during this period will give us leverage to detect changes in living arrangements due to changes in $D(x,t)$. Although the interval between 1991 and 2001 is wide enough to capture time lags inherent in the progression of the epidemic and address the second identification condition, it may not be short enough to contribute to the third identification condition. In fact, we may not be able to fend off the threats to identifiability originating in the reciprocal relations between demographic availability and propensities. However, our inability to distinguish changes in living arrangements due to changing propensities from changes due to demographic availability will be a less serious issue if we are interested in assessing the *overall* effect of HIV/AIDS. It will be a problem only if the propensities are changing due to exogenous factors (e.g., modernization).

Third, to address the first identification condition and distinguish the effects of HIV/AIDS on the living arrangements of the elderly from those of migration, our analyses will compare conditions across South African provinces, which differ in levels of HIV/AIDS prevalence and magnitude and direction of migration flows. By contrast, there is no similar strategy to reduce the confounding effects of the pension system on patterns of elderly coresidence. Fortunately, changes in pension laws are more likely to affect certain types of coresidential arrangements than others. While coresidence with adult children could be easily related to the issuance of pension receipts, changes in the coresidence of the elderly with grandchildren (but not their parents) are less likely to be related to availability of pension payments to the elderly.

DATA ON LIVING ARRANGEMENTS

Data Sources

Our observation of changes in $P(x)$ relies primarily on the analysis of the last apartheid census taken in 1991, the 10-percent public sample of the first postapartheid census taken in 1996, and the 10-percent public sample of the 2001 census.

The 1991 census is well known for its apartheid-induced distortions in coverage, which produced significant underenumeration, especially in the self-governing territories, that is, the six homelands that remained part of South Africa after "independence" was granted to the four TBVCs (Orkin, 2000).[6] Even after various adjustments, the underenumeration of the African population was estimated at 17 percent (Zuberi and Khalfani, 1999). The granting of "independence" to the TBVCs further complicates the comparability of data sources in the 1990s, because in 1991 the TBVCs conducted their own censuses.

As the first and second postapartheid censuses, the censuses of 1996 and 2001 were conducted after reintegration of the TBVCs into South Africa. These censuses standardized methodologies of data collection for all areas (Cronje and Budlender, 2004). We use the 10-percent public samples of both censuses, based on a systematic sample of households stratified by district and province.

Statistics South Africa offers users of 2001 census data a combination of two kinds of imputations for the 2001 data: "logical" imputations, in which "a consistent value is calculated or deduced from other information relating to the individual or household" and "hotdeck" imputations (Statis-

---

[6]In many urban townships, informal settlements, and rural areas that fell into the homelands, where residents were overwhelmingly African, mapping was not uniformly available and many areas were not demarcated into census enumeration areas. Teams of enumerators swept through some of these areas without prior demarcation or lists. In other areas, considered inaccessible due to political unrest or other reasons, dwellings were counted using aerial photographs, and population characteristics imputed using household densities obtained from sample surveys. In perhaps the most extreme demonstration of the impact of apartheid on official statistics, when areas covered by aerial photographs and sample surveys were found with an unexpected number of women (wives and children of male migrant workers were barred from cohabiting with their husbands in areas of migration destination), women were reclassified as men. This resulted in the reclassification of 250,000 women in these areas (Orkin, 2000).

tics South Africa, 2001). No imputation of missing data was undertaken to correct the 1996 census data (Kevin Parry, Statistics South Africa, personal communication, April 21, 2005). For the present analysis, we accept the logical imputations but code as missing the observations with values imputed by hotdeck procedure. This approach resulted in comparable fractions of missing values in the 1996 and 2001 censuses on the variables of interest to this analysis.

Issues of Census Comparability

Important issues affect the ability to compare censuses over time. First, the empirical geographic basis of the 1991 census is different from those of the 1996 and 2001 censuses. Whereas the 1996 and 2001 censuses covered the entire country, the 1991 census excluded the former TBVCs. Where needed, we were able to use a version of the 1996 census subsetted to the same geographic areas as the 1991 census, which excludes the population residing in the former TBVC states, to compare the 1991 census population with the 1996 population purged of the fraction of the population enumerated in the former TBVCs. Moreover, because the different sizes of the territory covered and different provincial boundaries complicate the comparison of the population enumerated in the 1991 and 1996 censuses, we use a version of the 1991 census, which allots the population to the same geographic areas of the nine South African provinces in the 1996 census.

Second, all three data sets contain information on the relationship of each household member to the household head. This information is necessary to calculate the distribution of living arrangements of the elderly, widowhood and orphanhood rates, and other indicators pertaining to the residential arrangements of the elderly. But the number of relationships to household head provided in each census varies. The 1991 census has the smallest number (spouse, child, other family, unrelated), with the most notable absence being the category of grandchild. The 1996 and 2001 censuses are richer in details.[7]

To increase our ability to capture key living arrangements of the elderly by successfully identifying grandchildren in the 1991 census, we imputed the relationship of grandchildren of head in the 1991 census by estimating the proportion of "other family" who are grandchildren of head in a nationally representative survey conducted on a date close to 1991 and apply-

---

[7]The 1996 census question on relationship to household head includes head/acting head of household, husband/wife/partner, son/daughter/stepchild/adopted child, brother/sister, father/mother, grandparent, grandchild, other relative (e.g., in-laws), and nonrelated person. In addition to these categories, the 2001 census has three additional categories for parent-in-law, son/daughter-in-law and brother/sister-in-law.

ing this proportion to 1991 data to obtain grandchild status.[8] We then degraded the 1996 and 2001 data by ignoring information unavailable in the 1991 census, so that, beside household head, the only relations to head used to construct household types were spouse, child, grandchild, other family, and unrelated.

Third, the definition of what constitutes a household changed over time. A household in the 1991 census was defined as "a person or a group of persons (*whether related or not*) who usually occupy a dwelling or part thereof and who provide themselves with food and other essentials for living or have made arrangements for such provision" (Republic of South Africa Central Statistical Service, 1991). Live-in domestic workers were classified alongside their employers' households as unrelated members. In the 1996 and 2001 censuses, a household was "a person or a group of persons who occupy a common dwelling and who provide themselves jointly with food and other essentials for living." Domestic workers were classified as separate households (Statistics South Africa, 1998a, 2004).

Fourth, each census adopted different procedures to enumerate individuals living in hostels and the institutionalized elderly. In the 2001 census, every individual (or household) living in a workers' hostel, student residence, residential hotel, or home for the independent elderly was enumerated on a household questionnaire. The 1991 census classified individuals living in hostels and the institutionalized elderly as "unrelated household members," regardless of whether they were enumerated at these locations along with one or more family member. In the 1996 census, only individuals living in hostels with their families were administered a household questionnaire. Individuals living in hostels as a single family unit were administered a personal questionnaire. Institutionalized elderly were individually enumerated with a special institution questionnaire, which prevents the tracing of household relations between spouses who are enumerated in the same institution.

---

[8]The closest data source to the 1991 census is South Africa's Living Standard Measurement Study (LSMS), conducted in 1993. The imputation procedure was carried out as follows: (1) We prepared a three-way table that cross-tabulates relation to head in 10-year age categories with 10-year age of head categories in the 1993 LSMS data. (2) For age-of-relation to age-of-head cells in which the proportion of grandchildren was greater than 80 percent in the 1993 data, a 100 percent grandchildren status was imputed to 1991 census data. (3) For cells in which the proportion of grandchildren was between 10 and 80 percent, logit regression models were fitted to 1993 data with the binary dependent variable 0/1 for grandchildren, and sex, marital status, and age as independent variables. The parameter estimates thus obtained were used to calculate the probability of being a grandchild in 1991. If the probabilities were greater than 0.5, grandchild status was imputed. The success rate of imputation of grandchild status was evaluated by implementing this procedure based on 1993 data on 1996 census data in which grandchild status is known. The success rate of imputation was 86.94 percent.

A PROFILE OF SOUTH AFRICA'S PROVINCES

In order to identify the effects of HIV/AIDS on the living arrangements of the elderly and separate them from those of migration, Table 4-1 displays a profile of South African provinces in the three census years. Most notably this table reports provincial levels of HIV prevalence and of migration. This information permits the assignment of provinces to two distinct regimes of HIV prevalence and migration, the former defined by the severity of HIV infection estimated from antenatal surveillance data, the latter defined by the proportion of households with an absent migrant member,[9] the level of urbanization, the sex ratio of the population, and the average per capita income. The most rapid increase in HIV prevalence over the 1990s has been experienced by KwaZulu-Natal, followed by Mpumalanga, Free State, Gauteng, and Northwest Province, while most of the increase of HIV prevalence in Eastern Cape occurred in the latter half of the 1990s. By 2001, six provinces displayed adult HIV prevalence rates higher than 20 percent. The remaining ones, Western Cape, Limpopo, and Northern Cape, displayed low to moderate levels of HIV.

As for migration, Gauteng and Western Cape, with the highest average incomes and levels of urbanization, are major destinations of rural migrants. These two provinces display the smallest fractions of African households with at least one absent migrant worker. In contrast, Limpopo, Eastern Cape, KwaZulu-Natal, Mpumalanga, and Northwest all display very large fractions of households with a migrant worker. Limpopo and Eastern Cape, which contain two of the former four TBVCs, are predominantly rural provinces and among the poorest. They are historically two major sending regions of labor migration. KwaZulu-Natal's major urban centers also receive migrants from Eastern Cape, especially from the former Transkei region (Percival and Homer-Dixon, 1995). But because of this province's good road and transportation system, KwaZulu-Natal also experiences significant internal migration flows. Mpumalanga and Northwest Province are predominantly rural but have large periurban settlements near the border, and Gauteng attracts large concentrations of rural migrants from the provinces' more remote corners (Kok, O'Donovan, Bouare, and van Zyl, 2003).

---

[9]No question on migration was asked in the 1991 census. Information on migration in 1996 was obtained from the 1996 census, which asked respondents to identify "any persons who are usually members of this household, but who are away for a month or more because they are migrant workers." In the 2001 census, however, no questions on migrant workers were included and it was not possible to identify migrant household members in their households of origin through other questions in the survey. Thus the proportion of households with an absent migrant worker was estimated for the 1998 October Household Survey.

Despite the value of this provincial categorization for our ability to identify the effects of HIV/AIDS on the living arrangements of the elderly and separate them from those of migration, the association between province and coresidential outcomes is fragile for at least one important reason. This is because we assign the consequences of HIV/AIDS mortality for the living arrangements of the elderly to provinces with high HIV prevalence and neglect to consider the indirect effects on provinces with low to moderate prevalence. Yet some of the consequences of HIV/AIDS are likely to be experienced by the elderly in low-prevalence regions as well as by those living in high-prevalence regions. Consider, for example, the hypothesized increased proportion of the elderly living with grandchildren but no adult children in areas with high HIV prevalence. Because of the well-established relation between mobility and the spread of high-risk sexual behavior leading to HIV infection (Hunt, 1989; Lurie, Harrison, Wilkinson, and Karim, 1997; Nunn, Wagner, Kamali, Kengeya-Kayondo, and Mulder, 1995; Pison, Le Guenno, Lagarde, Enel, and Seck, 1993; Quinn, 1994), migrant husbands may pass on the infection acquired in urban and periurban areas or in mining towns to their wives in rural areas. The death of both parents will entrust children to the care of grandparents in migration sending areas. Under this scenario, HIV mortality would be as likely to increase the proportion of skipped-generation households in low-prevalence areas, which are also sending areas of migration, thus complicating our ability to obtain the first identification condition.

THE DEMOGRAPHIC IMPACT OF HIV/AIDS: A SIMPLE MACROMODEL BASED ON BACKWARD AND FORWARD PROJECTIONS

Model

We focus on an elderly woman age x ($x \geq 60$) who is alive in a target year, say 1995.[10] Hereinafter we refer to this woman as the target or target person, and to the year 1995 as the target year. Our approach consists of back-projecting target women alive in the target year to the time when they

---

[10]We choose to work with female targets and her female children for convenience. However, as it happens, it is also a choice with nontrivial implications. First, relative to the male age pattern of HIV, the female age pattern is skewed towards younger ages. This simply means that our estimates of the burden of illness have a younger than average age profile and may understate the problems associated with the oldest targets. Second, it is grandmothers who are more likely to be burdened with the care of grandchildren left by ill or dying adult children. In this sense, the choice of female targets is justified for reasons other than computational convenience.

TABLE 4-1 Percentage Distribution of Population by Province and Selected Characteristics, South Africa 1991, 1996, and 2001

Census Year	Western Cape (WC)	Eastern Cape (EC)	Northern Cape (NC)	Free State (FS)
Census 1991				
African	16.6	57.3	29.8	83.3
Urban	54.3	53.5	52.2	51.4
Nonurban	45.7	46.5	47.8	48.6
Sex ratio	1.01	0.97	1.02	1.12
% age 60+	7.9	8.1	7.4	5.8
N	271,654	113,463	57,214	142,398
HIV %[a]	0.1	0.6	0.1	1.5
Census 1996				
African	21.1	86.4	33.1	84.5
Urban	88.9	36.6	70.1	68.6
Nonurban	11.1	63.4	29.9	31.4
Sex ratio	0.96	0.86	0.96	0.97
% age 60+	8.7	9.2	8.6	7.9
N	361,735	563,816	70,974	240,179
P.c. income 1996[b] in Rands	17,880	5,479	13,398	10,628
1996 % Afr hh w/ migr. worker	1.2	28.5	6.9	12.3
HIV %[a]	3.1	8.1	6.5	17.5
Census 2001				
African	26.7	87.6	36.2	87.8
Urban	89.7	38.1	80.2	74.8
Nonurban	10.3	61.9	19.8	25.2
Sex ratio	0.93	0.86	0.95	0.92
% age 60+	7.9	9.1	8.0	7.3
N	382,963	551,926	71,530	226,338
P. c. income 2000[c] in Rands	20,777	7,792	12,481	12,334
1998 % Afr hh with migr. worker[d]	1.0	35.3	10.5	14.9
2001 HIV %[e]	8.6	21.7	15.9	30.1

NOTE: All percentages from the 1991, 1996, and 1998 censuses reflect sampling weights, but the N rows report the unweighted denominators.

[a]South Africa Department of Health, cited in Ubomba-Jaswa (2000).

[b]Statistics South Africa (1998b).

[c]Bureau of Market Research (2000).

started reproduction and then projecting them forward to reproduce their childbearing experience. The forward projection exposes the target's children to the risk of HIV infection and death due to AIDS. This is done by applying rates of HIV incidence (transition from the healthy state to HIV+), rates of incubation (transition from HIV+ to AIDS), and mortality rates (transitions from any of healthy, HIV+, and AIDS to the absorbing state of

KwaZulu-Natal (KZN)	Northwest Province (NW)	Gauteng (GAU)	Mpumalanga (MPU)	Limpopo (LIM)	Total
81.7	75.5	61.7	88.3	96.4	70.2
49.6	50.8	55.5	48.9	46.6	51.4
50.4	49.2	44.5	51.1	53.4	48.6
0.90	1.21	1.18	1.02	0.85	1.00
6.6	5.4	6.7	5.0	5.4	6.5
499,295	88,582	331,959	187,819	313,555	2,005,939
2.2	1.5	1.1	1.2	0.5	1.0
81.8	91.2	70.2	89.4	96.6	76.7
43.1	34.8	97.0	38.9	10.9	53.7
56.9	65.2	3.0	61.1	89.1	46.3
0.89	0.97	1.04	0.91	0.84	0.92
8.0	7.5	7.6	7.6	8.4	8.2
735,832	304,384	660,722	246,319	437,240	3,621,201
8,070	7,944	25,281	12,921	3,159	11,421
17.9	17.1	1.6	16.4	31.7	17.2
19.2	13.8	15.5	15.8	8.0	14.2
85.0	91.4	73.9	92.5	97.2	79.2
45.2	41.0	96.3	39.1	10.5	56.3
54.8	59.0	3.8	60.9	89.5	43.7
0.88	0.99	1.01	0.92	0.84	0.92
6.9	7.4	6.2	6.1	7.8	7.3
738,655	310,109	726,517	264,193	453,424	3,725,655
10,592	9,693	25,988	11,088	6,021	13,502
26.5	25.3	2.7	26.8	42.0	23.5
33.5	25.2	29.8	29.2	14.5	24.8

dStatistics South Africa (1998c)
eDepartment of Health (2003).

SOURCE: South Africa 1991 census, 1996 census (10-percent sample), and 2001 censuses (10- percent sample).

death). Backward projection is carried out using estimates of AIDS-free mortality schedules and childbearing schedules for the period 1900 onward. Throughout we assume that childbearing and mortality are independent events for the subpopulation of target women.

Our goal is to calculate the following quantities: (a) the probability that a target's female children born alive when the target was age $x - y$ at time

$t - y$ have survived healthy to time t, or have not experienced HIV by time t, $SI(y,t)$; (b) the probability that they have survived to t but contracted HIV along the way and are alive but ill at time t, $QI(y,t)$; and, finally, (c) the probabilities that they have died due to HIV, $QID(y,t)$, or due to other causes, $Q(y,t)$. The time variable y varies from a minimum equal to $x - 50$ to a maximum equal to $x - 15$, thus constraining the childbearing period of the target to be within ages 15 and 50.[11] The expressions for each of these functions are defined in the appendix to this chapter. With knowledge of the time distribution of children ever born (or the age pattern of fertility to which women age x at time t were exposed during childbearing), $\phi(x - y, t - y)$, we can calculate the weighted probabilities of having a child in any of the four statuses defined above. This is achieved multiplying $\phi(x - y, t - y)$, for every permissible value of y, by each of the quantities defined above. These weighted values represent the average probabilities for an elderly woman age x at time t. In particular, $\phi(x - y, t - y) * QI(y,t)$ is the average fraction of all children born to the target person who are infected with HIV at age y at time t; $SI(y,t) \phi(x - y, t - y)$ is the average probability of having a child age y at time t who is healthy; and, finally, $\phi(x - y, t - y) * (QID(y,t) + Q(y,t))$ is the average probability of having lost a child to either HIV/AIDS or to mortality due to other causes.

Outcomes from the Model

The main outcomes from the model track the history of illness and mortality experienced by the target person's children. Calculations can be fine-tuned to project forward or to assess the target person's status some years ahead of the initial date of calculation.[12] In particular, we estimate the aforementioned quantities for the cohort of the elderly ages 60, 65, and 70 in 1995 and then project these forward 10 years to 2005, thus assessing the experience of these cohorts when they are ages 70, 75, and 80 in 2005. We also estimate the quantities for those ages 60, 65, and 70 in the year

---

[11]We assume that none of the target persons could have contracted HIV prior to age x. Because we use a minimum value for x of 60, the assumption is sensible but not entirely accurate, since some of these women could have been infected in the 10 years prior to 1995. But since the incidence rates between age 49 (approximately attained the year the epidemic started) and 60 (attained in the middle of the census year 1996) are extremely low, the assumption is not at all limiting. Even if the assumption departs from reality, our calculations will be in error only if the childbearing patterns to which targets not affected by HIV and the mortality and HIV incidence pattern of her children are different from those that apply to target persons who were infected prior to the target year.

[12]Throughout we start out with 1995 for convenience and for its closeness to 1996, the year of the first postapartheid census.

2000, and similarly project these forward to the year 2010. Thus, we are able to trace the experience of those ages 60, 65, and 70 in 1995, through the years 2000, when they are ages 65, 70, and 75, respectively, 2005, when they are ages 70, 75, and 80, respectively, and, 2010, when they attain ages 75, 80, and 85.

Armed with knowledge of the distribution of mothers by survival status of children ever born for a period, we can estimate the probabilities of having a given number of children alive and healthy or a given number of children alive with HIV or dead due to HIV or other causes. This extension is straightforward and relies on the quantities defined before and on the estimated distribution of mothers by number of children ever born. If, for example, we are interested in estimating the probability of r children alive and not affected by HIV for a target age x at time t, we use the following expression:

$$\tau_{xt}(r) = \sum_{\{\forall j > = r\}} w(j) * [C(r,j) * (\sum_{\{\forall y\}} \phi(x - y, t - y) * SI(y,t))^r * (\sum_{\{\forall y\}} \phi(x - y, t - y) * (1 - SI(y,t)))^{(j-r)}],$$

where $C(r,j)$ is the quantity $j!/(r! * (j - r)!)$, $\phi(x - y, t - y)$ is the standardized fertility rate (adding up to unity) at age $x - y$, $w(j)$ is the probability of having exactly j children ever born, and $SI(x,t)$ is as defined before. Simple modifications of this expression lead to the probability of exactly r children alive and infected, and r children dead due to non-HIV/AIDS-related causes or due to HIV/AIDS. Perhaps the most important quantity is the probability of having 0 children alive or 0 children alive and with no HIV. These are direct measures of demographic availability and the potential burden of illness, respectively.

Required Inputs

Estimation of model outcomes depends on six pieces of information. The first and most important are the yearly HIV incidence rates from the onset of the epidemic until time t. The second is the incubation function that determines the waiting time in the infected state. The third is mortality of healthy individuals, of individuals infected with HIV, and of those with full-blown AIDS. The fourth is the time distribution of children ever born or, equivalently, the fertility function approximating the childbearing experience of the target population. The fifth is the time distribution of targets by number of children ever born, $w(j)$. Finally, we need to have an approximation of the mortality schedule experienced throughout the childbearing period of the target persons. The nature of these inputs is described in the appendix to this paper.

RESULTS FROM THE MODEL

Prevalence and Incidence at the National and Provincial Levels[13]

Figure 4-1a displays observed, fitted, and "adjusted-fitted" values of cumulated incidence for South Africa. The adjusted-fitted values obtain after correcting the associated post-peak incidence using a model-based procedure outlined in the appendix. Figure 4-1b shows the fitted and adjusted values of annual incidence rates consistent with estimated cumulated prevalence.[14] Two points are worth mentioning. First, the fitted cumulated incidence shows a peak of about 0.45, a value lower than those utilized by the Joint United Nations Programme on HIV/AIDS (UNAIDS) (Zlotnik, personal communication). However, after adjusting the post-peak incidence rates we obtain a ceiling of about 0.53, a value more consistent with those imputed by other researchers. Second, although fitted and observed values are hard to distinguish from each other, we downplay this feature since the "observed" values are the result of operations that are of unknown nature to us.

Figure 4-2 shows adjusted incidence for South Africa and contrasts these with two provinces representing high and low HIV prevalence, KwaZulu-Natal and Limpopo. Note that the incidence rates in all three settings peak around the same year but at different levels, suggesting heterogeneity of ceilings and of stable incidence rates but not a different timing for the epidemic.

Households of the Elderly and HIV/AIDS Prevalence

Estimates of HIV prevalence can be used in simple ways to calculate the prevalence of elderly households with at least one HIV-infected adult child. The estimates are calculated by province and obtained as follows:

$$\rho_k = \Sigma_{(r)}\, g_k\, (r)\, (1 - p_k)^r,$$

where k denotes the province, r denotes the number of adult (ages 15-49) members in the household, p_k is the observed HIV prevalence among adults

---

[13]To simplify the illustration of the model results, we discuss information for South Africa as a whole and for the provinces of KwaZulu-Natal and Limpopo only, to represent the expected patterns in a province with very high HIV prevalence and in one with low or moderate levels.

[14]In all cases, and unless explicitly stated, we use the concept of incidence rates to refer to an occurrence-exposure rate, in strict analogy to a force of mortality. We discard the definition of incidence rate that contains in the numerator all the events of interest and in the denominator the entire population, exposed or not, as is frequently done in the literature.

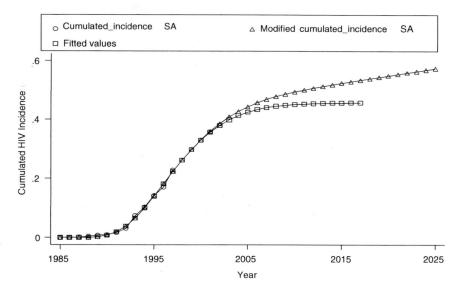

FIGURE 4-1a Observed and expected cumulated adult HIV incidence.

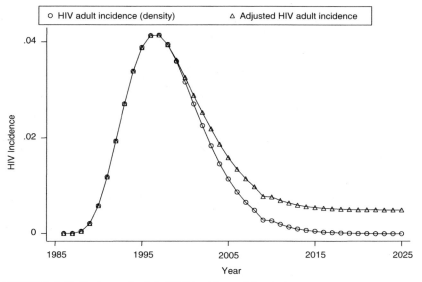

FIGURE 4-1b Estimated adult HIV incidence (density).

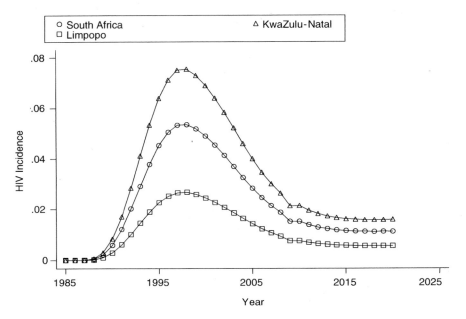

FIGURE 4-2 Estimated adult HIV incidence (density): KwaZulu-Natal, Limpopo, and South Africa.

in the province, and $g_k(r)$ is the fraction of all households containing an elderly member that include exactly r adult members. The values of ρ_k are displayed in Table 4-2. Although the table is suggestive, the estimates rest on an assumption of independence that is likely to be violated. To the extent that infection of one adult member of the household is a marker for exposure for all other members of the same households (spouses and children), the quantities in Table 4-2 will overestimate the fraction of households with infected members. A bias in the same direction is possible due to the fact that the epidemic tends to cluster in social and ethnic groups. Since the expression overlooks such heterogeneity, it will generate overestimates of households' HIV/AIDS prevalence, more so in provinces where heterogeneity of social groups is paramount. Provinces with higher average adult household size will tend to show a higher probability of at least one member's being infected with HIV/AIDS even if the overall prevalence is relatively low. The figures in Table 4-2 show that in KwaZulu-Natal one should expect about 37 percent of households (with at least one adult member) having at least one infected adult. This is a remarkably high value, even

TABLE 4-2 Estimates of the Proportion of Households Containing at Least One Elderly Person with at Least One HIV-Infected Adult Member (by province, 1996)

Province	HIV Prevalence (1996)	Proportion
Western Cape	.031	.05
Eastern Cape	.081	.15
Northern Cape	.065	.13
Free State	.180	.28
KwaZulu-Natal	.199	.37
NorthWest	.138	.27
Gauteng	.155	.24
Mpumalanga	.158	.29
Limpopo	.080	.14
Total	.142	.26

SOURCE: South Africa 1996 census, 10-percent sample.

if upwardly biased. Still, there are provinces that are hardly touched by the epidemic, for example Western Cape.

Children of the Elderly and Their Experience with HIV/AIDS

Figure 4-3a displays the functions $SI(y,t)$ evaluated in 1995 and 2005 (prob_healthy_1995 and prob_healthy_2005). In addition, the figure includes the probabilities of surviving to age y in the absence of HIV/AIDS (prob_survival_1995). The two $SI(y,t)$ curves trace the probabilities that adult children born y years before the target year (values of y in the x-axis: 10, . . . , 55) are alive and healthy (uninfected) in years 1995 and 2005; the third set of plotted values represents the probabilities that the adult children will be alive in the absence of HIV/AIDS. Note that because all values of $SI(y,t)$ are associated with real cohorts of adult children, they need not be monotonically decreasing. In fact, they should not be, since they must reflect, on one hand, the combined effects of mortality and of HIV incidence on the other. For example, in 2005 slightly more than 40 percent of the adult children age 20 were expected to survive with no HIV infection, whereas about 50 percent of those aged 50 will do so. This is because the burden of HIV weighs more heavily among the younger cohorts than among the older ones. While in the absence of HIV/AIDS an elderly parent could expect that almost 80 percent of her adult children born 30 years before would have survived to target year 2005, only 48 percent will survive healthy, not infected, as a result of the epidemic. This is a formidable load of illness that could potentially translate into reduced transfers of assets and

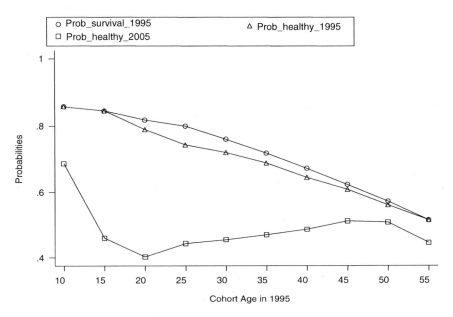

FIGURE 4-3a Survival and healthy survival, South Africa, 1995-2005.

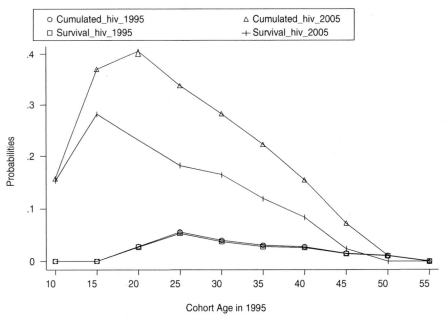

FIGURE 4-3b Cumulated HIV and HIV survival, South Africa, 1995-2005.

income to the elderly, additional labor, added burden to grandparents in the form of care for adult children and grandchildren, and, finally, reorganization of residential arrangements.

Figure 4-3b shows another face of the impact of the epidemic: the cumulated incidence of HIV by cohort of children (cumulated_hiv_1995 and cumulated_hiv_2005) and the cumulated survival among adult children who experience HIV (survival_hiv_1995 and survival_hiv_2005). The difference between these two sets of curves for each target year is a measure of the bereavement load on the elderly, the cumulated mortality among their adult children due to HIV/AIDS. Note that, as it should be given the youth of the epidemic, the bereavement load is trivial in 1995 (the lowest pairs of curves), but it grows to be as large as 0.20 among those in cohorts ages 20-35 in 2005: this implies that the probability of an adult child dying of HIV/AIDS before attaining ages 20-35 in 2005 is on the order of 0.20 or, equivalently, that a fifth of all daughters belonging to these cohorts will experience mortality due to HIV/AIDS.

Figures 4-4a and 4-4b are analogous to Figures 4-3a and 4-3b but correspond to evaluations in 2000 and 2010, respectively. The cumulated impact of the epidemic is quite visible in Figures 4-4a and 4-4b: only 35 percent of the cohorts born 20-30 years before 2010 will reach the target year without having been infected by HIV/AIDS. The bereavement load for elderly associated with adult children ages 20-30 in 2010 grows from 0.20 in 2005 to a staggering 0.35 in 2010. This means that the probability of an adult child dying of HIV/AIDS before attaining ages 20-35 in 2010 is on the order of 0.35. More than a third of all daughters belonging to these cohorts will die due to HIV/AIDS.

Table 4-3 displays summary measures for South Africa nationwide and two provinces with stark contrasts in the HIV/AIDS epidemic, KwaZulu-Natal and Limpopo. These figures contain the probabilities that the elderly ages 60, 65, and 70 will have children who are alive and healthy, infected, and dead to HIV/AIDS in selected target years. The numerical evaluation is for the pair of years 1995-2005 and for 2000-2010. The table sections associated with 1995 and 2005 trace the experience of the elderly ages 60, 65, and 70 in 1995 over 10 years until 2005. A similar interpretation applies to the sections associated with the years 2000 and 2010.[15]

---

[15]Figures on these tables are calculated from the set of values $SI(y,t)$, $QI(y,t)$, etc. and the time distribution of children ever born associated with the elderly ages 60, 65, and 70 in the target years. The latter correspond to the values of $N(x - y, t - y)$ referred to in the expressions for the main functions.

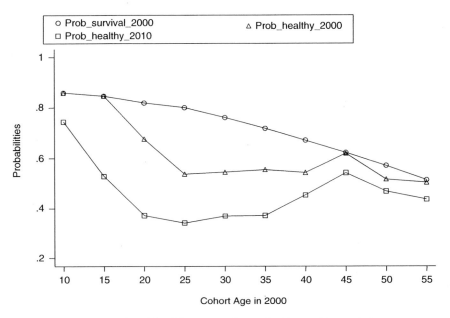

FIGURE 4-4a Survival and healthy survival, South Africa, 2000-2010.

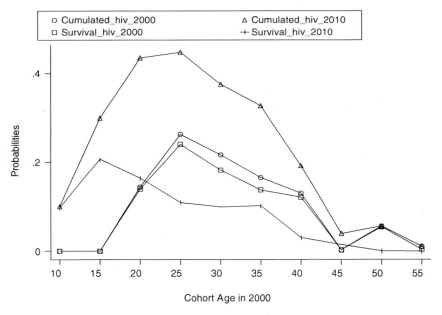

FIGURE 4-4b Cumulated HIV and HIV survival, South Africa, 2000-2010.

TABLE 4-3 Proportion of the Elderly Ages 60, 65, and 70 Who Will Have an Adult Child Infected with HIV or Dead Due to AIDS, 1995-2010

Province and Age	Infected 1995	Died 1995	Infected 2000	Died 2000	Infected 2005	Died 2005	Infected 2010	Died 2010
South Africa								
60	.032	.01	.14	.02	.15	.02	.28	.20
65	.026	.002	.11	.01	.12	.013	.20	.15
70	.019	.001	.08	.01	.08	.01	.13	.10
KwaZulu-Natal								
60	.040	.01	.19	.022	.28	.13	.34	.25
65	.032	.002	.14	.002	.19	.09	.25	.19
70	.022	.001	.10	.001	.12	.06	.16	.011
Limpopo								
60	.022	.002	.089	.012	.14	.02	.19	.13
65	.019	.001	.07	.01	.10	.01	.13	.10
70	.019	.001	.05	.01	.08	.01	.09	.06

NOTE: All calculations represent weighted averages of the functions $QI(y,t)$ and $QID(y,t)$ for elderly of the specified age. The weights are the time distribution of children ever born for elderly of the specified age.

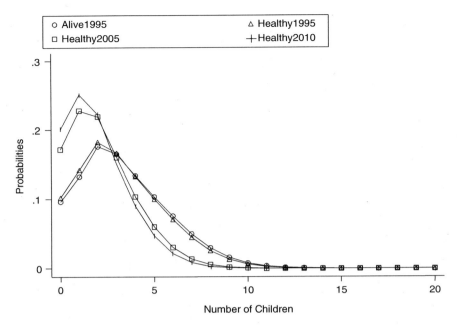

FIGURE 4-5 Problems of adult children alive-healthy, South Africa, 1995-2010.

Constraints on the Availability of Healthy Adult Children
Imposed by HIV/AIDS

An outcome computable from the results of the model is the distribution of the elderly by number of children alive and healthy, infected with HIV, or dead due to AIDS. These estimates are indicators of demographic availability and of the potential burden of disease on the elderly. Figure 4-5 displays the estimated distribution of children surviving in 1995 in the absence of HIV/AIDS (alive1995) uninfected and alive in 1995 (healthy1995), and uninfected and alive in 2005 and in 2010 (healthy2005 and healthy 2010) for the elderly between ages 60 and 70 in the target year. The impact of HIV is remarkable: the distributions of healthy children narrows down considerably and drifts toward much lower means. The fraction of elderly with no surviving children (in the absence of HIV) is around 10 percent in 1995 but balloons to 18 and 20 percent in 2005 and 2010, respectively.

But the damage caused by the epidemic may be even larger than what these figures suggest. In fact, although the increase in the number of the elderly with no surviving children is a key determinant of the probability of the elderly living alone (Palloni, 2000; Wolf, 1994), the fall in the mean number of healthy children may produce effects that are not captured by the results of the model. Indeed, while the model results indicate the magnitude and direction of demographic constraints placed on the elderly, they do not remove the uncertainty associated with endogenous effects, whereby demographic constraints may shift and alter residential propensities. Thus, while in some social settings the drop in the number of healthy children may increase the elderly's propensities to live with adult children, because joint residential arrangements are a mechanism to cope with a sick adult child, in other settings it may increase the propensity of grandparents to take in their grandchildren to ease the burden on their sick adult children. A third social reaction could be more perverse, as elderly parents shy away from sick adult children to avoid social stigma and preference for coresidence is reduced. If the first mechanism were to prevail, we should expect an increase in the proportion of the elderly living with adult unmarried and widowed children. If instead the second mechanism dominates, we should observe an increase in living arrangements involving skipped-generation households. The third mechanism, together with the sheer pressure on the availability of surviving children produced by HIV/AIDS mortality, should lead to sharp increases in the proportion of the elderly living alone or with their spouse.

Our model results provide only benchmark estimates of the constraints in demographic availability but cannot tell us anything about actual residential arrangements. In order to investigate these, we turn now to results from the 1991, 1996, and 2001 data.

ANALYSIS OF CENSUS DATA

Orphanhood and Widowhood

Before turning to an examination of the observed living arrangements of the African elderly from the three South African censuses, we calibrate our ability to detect gross effects of HIV/AIDS from each data source. We do this by examining patterns of orphanhood and widowhood among African children and women. If the empirical results we obtain are broadly consistent with expected results, we have prima facie evidence that the three data sources reflect the impact of HIV/AIDS and that they can be used to inquire about other outcomes, such as the living arrangements of the elderly. Inconsistency between expected and observed results could mean one of two things: either that the epidemic has not yet gathered enough momentum to produce visible effects or, alternatively, that adjustment mechanisms obscure what should otherwise be clearly observed effects. If the first interpretation is correct, we should not expect to find large effects on residential arrangements, either. If the second explanation is more appropriate, our ability to observe effects at the level of elderly residential arrangements will be a function of how effective adaptive mechanisms are, such as fosterage in the case of orphanhood and remarriage in the case of widowhood, in offsetting the impact of the epidemic.

To facilitate comparisons with other research (Zaba and Gregson, 1998) and because information on parental survival was not collected in the 1991 census, we estimate linear regressions of the logarithm of the proportion of orphans on the logarithm of prevalence by provinces from 1996 and 2001 census data. The estimated regression coefficients can be interpreted as elasticities or, equivalently, as the proportionate change in orphanhood relative to a proportionate change in HIV prevalence. Each regression is based on nine observations, one for each province.

To ensure consistency with other research, in each year we focus on three types of orphanhood (maternal, paternal, and dual orphans) in the age groups 0-4, which we regress on contemporaneous HIV prevalence.[16] The R-squares fluctuate between 0.004 for paternal orphans in 2001 and 0.59 for maternal orphans in 2001. The elasticities for maternal and paternal orphanhood are 0.17 and -0.11 in 1996, and 0.64 and 0.04 in 2001. Estimates of relative changes in maternal orphanhood obtained from data collected elsewhere in Africa suggest elasticities in the range between 0.10 and 0.90 (Zaba and Gregson, 1998). Thus, our results fall within an expected, albeit fairly liberal, range. The estimated coefficient for maternal orphanhood for 2001 is, as expected, higher than for 1996, and it is statistically significant (p < 0.001). Differential fosterage practices, documented elsewhere in Africa (Ntozi et al., 1999b), may explain the much lower elasticities for paternal than maternal orphanhood. The elasticities of the proportion of dual orphans in 1996 and 2001 are 0.07 and 0.45, respectively: the change is in the expected direction and the higher 2001 coefficient is marginally significant (p = 0.09). These estimates are, respectively, 0.10 lower and 0.25 higher than estimates obtained from macrosimulation models (Palloni and Lee, 1992).

Because of the dynamics of HIV transmission and sex differences in the

---

[16]Two remarks are important. First, estimation was carried out alternatively assuming parents identified as missing in a household roster were alive and dead. The results presented here correspond to the conservative definition of orphanhood (when information on parent is missing, the parent is considered alive). Estimates corresponding to this more conservative definition are slightly lower in all cases. Second, because of the long incubation period between the onset of HIV infection and AIDS death, ideally we would have preferred to use lagged values of HIV prevalence instead of contemporaneous values. However, this is complicated by the fact that past HIV estimates are less reliable than more recent ones, and by the difficulty of determining precisely the right lag for the prevalence. Contemporaneous HIV prevalence should be highly correlated with true past prevalence that gives rise to orphanhood.

age-specific incidence curve of HIV/AIDS, the progression of the HIV/AIDS epidemic is expected to increase first the proportion of women who are widowed. To assess the responsiveness of widowhood to HIV/AIDS, we estimate the elasticity of widowhood among women ages 15-59 with respect to HIV prevalence between 1991 and 2001. The focus on female widowhood in this age group is consistent with the age selectivity of AIDS mortality among men and the documented South African decline in mortality at the older ages over the 1990s (Dorrington et al., 2001). Elasticities for 1991, 1996, and 2001 are –0.006, 0.07, and 0.18, respectively. The increase in the elasticities is in the expected direction, but their values are low and not statistically significant, suggesting a weaker relationship between HIV/AIDS and widowhood than between HIV/AIDS and orphanhood. This may be partly explained by remarriage patterns, but also by the fact that widowhood itself is likely to be of short duration, truncated by the death of the surviving partner, since the infectious status of one of the partners is highly correlated with the infectious status of the other (Palloni and Lee, 1992). Paradoxically, the dynamics of HIV transmission censors the widowhood experience of the surviving partner and weakens one effect of the epidemic.[17]

In sum, these aggregate results reveal the signature of HIV/AIDS, as the epidemic progresses over time. The magnitude of the elasticity coefficients are also within the bounds of empirical or model-based estimates. However, the observed effects of the epidemic may be dampened by sociocultural responses, especially in the case of paternal orphanhood and female widowhood.

Patterns of Living Arrangements of the African Elderly

The taxonomy of living arrangements of the elderly adopted here is suggested by the outcomes of the macrosimulation model. We focus on four main residential arrangements of the elderly: (1) living alone or with a spouse,[18] (2) living with unmarried or widowed adult children with or with-

---

[17]Levels of widowhood are particularly low in the 1991 and 1996 censuses. The low level in 1996 is especially surprising, because the epidemic is more advanced in 1996 than in 1991 and, unlike the 1991 census, the 1996 census enumerated the population of the former TVBCs, where widowhood is expected to be higher due to worse socioeconomic conditions compounded by political violence. We strongly doubt the quality of the 1996 census data on marital status. A comparison of the female age-specific widowhood rates estimated from the 1991 census, the 1996 census, and the 1996, 1997, 1998 October Household Surveys has shown lower female widowhood rates in 1996 than in any of the other data sources, leading us to suspect underreporting of widowhood in the 1996 census.

[18]Individuals living in institutions for the aged in the 1991 and 1996 censuses and those living in hostels in the 1991 census were reclassified as living alone.

out grandchildren, (3) living with grandchildren but no adult children, and (4) living with one or more orphaned grandchildren.

Similar to our previous analysis of orphanhood and widowhood, we explore the relationship between living arrangements of the African elderly age 60 and above and HIV prevalence across the nine South African provinces by estimating a linear regression of the logarithm of each type of living arrangement of the elderly in 1991, 1996, and 2001 on the logarithm of HIV prevalence. For each relationship, the data are shown by means of scatterplots of the values of the nine provinces together with the regression line that best fits the data, the estimated regression equation, and the associated R-square. While an increase in the size of the regression coefficient over time implies a stronger relationship between HIV and a given living arrangement, the movements of the regression line along the y axis imply a change in the proportion of the elderly living in a given living arrangement. Besides gauging the responsiveness of each type of living arrangement of the elderly to HIV prevalence, this approach also allows identification of patterns across provinces grouped according to their shared level of HIV prevalence and migration characteristics. 1991 provides the baseline observation for the period before the onset of the HIV/AIDS epidemic in South Africa, while the observations for 1996 and especially 2001 are for a period when the impact of HIV/AIDS should already be felt.[19]

Figure 4-6 shows the relationship between the fraction of the elderly living alone or with a spouse and HIV prevalence in 1991, 1996, and 2001. Based on model predictions, we expect the proportion of the elderly living alone or with a spouse to increase over the 1990s with increasing levels of HIV prevalence as a result of harsher constraints on the availability of adult children. However, although the fraction of the elderly experiencing solitary living has increased over time in most provinces, the association between this living arrangement and HIV is negative in all years. Rather than by changes in demographic availability of adult children, these patterns may be explained by forces of modernization, which, especially in the most urbanized provinces of Western Cape and Gauteng, may have weakened emotional ties that sustain traditional adherence to coresidence of the eld-

---

[19]To facilitate the comparison between 1991 and 1996, regression estimates were produced for the full 1996 sample as well as a smaller sample of the 1996 subsetted to the same geographic areas of the 1991 census, which did not enumerate the population of the four TBVCs. Because the two sets of estimates for 1996 were similar, we conclude that the exclusion of the population residing in the former TBVCs in the 1991 census did not significantly affect the comparison between 1991 and 1996 census data. Here we present only estimates drawn from the full 1996 census sample.

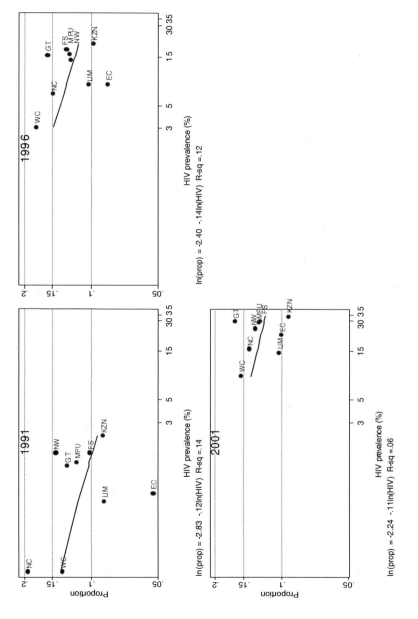

FIGURE 4-6 Proportion of African elderly living alone or in a couple and HIV prevalence.
SOURCES: South Africa 1991, 1996, 2001 censuses, 10-percent samples.

152

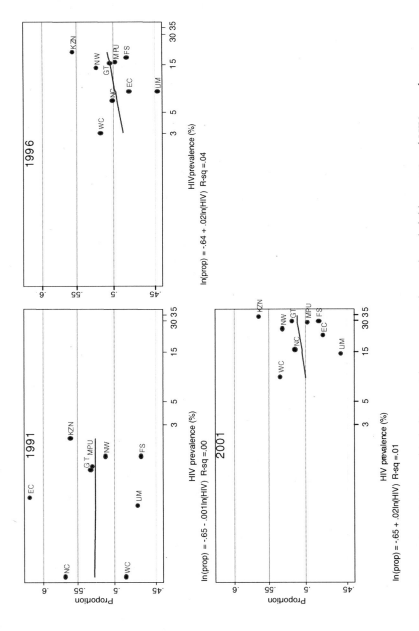

FIGURE 4-7 Proportion of African elderly living with an unmarried or widowed child over 15 and HIV prevalence.
SOURCES: South Africa 1991, 1996, 2001 censuses, 10-percent samples.

erly with their children and prevent the identification of the effects of HIV/AIDS.

Similarly, in Figure 4-7, although model results predicted that increases in HIV/AIDS will be associated with increasing proportions of the elderly providing care for their sick adult children in the form of coresidence, the data show only very small increases in this type of living arrangement over time with the absence of an association between this type of living arrangement and HIV/AIDS.

The macromodel further predicted an increase in the number of grandparents who live with a young grandchild to relieve the burden on their sick children or to provide care for their orphaned grandchildren. Indeed, in Figure 4-8 the fraction of the elderly living in skipped-generation households rises over time in all provinces. But if the rise in skipped-generation households were associated with HIV, we would expect to see a strengthening of the association over time. On the contrary, the association is weaker in 2001 and 1996 than it is in 1991. Like HIV/AIDS, migration is likely to provide the conditions for grandparents to take in their grandchildren. In fact, introducing controls for the levels of migration gauged by the proportion of households with at least one migrant worker in 1996 and 2001, the association between prevalence of skipped-generation households and HIV further weakens, while that with migration is strong. In 1996, the HIV coefficient drops to .04, while the coefficient for migration is high (.31) and statistically significant ($p < 0.001$). In 2001, the HIV coefficient drops to −.10 and the coefficient for migration is .26 ($p < 0.001$).

In order to unequivocally associate changes in the living arrangements of the elderly with the impact of HIV/AIDS, Figure 4-9 shows the relationship between HIV and the fraction of the elderly living with a dual orphaned grandchild in 1996 and 2001. The prevalence of this type of living arrangement does indeed rise between 1996 and 2001, and the size of the coefficient in 2001 is much larger than in 1996. In 2001, a 1 percent increase in HIV is associated with a 0.75 percent increase in the proportion of the elderly living with orphaned grandchildren ($p < 0.01$). The strong relationship between this type of living arrangement and HIV is suggestive of the elderly's coping mechanisms with increased mortality due to HIV/AIDS.

CONCLUSION

We have focused on the effects of the HIV/AIDS epidemic on the living arrangements of the African elderly in South Africa, a country that over the last decade has experienced an exceptionally rapid spread of HIV/AIDS. We have proceeded in two steps. First, we combined results from macrosimulation models of the epidemic with backward and forward projections of HIV incidence and related mortality to estimate expected current

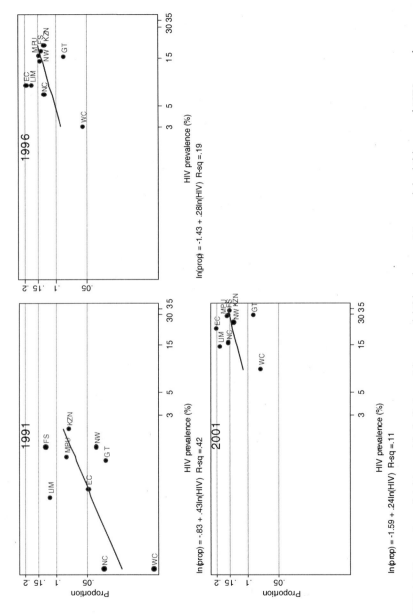

FIGURE 4-8 Proportion of African elderly living with a grandchild under age 15, no adult children, and HIV prevalence.
SOURCES: South Africa 1991, 1996, 2001 censuses, 10-percent samples.

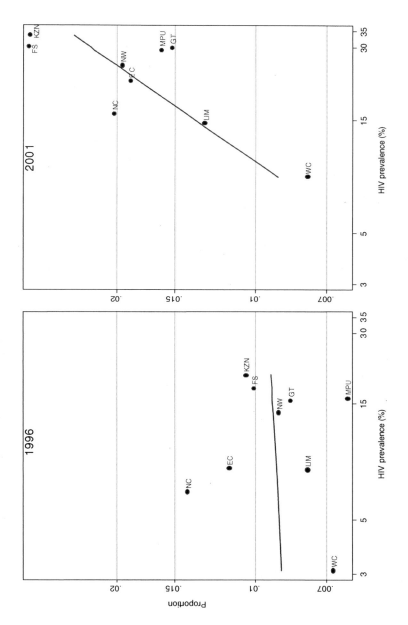

FIGURE 4-9 Proportion of African elderly living with dual orphan under age 15, no adult children, and HIV prevalence.
SOURCES: 1996 and 2001 censuses, 10-percent samples.

availability of adult children for the elderly, prevalence of sickness among the children born to elderly people, and to project changes in availability and sickness over the next 10 to 15 years. We then used the macromodel as a heuristic tool and compared expected outcomes with observed changes in the living arrangements of the elderly over time and across provinces, using three consecutive South African censuses conducted before and after the onset of the HIV/AIDS epidemic, in 1991, 1996, and 2001.

Because the progression of HIV/AIDS is expected to increase the proportion of children who are orphaned and the proportion of women who are widowed, we calibrated our ability to detect gross effects of HIV/AIDS by examining the association between patterns of orphanhood and widowhood among African children and women and HIV/AIDS in each data source. The examination of orphanhood and widowhood indeed revealed the signature of HIV/AIDS as the epidemic progresses over time.

The results from the macromodel suggested that the fall in the number of healthy children and the growing loss of children to AIDS may leave the elderly with fewer or no surviving children to live with and may increase the propensities of grandparents to take in their grandchildren to ease the burden on their sick adult children or to care for their orphaned grandchildren. Our descriptive analysis of changes in the living arrangements of the elderly as they relate to the growth of HIV prevalence has revealed flickers of evidence suggesting the effect of HIV/AIDS. Some of the outcomes we analyzed have changed in the way expected by models of availability, whereas some others have done so in accordance with what one would expect given hypothesized changes in preferences.

Most notably, in support of the expected decline in demographic availability of adult children due to HIV/AIDS, we have observed an increase in the proportion of the elderly who live with an orphaned grandchild in provinces that have experienced the fastest rise of HIV/AIDS prevalence. Where the record is inconclusive, it may be because the epidemic has not worked its way through with sufficient force, because individuals and groups react in ways that conceal the trail left by HIV/AIDS, or because we may be unable to distinguish the effects associated with HIV/AIDS from those triggered by migration, which mimics the effects of HIV/AIDS on the availability of kin, or those induced by modernization, which changes preferences for coresidence. As shown by the data, the observed growth of skipped-generation households is more likely to reflect levels and changes of provincial migration flows than the growth of HIV/AIDS. Similarly, our inability to detect the effects of HIV/AIDS on solitary living is overwhelmed by the tug of modernization, which may increase the elderly's propensity for solitary living.

Establishing benchmarks using model-based approaches as we have done here is useful but insufficient. Unless all the minimal identification conditions are simultaneously met, conventional cross-sectional data sources, such as censuses, can sustain only weak inferences, because they reduce the analytical options to a handful of indicators, for example, household distributions and the living arrangements of the elderly, which do not reveal the processes that produced them.

More promising ways to address the problem of identification of causal pathways include obtaining richer and better data, such as those provided by longitudinal studies or demographic surveillance systems performed at lower levels of aggregation. These data collection efforts can elicit direct information on residential preferences, changes in availability, and changes in actual living arrangements in subgroups affected and not affected by HIV/AIDS.

Another promising approach to enhance knowledge of the effects of the HIV/AIDS epidemic on the elderly and to isolate the most important contributors to observed patterns in living arrangements is the implementation of microsimulations that combine the realistic modeling of the HIV/AIDS epidemic, of kin availability, and of coresidence. The realism of the simulations hinges on the availability of demographic information (such as marriage, fertility, and mortality), epidemiological information to estimate parameters governing the spread of the epidemic (such as transmission probabilities, rates of partner change, incubation times), and information that enables the estimation of explicit rules of coresidence, such as the timing of children's leaving home and types of destination households. While censuses and cross-sectional surveys provide information on realized residential arrangements, longitudinal studies and demographic surveillance systems are the ideal sources of quantitative information on residential rules and preferences and would easily accommodate questions aimed at the explicit identification of residential rules and preferences under AIDS and non-AIDS regimes.

APPENDIX TO CHAPTER 4

Assume we focus on an elderly woman age x who is alive in the census year 1995. This will be the target or target person and the year the target year. The main objective is to derive expressions for the following probabilities applicable to the female children born alive when the target was age $x - y$ at time $t - y$: (a) that these female children have survived healthy (no HIV) to time t; (b) that they survived to t but contracted HIV along the way; and (c) that they have died due to HIV and other causes. In all these cases, the index variable y varies from a minimum equal to $x - 50$ to a maximum equal to $x - 15$, thus bounding the childbearing period of the target between ages 15 and 50. We assume that none of the targets contracted HIV prior to age x or that the fraction that does is trivial and can be dismissed. Because we use a minimum value for x of 60, this assumption is sensible but not entirely accurate, since some of these women could have been infected in the 10 years prior to 1995. However, since the HIV incidence rates between ages 49 (attained the year the epidemic started) and 60 (attained in the middle of the census year 1996) are very low, the assumption is highly realistic. Furthermore, to the extent the assumption departs from reality, our calculations will be in error only if the childbearing patterns to which targets not affected by HIV and the mortality and HIV incidence pattern of her children are different from those that apply to targets who were infected prior to the target year.

To derive expressions for these probabilities, we rely on the following simplified scheme: let $\mu(z, t^*)$ be the force of mortality (in the absence of HIV) at age z at year t^*, the year when the target's child attained age z, let $\iota(z, t^*)$ be the rate of HIV infection at age z and time t^*, and finally let $\gamma(d)$ be the joint rate of incubation and mortality due to HIV/AIDS and other causes for individuals who have been infected d years. The set of all the target's children born $x - y$ years ago who could be age y at time t is the union of several disjoint subsets: one containing individuals who will not reach age y due to mortality in the absence of HIV, $Q(y,t)$; another subset containing those who will attain age y at time t but are infected with HIV, $QI(y,t)$; a third subset containing those who will die of HIV/AIDS-related causes, $QID(y,t)$; and, finally, a subset including those who will attain age y at time t as healthy individuals (not infected), $SI(y,t)$. The expression for the corresponding probabilities, referred to a target age x at time t, are as follows:

$$SI(y,t) = exp(-\int_{[0, y]} (\mu(v, t-v) + \iota(v, t-v))dv)$$
$$QI(y,t) = \int_{[0, y]} [exp(-\int_{[0, w]} (\mu(v, t-v) + \iota(v, t-v))dv)) * \iota(w) *$$
$$exp(-\int_{[w, y]} \gamma(z-w) \, dz] \, dw$$
$$Q(y,t) = \int_{[0, y]} [exp(-\int_{[0, w]} (\mu(v, t-v) + \iota(v, t-v))dv) * : (w)]dw$$
$$QID(y,t) = 1-[SI(y,t)+Qi(y,t)+QID(y,t)].$$

If one knows the time distribution of children ever born reflected in the age pattern of fertility to which women age x at time t were exposed during childbearing, $\phi(x - y, t - y)$, it is possible to calculate the weighted probabilities of having a child in any of the four statuses defined above. This is achieved multiplying $\phi(x - y, t - y)$ by each of the quantities defined above for every permissible value of y. These weighted values represent the average probabilities for an elderly woman age x at time t. In particular, $\phi(x - y, t - y) * QI(y,t)$ is the average fraction of all children born to the target elderly women who are infected with HIV at age y at time t; $SI(y,t) \phi(x - y, t - y)$ is the average probability of having a child age y at time t who is healthy; and, finally, $\phi(x - y, t - y) * (QID(y,t)+Q(y,t))$ is the average probability of having lost a child to either HIV/AIDS or to mortality due to other causes.

In addition to the assumptions discussed above, we rely on the simplification that one can follow the progression to mortality of infected individuals by combining the force of mortality due to other causes, the incubation function, and AIDS-related mortality in a single synthetic superfunction, $\gamma(d)$, which depends only on duration since infection and not at all on age.

Estimation of the Model

Estimation of the model depends of five pieces of information. The first and most important are the yearly HIV incidence rates from the onset of the epidemic until time t. The second is the incubation function that determines the waiting time in the infected state. The third is the mortality of healthy individuals, of individuals who are HIV+, and of those with full-blown AIDS. The fourth piece of information is the time distribution of children ever born or, equivalently, the fertility function approximating the child-bearing experience of the target population. Finally, we also need the distribution of targets by number of children ever born, $w(j)$. Below we briefly define the nature of these inputs.

Estimation of HIV Incidence

A most difficult task is to derive estimates of HIV incidence for the period 1985-2010. We proceed in several stages. In a first stage, we obtain a time series of prevalence estimates for each province during the period 1990-1999. These estimates were obtained from calculations made at Statistics South Africa using the estimates prepared by the UNAIDS and independent estimates obtained from surveillance sites and gathered at the U.S. Census Bureau. The second stage consisted of fitting a curve to the estimated cumulative prevalence, $Pre(t)$. We used a Gamma function of the form

$$Pre(t)= (k/\Gamma(\alpha)) \int_{\{0,\, \beta d(t)\}} exp(-\lambda d(t))\, [d(t)]^{(\alpha-1)}\, dd(t),$$

where $d(t)$ is the duration of the epidemic at year t and k, α, and λ are parameters to be estimated.[20] Our motivation in using this expression is more a matter of adherence to convention than of logical reasoning or empirical judgment; there is no compelling reason to prefer this function over

---

[20]In all cases it was assumed that $t(d)$ was equal to $t - 1985$, that is, that the epidemic started in earnest in 1985.

a virtually infinite set of equally plausible ones. Indeed, the utilization of this function leads to serious problems that require ad hoc solutions. The most important of these problems is that, by its own nature, the associated incidence curve—the density function associated with the cumulative Gamma function—will tend to peak very early and taper off and drift to zero very rapidly. For starters, this type of behavior is inconsistent with the possibility that HIV/AIDS becomes endemic with a constant level of incidence, a possibility that is not only mathematically feasible but also quite likely. Second, systematic comparisons with a number of simulated results using one detailed macromodel of HIV/AIDS (Palloni and Lamas, 1991) demonstrate that almost always, and regardless of the nature of input parameters, the Gamma incidence drops too fast and does not reflect at all the post-peak course of the epidemic.

To resolve this problem, other researchers have adopted arbitrary solutions. They cannot be otherwise, since there are no observations beyond the peak of the epidemic. Estimates exceeding that point are anybody's guess. In this paper we adopt a rather sui generis solution: we take a large set of simulated results using parameters that are deemed to represent well the situation in South Africa (with respect to mortality, fertility, number of partners per person per year, etc.) and then retrieve the estimated incidence curves after the onset of the simulated epidemics. We then fit a Gamma function to the simulated cumulated prevalence, derive estimates of incidence, and calculate the difference between the simulated and estimated incidence rates. These differences are tantamount to "Gamma-adjustment factors." To modify the post-peak estimated incidence for South Africa, we search for the set of Gamma parameters estimated in the simulated model that most closely resemble those observed in South Africa and adopt the corresponding Gamma-adjustment factors. We do not adjust the pre-peak estimates, which are heavily determined by the observed prevalence, but only the post-peak profile of incidence rates. In all provinces and in South Africa nationwide, the adjustments apply to the years after 2003, not before. In this sense, the uncertainty surrounding the estimates of HIV incidence is larger in the post-2003 period than before, when the estimates are at least more closely anchored to the trajectory of observed prevalence.[21] This fact makes the calculations of the key quantities via forward projections less sensitive to errors associated with the use of incorrect Gamma-adjustment factors because post-peak epidemic incidence rates will affect

---

[21]This is a generous statement, for the "observed" prevalence is not so: it is estimated via procedures that are not always reproducible and rest on observed prevalence in small and selected samples of pregnant women.

only the cohorts who reach age 15 some time after 2005. All our calculations refer to periods before 2010.[22]

Estimation of the Incubation Function

We assumed that $\gamma(d)$ follows a Weibull hazard function with parameters $\alpha = .08$ and $\beta = 3.2$, dictating a survival distribution with a median survival time of approximately 10 years. Given the fact that mortality among HIV-infected individuals in Africa is likely to be much higher than normal even in the absence of full-blown AIDS, this assumption does not seem unrealistic. It is also consistent with reports suggesting that the median survival time of HIV-infected individuals in Africa is of the order of 7.5 years (Boerma et al., 1998).[23]

Estimation of Healthy Mortality Levels

We use mortality levels estimated for South Africa by the United Nations (UN) for the period 1950-2000 and then the projected life expectancies through the year 2010 corresponding to the UN medium projections. For the years before 1950 we estimate life expectancy linearly, extrapolating backward from 1960. In all cases, we use the North female pattern of mortality from the Coale-Demeny model life tables.[24]

Estimation of Fertility and of ϕ and w

Estimates of ϕ were obtained from the age pattern of fertility implicit in the Coale-Demeny stable models. We made no extra efforts to approximate

---

[22]An important limitation of our estimates is that the estimated incidence curve depends heavily on the provincial antenatal clinic-based estimates of HIV prevalence that we found published. To the extent that these are in error (Bignami-Van Assche, Salomon, and Murray, 2005), our calculations will yield erroneous estimates of the key quantities describing the family burden of HIV/AIDS.

[23]It is unlikely that either the median incubation time or the median survival time since from the onset of HIV were any longer than these figures in the pre-2000 period. Longer incubation and survival times can be attained but in disease environments quite different than those prevailing in Africa. In any case, our calculations are only mildly sensitive to errors of + or – 3 years on either side of the estimates we used.

[24]The use of the North model to represent the HIV-free mortality patterns of sub-Saharan Africa has a long and distinguished tradition in demography. This tradition is critically based on the observed relations between adult and child mortality, not on the pattern of adult mortality alone. It is highly unlikely that our estimates would differ by much had we used a different pattern but holding constant the level of mortality, for in our calculations what matters most is the latter, not the former.

closely a fertility scheduled for South Africa since what mattered in our calculation was the experience of women who are now 60 and above, that is, the childbearing experience pertaining to years as late as 1980 and as early as 1945. The fertility pattern between 1945 and 1975 at least is a matter of guesswork, and instead of deriving original estimates we chose to adhere to accepted age patterns that have been widely applied.

Estimates of $w(j)$ were obtained directly from the observed distribution of children ever born to mothers age 50 at the time of the 1996 census. Although this distribution may differ from the one that applies to mothers age 60 and above in 1995, it is unlikely that the difference will be major, since substantial fertility changes are unlikely to have been experienced by women younger than 30 or 35 in 1996.

REFERENCES

Ainsworth, M., and Dayton, J. (2001). *The impact of the AIDS epidemic on the health of the elderly in Northwestern Tanzania.* Presented at the 2001 meeting of the Population Association of America, Washington, DC.

Ainsworth, M., and Over, M. (1999). *Confronting AIDS: Public priorities in a global epidemic.* New York: Oxford University Press.

Ainsworth, M., and Semali, I. (1998). *The impact of adult deaths on the nutritional status of children.* Presented at the Workshop on the Consequences of Maternal Morbidity and Mortality, October 19-20, Committee on Population, National Research Council, Washington, DC.

Barnett, T., and Blaikie, P. (1992). *AIDS in Africa: Its present and future impact.* New York: Guilford Press.

Bignami-Van Assche, S., Salomon, J.A., and Murray, C.J.L. (2005). *Evidence from national population-based surveys on bias in antenatal clinic-based estimates of HIV prevalence.* Presented at the 2005 meeting of the Population Association of America, March 31-April 2, Philadelphia, PA.

Boerma, T., Nunn, A.J., and Whitworth, A.G. (1998). Mortality impact of the AIDS epidemic: Evidence from community studies in less-developed countries. *AIDS, 12*(Suppl. 1), S3-S14.

Boerma, T., Urassa, M., Senkoro, K., Klokke, A., and Ng'weshemi, J.Z.L. (1999). Spread of HIV infection in a rural area in Tanzania. *AIDS, 13,* 1233-1240.

Bray, R. (2003). Predicting the social consequences of orphanhood in South Africa. *African Journal of AIDS Research, 3,* 39-55.

Bureau of Market Research. (2000). *The South African provinces: Population and economic welfare levels.* (Report 276). Pretoria: BMR, University of South Africa. Available: http://www.unisa.ac.za/Default.asp?Cmd=ViewContent&ContentID=2456 [accessed May 5, 2004].

Burman, S. (1996). Intergenerational family care: Legacy of the past, implications for the future. *Journal of Southern African Studies, 22,* 585-598.

Case, A., and Deaton, A. (1998). Large cash transfers to the elderly in South Africa. *Economic Journal, 108,* 1330-1361.

Collinson, M., Tollman, S., Kahn, K., and Clark, S. (2003). *Highly prevalent circular migration: Households, mobility, and economic status in rural South Africa.* Presented at the Conference on African Migration in Comparative Perspective, June 4-7, Johannesburg, South Africa.

Cronje, M., and Budlender, D. (2004). Comparing census 1996 and census 2001: An operational perspective. *South African Journal of Demography, 9*(1), 67-89.

Department of Health. (2003). *National HIV and syphilis antenatal seroprevalence survey in South Africa, 2002.* (Summary report). Pretoria, South Africa: Department of Health.

Dorrington, R., Bourne, D., Bradshaw, D., Laubscher, R., and Timaeus, I.M. (2001). *The impact of HIV/AIDS on adult mortality in South Africa.* (Technical report). Cape Town, South Africa: Burden of Disease Research Unit, South Africa Medical Research Council.

Foster, G., Makufa, C., Drew, R., and Kralovec, E. (1997). Factors leading to the establishment of child-headed households: The case of Zimbabwe. *Health Transition Review, 7*(Suppl. 2), 155-168.

Foster, G., Shakespeare, R., Chinemana, F., Jackson, H., Gregson, S., Marange, C., and Mashumba, S. (1995). Orphan prevalence and extended family care in a peri-urban community in Zimbabwe. *AIDS Care, 7*(1), 3-17.

Groenewald, P., Nannan, N., Bourne, D., Laubscher, R., and Bradshaw, D. (2005). Identifying deaths from AIDS in South Africa. *AIDS, 19*, 193-201.

Hosegood, V., Vanneste, A.M., and Timaeus, I.M. (2004). Levels and causes of adult mortality in rural South Africa: The impact of AIDS. *AIDS, 18*, 663-671.

Hunt, C.W. (1989). Migrant labor and sexually transmitted disease: AIDS in Africa. *Journal of Health and Social Behavior, 30*, 353-373.

Kinsella, K., and Ferreira, M. (1997). *Aging trends: South Africa.* (International brief no. 97-2). Washington, DC: Bureau of the Census, U.S. Department of Commerce.

Knodel, J., VanLandingham, M., Saengtienchai, C., and Im-em, W. (2001). Older people and AIDS: Quantitative evidence of the impact in Thailand. *Social Science and Medicine, 52*(9), 1313-1327.

Kok, P., O'Donovan, M., Bouare, O., and van Zyl, J. (2003). *Post-apartheid patterns of internal migration in South Africa.* Cape Town, South Africa: Human Sciences Research Council Publishers.

Livi-Bacci, M. (1978). *La société italienne devant les crises de la mortalité.* Firenze, Italy: Dipartimento Statistico.

Lurie, M., Harrison, A., Wilkinson, D., and Karim, S.A. (1997). Circular migration and sexual networking in rural KwaZulu-Natal: Implications for the spread of HIV and other sexually transmitted diseases. *Health Transition Review, 7*(Suppl. 3), 17-25.

Martin, W.G., and Beitel, M. (1987). The hidden abode of reproduction: Conceptualizing households in Southern Africa. *Development and Change, 18*, 215-234.

Marwick, M. (1978). Household composition and marriage in a Witwatersrand African township. In W.J. Argyle and E. Preston-Whyte (Eds.), *Social system and tradition in Southern Africa* (pp. 36-53). New York: Oxford University Press.

Møller, V., and Devey, R. (1995). Black South African families with older members: Opportunities and constraints. *Southern African Journal of Gerontology, 4*(2), 3-10.

Møller, V., and Sotshongaye, A. (1996). My family eats this money too: Pension sharing and self-respect among Zulu grandmothers. *Southern African Journal of Gerontology, 5*(2), 9-19.

Mukiza-Gapere, J., and Ntozi, J.P.M. (1995). Impact of AIDS on marriage patterns, customs, and practices in Uganda. *Health Transition Review, 5*(Suppl.), 201-208.

Murray, C. (1980). Migrant labour and changing family structure in the rural periphery of Southern Africa. *Journal of Southern African Studies, 6*(2), 139-156.

Murray, C. (1987). Class, gender, and the household: The development cycle in Southern Africa. *Development and Change, 18*, 235-259.

Ntozi, J.P.M. (1997). AIDS morbidity and the role of the family in patient care in Uganda. *Health Transition Review,* 7(Suppl.), 1-22.

Ntozi, J.P.M., and Zirimenya, S. (1999). Changes in household composition and family structure during the AIDS epidemic in Uganda. In I.O. Orubuloye, J.C. Caldwell, and J.P.M. Ntozi (Eds.), *The continuing African HIV/AIDS epidemic in Africa: Response and coping strategies* (pp. 193-209). Canberra: Australian National University, National Centre for Epidemiology and Population Health, Health Transition Centre.

Ntozi, J.P.M., Ahimbisibwe, F.E., Ayiga, N., Odwee, J.O., and Okurut, F.N. (1999a). The effect of the AIDS epidemic on widowhood in northern Uganda. In I.O. Orubuloye, J.C. Caldwell, and J.P.M. Ntozi (Eds.), *The continuing African HIV/AIDS epidemic* (pp. 211-224). Canberra: Australian National University, National Centre for Epidemiology and Population Health, Health Transition Centre.

Ntozi, J.P.M., Ahimbisibwe, F.E., Odwee, J.O., Ayiga, N., and Okurut, F.N. (1999b). Orphan care: The role of the extended family in northern Uganda. In I.O. Orubuloye, J.C. Caldwell, and J.P.M. Ntozi (Eds.), *The continuing African HIV/AIDS epidemic* (pp. 225-236). Canberra: Australian National University, National Centre for Epidemiology and Population Health, Health Transition Centre.

Nunn, A.J., Wagner, H.U., Kamali, A., Kengeya-Kayondo, J.F., and Mulder, D.W. (1995). Migration and HIV-1 seroprevalence in a rural Ugandan population. *AIDS, 9*, 503-506.

Orkin, F.M. (2000). *From apartheid to democracy: Global lessons from a national experience.* Paper presented at the International Association for Official Statistics Conference 2000 on Statistics, Development, and Human Rights, September 4-8, Montreux, Switzerland.

Palloni, A. (1990). Assessing the levels and impact of mortality in crisis situations. In J. Vallin, S. D'Souza, and A. Palloni (Eds.), *Measurement and analysis of mortality: New approaches* (pp. 215-249). New York: Oxford University Press. Also in (1988) J. Vallin, S. D'Souza, and A. Palloni (Eds.), *Mesure et Analyse de la Mortalité: Nouvelles Approches.* Paris, France: Institut National Etudes Démographiques.

Palloni, A. (2000). *Living arrangements of older persons.* (CDE Working Paper No. 2000-02). Madison: Center for Demography and Ecology, University of Wisconsin.

Palloni, A., and Lamas, L. (1991). The Palloni approach: A duration-dependent model of the spread of HIV/AIDS in Africa. In *The AIDS epidemic and its demographic consequences* (pp. 109-118). New York: United Nations and World Health Organization.

Palloni, A., and Lee, Y.J. (1992). Some aspects of the social context of HIV and its effects on women, children, and families. *Population Bulletin of the United Nations, 33*, 64-87.

Percival, V., and Homer-Dixon, T. (1995). *Environmental scarcity and violent conflict: The case of South Africa.* (Occasional paper for Project on Environment, Population, and Security). Washington, DC: American Association for the Advancement of Science and the University of Toronto.

Pison, G., Le Guenno, B., Lagarde, E., Enel, C., and Seck, C. (1993). Seasonal migration: A risk factor for HIV infection in rural Senegal. *Journal of Acquired Immune Deficiency Syndromes, 6*(2), 196-200.

Posel, D., and Casale, D. (2002, September). *What has been happening to internal labour migration in South Africa, 1993-1999?* (DPRU Working Paper No. 03/74). Cape Town, South Africa: Development Policy Research Unit.

Potash, B. (Ed.). (1986). *Widows in African societies.* Stanford, CA: Stanford University Press.

Quinn, T.C. (1994). Population migration and the spread of types 1 and 2 human immunodeficiency viruses. *Proceedings of the National Academy of Sciences, 91*, 2407-2414.

Quinn T.C., Mann, J.M., Curran, J.W., and Piot, P. (1986). AIDS in Africa: An epidemiologic paradigm. *Science, 234*(4779), 955-963.

Republic of South Africa Central Statistical Service. (1991). *Census 91: 1991 population census*. Pretoria, South Africa: Central Statistical Service.

Ruggles, S. (1987). *Prolonged connections: The rise of the extended family in nineteenth-century England and America*. Madison: University of Wisconsin Press.

Russell, M. (1998). Black urban households in South Africa. *African Sociological Review*, 2(1), 174-180.

Sher, R. (1986, October). Acquired immune deficiency syndrome (AIDS) in the RSA. *Supplement to South African Medical Journal*, 23-26.

Smit, R. (2001). The impact of labor migration on African families in South Africa: Yesterday and today. *Journal of Comparative Family Studies*, 32(4), 533-548.

Spiegel, A., Watson, V., and Wilkinson, P. (1996). Domestic diversity and fluidity among some African households in greater Cape Town. *Social Dynamics*, 22(1), 7-30.

Statistics South Africa. (1998a). *The people of South Africa: Population census 1996, 10% sample of unit records*. (Report No. 03-01013, 1996). Pretoria: Author.

Statistics South Africa. (1998b). *Statistics for the calculation of the management echelon post provision for provincial administrations*. Pretoria: Author.

Statistics South Africa. (1998c). *October Household Survey (OHS), 1998*. Pretoria: Author.

Statistics South Africa. (2001). *Census 2001 10% sample*. Pretoria: Author.

Statistics South Africa. (2004). *Census 2001: Concepts and definitions* (Report No. 03-02-26, 2001). Pretoria: Author.

Ubomba-Jaswa, P. (2000). *The dying game: HIV/AIDS in South Africa*. Unpublished manuscript, School of Development Studies, University of Natal-Durban, Durban, South Africa.

Urassa, M., Boerma, J.T., Ng'weshemi, J.Z.L., Isingo, R., Schapink, D., and Kumugola, Y. (1997). Orphanhood, child fostering, and the AIDS epidemic in rural Tanzania. *Health Transition Review*, 7(Suppl. 2), 141-153.

Urassa, M., Boerma, J.T., Isingo, R., Ngalula, J., Ng'weshemi, J.Z.L., Mwaluko, G., and Zaba, B. (2001). The impact of HIV/AIDS on mortality and household mobility in rural Tanzania. *AIDS*, 15, 1-7.

Wachter, K.W., Hammel, E.A., and Laslett, P. (1978). *Statistical studies of historical social structure*. New York: Academic Press.

Wachter, K.W., Knodel, J.E., and VanLandingham, M. (2002). AIDS and the elderly of Thailand: Projecting familial impacts. *Demography*, 39, 25-41.

Wolf, D.A. (1994). The elderly and their kin: Patterns of availability and access. In National Research Council, *Demography of aging* (pp. 146-194). L.G. Martin and S.H. Preston, Eds. Committee on Population, Commission on Behavioral and Social Sciences and Education. Washington, DC: National Academy Press.

Zaba, B., and Gregson, S. (1998). *Impacts of HIV on fertility and family structure*. Prepared for the World Bank/UNAIDS Seminar on Demographic Impacts of HIV.

Zuberi, T., and Khalfani, A.K. (1999). *Racial classification and the census in South Africa, 1911-1996*. (ACAP Working Paper No. 7). Philadelphia: University of Pennsylvania.

5

Older Adults and the Health Transition in Agincourt, Rural South Africa: New Understanding, Growing Complexity

Kathleen Kahn, Stephen Tollman, Margaret Thorogood,
Myles Connor, Michel Garenne, Mark Collinson,
and Gillian Hundt

INTRODUCTION

The population living in less developed regions of the world is growing rapidly, with the fastest growth projected for Africa. With declining mortality and fertility, the age structures of developing countries have aged. Subject to the same mortality and fertility declines, the percentage of people over age 50 will continue to rise, with large increases in the numbers of older people (Heligman, Chen, and Babkol, 1993). United Nations projections for South Africa indicate that the percentage of the population over age 60 will more than double from 6 percent in 1999 to 14 percent in 2050, estimates that are lower than those computed for less developed regions as a whole (United Nations, 1999).

While mortality levels are projected to decrease, the absolute number of deaths in the less developed regions will increase, with a shift to an older age distribution. As the population structure ages, so the age structure of deaths changes to one in which the greatest proportion of deaths is at the oldest ages. This is due to the fact that a greater proportion of the population has reached older ages as well as the lower probability of dying at younger ages. Such change in population age structure shifts the mortality profile from one dominated by the infectious diseases more common in children, toward one dominated by the noncommunicable diseases that affect older adults and the elderly. Despite the relatively young distribution of African mortality compared with other less developed regions, the number of deaths in Africa has increased more at the older ages; this reflects both the changing age structure and the relative success of improvements in child health and reductions in child mortality.

Without HIV/AIDS, 19 percent more deaths are expected to occur during 2010-2015 compared with 1985-1990, with the entire increase occurring in the adult population (Heligman et al., 1993). However, high levels of HIV/AIDS characterize much of sub-Saharan Africa, including South Africa, and are altering the expected age distribution of these populations as a result of dramatically increasing mortality in the young and middle adult age groups (Dorrington, Bourne, Bradshaw, Laubsher, and Timaeus, 2001; Heligman et al., 1993; Joint United Nations Programme on HIV/AIDS, 2002; Timaeus, 1998), together with decreasing fertility (Gregson, 1994; Gregson, Zaba, and Garnett, 1999).

Almost half the South African population resides in rural and semirural settings, comprising the majority of the country's poor. The past decade has been one of momentous sociopolitical change in South Africa, with the population undergoing dramatic changes in patterns of health and disease. Yet the evidence base on which to premise interventions in support of rural health and development remains deeply inadequate. Characterizing and understanding the transitional process, let alone managing it effectively, are difficult tasks. This is apparent in the mixed results from policies to date, the concerns of leaders in the public sector, and a renewed government initiative to launch an integrated rural development strategy.

An overarching concern in the country, mirrored in many other settings, focuses on how best to apply society's limited resources to a rapidly unfolding health and social transition in the face of escalating HIV/AIDS and continuing high levels of violence and injury. To do this, knowledge is needed about trends in rural health status and population dynamics, insight into the complex interplay between poverty-related diseases and emerging "chronic diseases of lifestyle," understanding of the socioeconomic pressures imposed on households by severe illness and death, and evidence for medical, health, and social interventions that can enhance individual and household resilience.

Such understanding is vital to effective decision making at different levels of the health service. Understanding of changing mortality patterns is of real consequence for intervention programs, development of "essential packages" of care and the impact that can be expected, and resource allocation and human resource development. As reflected in the report of the Commission on Health Research for Development, drafted more than a decade ago, research on the problems of rural health and development remains essential to an effective societal response and may well prove the "essential link to equity in development" (Commission on Health Research for Development, 1990).

This paper is divided into three parts. First, we review the theory of epidemiological transition and its evolution over more than 30 years. Next, we examine, as a case study, changing mortality in the Agincourt subdistrict of rural South Africa, focusing particularly on older adults and on stroke and its risk factors. We contend that the early conceptions of epidemiological transition theory are inadequate to explain the changes observed, and we locate the empirical findings in a more contemporary analysis of the health transition. Finally, we raise some implications of the transition for the provision of health care.

THE THEORY OF EPIDEMIOLOGICAL TRANSITION

The first recorded discussion of changing population patterns and their impact, espoused by Thomas Malthus, dates back more than 200 years (Caldwell, 2001; Cappuccio, 2004). Since then, ideas concerning a health transition framework have evolved to explain the changes in levels and causes of illness and death occurring in most countries (Feacham, Phillips, and Bulatao, 1992), and to attempt to predict the trajectory of future change. The limitations of the demographic transition, with its focus on change from high mortality and fertility in traditional societies to low rates in more modern societies, was recognized by Abdel Omran, who in 1971 wrote about his theory of "epidemiologic transition." Conceptually, this broadened the scope of "mortality transition" to include changing morbidity patterns—from pandemics of infection to degenerative and manmade diseases—and the interaction of these with their socioeconomic determinants and consequences (Omran, 1971).

Omran proposed three stages through which societies move sequentially: the era of pestilence and famine, the era of receding pandemics, and the era of degenerative and manmade diseases. The first stage is characterized by exceedingly high mortality, particularly in children, due largely to infectious diseases, nutritional disorders, and complications of pregnancy and childbirth. The second stage sees declining mortality and sustained population growth, and the third stage has lower overall mortality that peaks at older ages and results from noncommunicable disease and injuries. In this stage, life expectancy is higher for women than men, in contrast to the era of pestilence and famine, which has higher male life expectancy. Omran also described three basic models of the epidemiological transition differentiated by variations in the pattern, pace, determinants, and consequences of population change: the classical or Western model, in which progressive mortality and fertility declines followed socioeconomic development (seen in most Western European societies); the accelerated model, which started later and was more rapid (experienced in Japan and Eastern Europe); and the contemporary or delayed model, which attempts to describe the unfinished transition of most developing countries. The accelerated model was also determined by socioeconomic advances but enhanced by developments in medical technology, whereas the delayed model was largely driven by the spread of medical and public health interventions (Gaylin and Kates, 1997; Omran, 1971).

While regarded as having made a groundbreaking contribution to public health through concentrating on the mortality side of the demographic transition, placing health change as part of social change, leading public health practitioners to value the importance of their activities, and stimulating debate and enquiry (Caldwell, 2001; Cappuccio, 2004), Omran's theory is not without criticism. Caldwell (2001) points out that while epidemiological transition theory emphasizes the role of social, economic, ecobiological, and environmental change, it understates the contributions of scientific discovery, medical technology, and public health interventions, such as water purification, sewage disposal, and immunization. Defining just three stages of the epidemiological transition is thought too restrictive, a limitation identified by Omran and others in the 1980s who have added a subsequent stage dealing with the reduction of age-specific death rates due to degenerative diseases (Beaglehole and Bonita, 2004; Olshansky and Ault, 1986; Omran, 1982). Their sequential relationship, moving through one stage and then the next, has been challenged, too (Beaglehole and Bonita, 2004; National Research Council, 1993). "The ephemeral nature of health trends in developed countries seriously undermines widely held notions of epidemiologic transition as a stable march of progress" (Gaylin and Kates, 1997:615).

Frenk, Bobadilla, Sepulveda, and Cervantes (1989) propose modifications to the original theory through examination of the transition in middle-income countries. They find that the eras are not necessarily sequential but may overlap, patterns of morbidity and mortality may be reversed (a so-called counter transition), change may not occur fully, and infectious and noncommunicable diseases may coexist (a protracted or prolonged transition). Epidemiological polarization is seen in places where the poorest experience the highest death rates from more pretransitional diseases, including infections and nutritional disorders. Gaylin and Kates (1997) argue that the two key limitations of epidemiological transition theory are its generalized formulation and failure to differentiate among population subgroups and its suggestion that infectious diseases can be eliminated and are replaced by degenerative diseases. The emergence of HIV/AIDS as a new infectious disease challenges the latter assumption, exacerbating mortality differentials among particular subgroups.

Although further theoretical development has been called for (Frenk, Bobadilla, Stern, Frejka, and Lozano, 1994), ongoing conceptual advances do begin to address the critique that bodies of understanding derived from demographic and epidemiological transition theory project too linear and unidimensional a developmental path, which is inadequate to explain the transitions under way today in rural and developing settings (Beaglehole and Bonita, 2004; National Research Council, 1993). The concept of a health transition attempts to extend classical transition theory to include the social and behavioral changes that parallel and drive the changes in mortality, fertility, and patterns of illness, disability, and death. While this makes it the most appropriate framework for describing changing mortality patterns, limitations remain. It can describe differences in death rates from country to country but cannot explain these differences, its ability to predict changing patterns of disease precipitated by development is limited, it minimizes the interaction between infectious and noncommunicable diseases, and it takes insufficient account of the major social and economic changes that drove the transition (Beaglehole and Bonita, 2004).

While these transition frameworks are helpful in thinking about changing patterns of illness and death, actual information on the direction and scale of change is required, with empirical data best, for developing appropriate policy in response to the health needs of populations.

OLDER ADULTS AND THE HEALTH TRANSITION IN AGINCOURT: A CASE STUDY

The Agincourt Study Site

Geographic, Social, and Economic Characteristics of Agincourt

The Agincourt subdistrict site covers 390 sq km of the Bushbuckridge district of Mpumalanga Province, lying just south of Limpopo Province, adjacent to Mozambique's western boundary (separated by the Kruger National Park). The area is reasonably typical of the densely settled former Bantustan areas (homelands) in South Africa's rural northeast (about 170 persons per sq km), with some 69,000 people in 11,500 households across 21 villages that range in size from 100 to 1,100 households. Nearly one-third of the population are Mozambican immigrants, largely displaced in the early to mid-1980s during the civil war, who fled into South Africa across its eastern border and dispersed within host communities or settled on land allocated to them by local tribal authorities.

The geoecological zone is semiarid savannah, dry (annual rainfall 550-700 mm), and better suited to cattle and game farming than agricultural development. A high variability in interseasonal rainfall patterns renders the area vulnerable to drought—some 80 percent of the rain falls during summer months (Collinson et al., 2002). In addition, household plots are generally too small to support subsistence agriculture, although crops supplement the family diet (Tollman, Herbst, and Garenne, 1995). Despite recent development activities, water shortage is a serious problem and household sanitation is generally limited to pit latrines (Dolan, Tollman, Nkuna, and Gear, 1997). The paving of gravel roads is beginning, however, and electricity is now widely available in the area, although few people can afford the service. While most children reach secondary school, few obtain any form of tertiary education (Tollman et al., 1995). Health care is based on the Agincourt Health Centre and five fixed clinics, all government facilities that provide free consultation and treatment. Referral is to three district hospitals (Mapulaneng, Matikwane, and Tintswalo) 25-60 km away. Private allopathic providers, traditional healers, and faith healers also provide services in or close to the study site.

Formal-sector employment is limited in the area. Migrant labor, involving work in the mines, in larger towns, and on nearby farms, continues to dominate, with remittances critical to local livelihoods. The permanent population is 80.5 percent of the total, the balance temporarily absent for more than 6 months in a year. The sex ratio is 93 for the whole population and 80 for the permanent population. While temporary labor migration rates of men are substantially higher than those of women, increasing numbers of women are joining the migrant labor force, a pattern that probably reflects new economic opportunities. South Africa has a system of state-supported social welfare unique in sub-Saharan Africa, which includes an old-age pension payable to women from age 60 and men from age 65.

Population Growth and Age Structure, 1992-2000

The foundation of the work in the Agincourt study site is a Health and Demographic Surveillance System (HDSS). A baseline census on the entire Agincourt population was conducted in 1992, with registration of every household and individual, including date of birth, sex, nationality, residence status, education, and relationship to household head. Since then, rigorous annual updates have been conducted, with information on all births, deaths, and in- and out-migrations collected in the population under surveillance. The update involves a household visit during which a fieldworker verifies existing information, adds new individual- or household-level data, and records the demographic events that have occurred since the preceding year's census update. Additional information is collected on all pregnancy outcomes, movements in and out of households, and deaths; maternity histories are also conducted. The result is a longitudinal database, dating back to 1992, containing empirical numerator and denominator data, used for the examination of trends in population size and structure and the calculation of rates. Details of the Agincourt HDSS approach and methods have been published elsewhere (Collinson et al., 2002).

The Agincourt population has increased in size from some 57,600 people in 1992 to close to 69,000 at the end of the decade, an increase of 8 percent despite declining fertility (Garenne, Tollman, and Kahn, 2000) and worsening mortality (Kahn, Garenne, Tollman, and Collinson, in press; Tollman, Kahn, Garenne, and Gear, 1999). Ten percent of the population is age 50 and over, a proportion similar at the beginning and the end of the decade. The proportion of elderly ages 75 to 85, however, has doubled from 1 to 2 percent of the population. This translates into a 60 percent increase in the number of elderly.

Findings

Changing Age- and Cause-Specific Mortality, 1992-2000

As part of the Agincourt HDSS, a verbal autopsy (VA) is conducted for every death recorded in the study site. This involves an interview with the closest caregiver of the deceased to elicit details on the clinical signs and symptoms of the terminal illness. Additional information is collected on lifestyle practices (alcohol, smoking, physical activity), health-seeking behavior, and occupation. Verbal autopsy review entails assessment by two medical practitioners, blind to each other, who assign a probable cause to each death. When these correspond, the diagnosis is accepted. When they differ and consensus is not achieved, a third practitioner assesses the verbal autopsy blind to the earlier findings. If this assessment is congruent with one other, it is accepted as the probable cause of death; if not, the cause is coded as "ill-defined." Whenever possible, a main (or underlying) cause, immediate cause, and contributory factors are identified; classification is consistent with the International Classification of Diseases (ICD-10) (Kahn, Tollman, Garenne, and Gear, 1999). The Agincourt VA tool and assessment approach has been validated by comparing VA diagnoses with hospital reference diagnoses. This procedure concluded that the Agincourt VA yielded reasonable estimates of cause-of-death frequencies in all age groups and that the findings could reliably inform district health planning (Kahn et al., 1999).

Trends in Older Adult Mortality, 1992-2000

As expected, mortality rates increase with age, with those over age 75 experiencing higher mortality than those in their 50s and 60s, in both men and women. However, mortality change across the decade reveals age and gender differences (Table 5-1). During ages 75-84, male mortality remained stable while female mortality decreased. During ages 65-74, female mortality remained stable while male mortality increased. These changes were

TABLE 5-1 Change in Mortality Rates by Age and Sex, Agincourt 1992-2000

Gender and Age Group	Period		Change		
	1992-1994	1998-2000	1992-1994 / 1998-2000	P-value	Significance
Men					
0-4	0.03169	0.05637	2.21	0.0000	–
5-14	0.00911	0.00766	0.56	0.5849	NS
15-29	0.02920	0.03464	1.15	0.4059	NS
30-49	0.11893	0.20565	2.36	0.0001	*
50-64	0.25108	0.19948	0.65	0.1649	NS
65-74	0.28233	0.34651	1.18	0.1672	NS
75-84	0.58817	0.58540	1.06	0.9797	NS
Women					
0-4	0.03179	0.05335	1.97	0.0002	–
5-14	0.00616	0.00532	0.55	0.7063	NS
15-29	0.01766	0.04413	3.12	0.0000	–
30-49	0.06728	0.12356	2.50	0.0002	–
50-64	0.09537	0.15114	2.29	0.0227	–
65-74	0.20834	0.20700	0.98	0.9653	NS
75-84	0.42415	0.32092	0.65	0.1603	NS

* Significant change, P < 0.05.

not significant. Notable, however, are trends in the 50-64 age group. Comparing the first 3 years with the final 3 years of the study period, female mortality increased significantly from 95 per 1,000 in 1992-1994 to 151 per 1,000 in 1998-2000, while male mortality decreased from 251 to 199 per 1,000. By 2000, female mortality levels had reached those of men at 182 per 1,000.

Why women appear to be losing their survival advantage in this population is a critical question. Verbal autopsy data indicate that women are bearing the brunt of emerging noncommunicable diseases: for all ages, female mortality from stroke, diabetes, and hypertension combined increased significantly over the 1992-2000 period (Figure 5-1). Female death rates from diabetes (Figure 5-2) and hypertension independently also increased significantly, exceeding male rates beginning from 1996. Divergence in the male and female trends for these conditions, as well as for stroke mortality (Figure 5-3), tested significant.

The profile of causes of death for women ages 50-64 indicates the contribution not only of cardiovascular and other noncommunicable diseases, but also of HIV/AIDS and cervical cancer to the observed mortality increase. Stroke, the top cause of death in this age group, together with diabe-

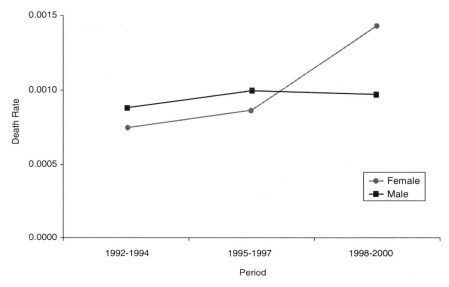

FIGURE 5-1 Death rate from noncommunicable diseases, all ages, Agincourt 1992-2000.
NOTE: Noncommunicable diseases include hypertension, diabetes, stroke, and cerebrovascular accident.

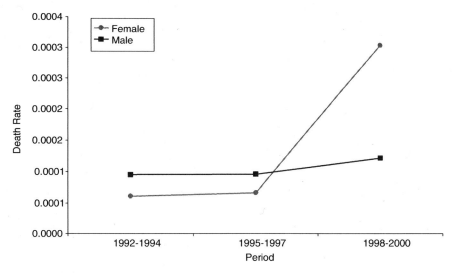

FIGURE 5-2 Trends in overall death rates from diabetes, Agincourt 1992-2000.

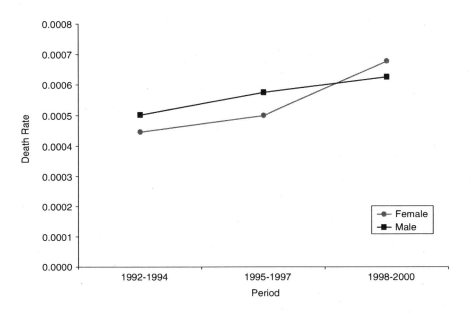

FIGURE 5-3 Trends in overall death rates from stroke, Agincourt 1992-2000.

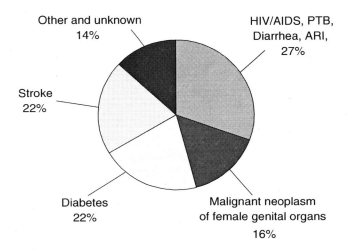

FIGURE 5-4 Causes of deaths responsible for the *increase* in mortality among women ages 50-64, Agincourt 1992-2000.
PTB = pulmonary tuberculosis; ARI = acute respiratory infection.

tes contributed 44 percent of the mortality increase, HIV/AIDS and related diseases a further 27 percent, and female genital malignancies (largely cancer of the cervix) 16 percent (Figure 5-4).

While the focus of this paper is on older adult mortality, it is necessary to briefly examine mortality at younger adult ages, because changes may affect the role and lifestyles of older adults, particularly women (discussed later in the chapter). In Agincourt, mortality rates are increasing dramatically in men and women ages 15-49. As in older women, a shift in gender balance is evident in the 15-29 age group, with female mortality exceeding that of men from about 1998. Increases in mortality for men and women ages 30-49 are similar.

Emerging Noncommunicable Diseases: The Case of Stroke

As populations undergo health and economic transitions, their disease patterns change, with cardiovascular disease (stroke, ischemic heart disease, and peripheral vascular disease) increasing. Hypertension is seen to increase first, followed by hemorrhagic stroke, and later peripheral vascular disease, ischemic heart disease, and ischemic stroke due to atherosclerosis (Pearson, 1999). Mortality data in Agincourt demonstrate this pattern, with stroke a top cause of death in adults ages 50-64 and age 65 and older (Kahn et al., 1999; Kahn and Tollman, 1999). However, a comprehensive picture of the current burden requires knowledge of the prevalence, incidence, and case fatality rates of stroke. Policies and programs to improve prevention and treatment of stroke, whether at the community or health facility level, require an understanding of the risk factors as well as the lay beliefs and practices that determine health-seeking behavior.

Source of Data

The Southern Africa Stroke Prevention Initiative (SASPI) is an Agincourt-based multidisciplinary research project, including public health, epidemiology, neurology, and anthropology. The project aims to measure the current burden of stroke, to investigate the causes and social context of stroke, and to lay the groundwork for a program of intervention research. Between 2001 and 2003, the project employed multiple methods to quantify the community impact of stroke, understand the social setting of stroke, understand the nature of stroke and its risk factors in hospitalized patients and in stroke survivors in the community, and identify problems related to the prevention, diagnosis, and management of stroke (SASPI Project Team, 2003).

Stroke Prevalence and Risk Factors

A crude stroke prevalence of 290 per 100,000 people age 15 and over was found on the basis of clinical examination of all adults in the Agincourt study site who reported one-sided weakness or a history of stroke. This level is lower than that found in New Zealand, but higher than figures reported for Tanzania. A total of 66 percent of stroke survivors needed help with at least one activity of daily living, a prevalence of 200 per 100,000, which is higher than the rates previously reported for both New Zealand and Tanzania (Table 5-2) (SASPI Project Team, 2004a).

From their findings, the SASPI Project Team (2004a) suggests that Agincourt may be at an earlier stage of the health transition than New Zealand and further along than Tanzania. Alternatively, case fatality in Agincourt may be higher than in New Zealand but lower than in Tanzania. The high levels of disability could result from poor levels of care after strokes, or they could suggest more hemorrhagic than occlusive strokes. Population-based incidence studies with stroke-typing are needed to address these questions.

Risk Factors for Stroke

Little research has been done on risk factors for stroke in African populations, or on the relevance of Western population risk factors for develop-

TABLE 5-2 Comparison of Age-Standardized Rates (Segi population per 100,000) in Three Prevalence Studies

	New Zealand[a]	Tanzania[b]	SASPI (Agincourt)
All Stroke Survivors	833	NA	290
Men	991	154	281
Women	706	114	315
Male/female ratio	1.4	1.4	0.9
Stroke Survivors "Needing help with at least 1 activity of daily living"	173	NA	200
Men	156	69	218
Women	188	90	188
Male/female ratio	0.8	0.8	1.2

NOTE: NA = not available.
[a]Bonita, Solomon, and Broad (1997).
[b]Walker et al. (2000).

SOURCE: SASPI Project Team (2004a).

ing countries. In order to develop and implement appropriate interventions, it is important to identify the risk factors for stroke prevalent in the Agincourt population. Among stroke survivors, hypertension was the main risk factor found (84 percent were hypertensive or had evidence of organ damage resulting from hypertension), suggesting that rural South Africans are in the early transition stage. Evidence of atherosclerosis and myocardial infarction, which typically appear later in the transition, was absent (SASPI Project Team, 2004a). Cigarette smoking was not a major risk factor in stroke survivors (9 percent were smokers) (SASPI Project Team, 2004b).

In the general population, risk factor patterns for cardiovascular disease appear to be consistent with those proposed for a population in early transition (Pearson, 1999; Yusuf, Reddy, Ounpuu, and Anand, 2001). A cross-sectional risk factor survey of the general Agincourt population over age 35 (Thorogood, Connor, Tollman, Lewando Hundt, and Marsh, 2005) found that over 40 percent of subjects had hypertension (blood pressure >140/90 mmHg), and that obesity (body mass index and abdominal obesity) was a significant problem in women but not in men. The relationship between body mass index and blood pressure differed between men and women, with a positive relationship found in men but not in women. Cigarette and alcohol use was uncommon in women; a high prevalence of smoking was found in men, although the amount smoked was small. Consumption of fruit and vegetables was low (less than a quarter eat fruit or vegetables on a daily basis). About a quarter of the population had elevated blood lipids, and elevated blood glucose was rarely found (Thorogood et al., 2005).

Increasing Burden on Women

The decade of the 1990s saw steadily rising mortality in Agincourt adults up to age 65, with female mortality worsening relative to male mortality at both young (ages 20-49) and older ages (ages 50-64). Earlier transmission of HIV in women than in men is the most likely explanation at young adult ages, while data on cause of death in women over age 50 suggest that noncommunicable diseases are rising more rapidly in women, and that these may contribute to the pattern of female mortality at older ages. HIV/AIDS, while also propelling the worsening mortality in women ages 50-64, is affecting men and women similarly. Early evidence on cardiovascular risk factors indicates gender differentials in obesity, cigarette smoking, and alcohol consumption (Thorogood et al., 2005). More needs to be learned about gender differentials in risk factors, lifestyle behaviors, and genetic predisposition, if the burden on women is to be redressed through targeted health and social interventions.

The changing demography of young or prime-age adults affects older adults, particularly women, in ways that put them at great disadvantage. Increasing migration of young women to join the labor force affects their parents, who find themselves without the personal care and relief from responsibilities that are culturally expected at their stage of life. In addition, grandmothers often experience extension of their child care role to grandchildren and great-grandchildren. In the case of adult children leaving for reasons of employment, these negative impacts may be partially offset by remittances from the place of work back to the rural household. In contrast, adult children with AIDS become less able to work and consequently contribute less to household income at a time when their consumption of household resources, particularly health expenditures, increases (Gaylin and Kates, 1997). Widespread HIV/AIDS has resulted in older people left to fend for themselves, care for chronically ill and dying adult children, and raise and support grandchildren in circumstances of increasing poverty compounded by the burden of grief following the death of one or more of their children (Barnett and Whiteside, 2002).

IMPLICATIONS OF CHANGING ADULT HEALTH FOR PROVISION OF HEALTH CARE

During this early transitional stage of rural South African communities, what role does the health service currently play in hypertension control and secondary prevention of stroke? In South Africa, free primary health care has gone some way to increasing access for the poorest sectors of society and achieving greater equity. Despite this, evidence on outreach and quality of primary care services is not encouraging (Levitt et al., 1996). Other costs, particularly transport, remain a barrier, as do restricted opening hours for working adults. In the SASPI study, few stroke survivors were on antihypertensive treatment (8 percent whereas 84 percent had evidence of hypertension), with only one person adequately controlled and only one person taking daily aspirin (SASPI Project Team, 2004b). Only a quarter of those with hypertension in the general population were on treatment (75 percent of hypertensive people were thus untreated), and half of those on treatment still had an elevated blood pressure (Thorogood et al., 2005).

Do people's health beliefs result in inadequate utilization of Western health services, and does this partly explain the poor medical management found? In the Agincourt area, illnesses are generally understood as caused by biomedical problems (*xilungu*, white, Western) and by social problems (*xintu*, African traditional). Many conditions therefore need treatment from multiple sources. One-sided weakness is understood to be a biomedical condition (*xistroku*) but can also represent bewitchment or *xifulana*, a condition caused by humans through dysfunctional relations. *Xistroku* can be treated by allopathic methods, but *xifulana* requires intervention from churches or traditional healers. Most people access plural health care, visiting allopathic services, public clinics, and hospitals as well as private providers and also healers and prophets (Lewando Hundt, Stuttaford, and Ngoma, 2004). In fact, the majority (79 percent) of stroke survivors in Agincourt had sought allopathic care at some point after their stroke (SASPI Project Team, 2004b).

In South Africa and other developing countries, rapid demographic and epidemiological change has provided little time for health services to adjust to the needs of chronic care for older people (Bobadilla and Possas, 1993). Changing patterns pose a challenge to existing health services that are generally underresourced, inadequately skilled, and poorly organized and managed. In Agincourt, barriers to secondary prevention of stroke include cost of treatment, reluctance to use pills, difficulties with access to drugs, and lack of equipment to measure blood pressure (SASPI Project Team, 2004b), while problems with staff knowledge, attitudes, and practices have been identified in public-sector facilities providing primary care for diabetes in South Africa (Goodman, Zwarenstein, Robinson, and Levitt, 1996; Levitt et al., 1996).

There is concern that a move away from an infectious to a noncommunicable disease focus could be detrimental to poorer sectors of a population (Gwatkin and Guillot, 2000; Gwatkin, Guillot, and Heuveline, 1999), a concern relevant for rural South Africa, as disparities in child mortality by social class have been documented in Agincourt (Hargreaves, Collinson, Kahn, Clark, and Tollman, 2004). There is clear recognition that the development and financing of health systems to meet the needs of adults and address issues of chronic care delivery must occur without compromising services for women and children (Bobadilla and Possas, 1993; Phillips, Feachem, Murray, Over, and Kjellstrom, 1993; Unwin et al., 2001). In fact, the gains in health for children achieved through communicable disease prevention and control would be undermined if efforts were not also directed to noncommunicable disease prevention and control in adults (Mosely and Gray, 1993; Reddy, 1999).

The particular challenges for rural South African health services, and probably other parts of sub-Saharan Africa in the future, are substantial. There is need to effectively prevent and control the increasing burden of noncommunicable diseases, address HIV/AIDS transmission and treatment and provide home-based care for the terminally ill, while simultaneously maintaining and improving on gains in child and maternal health. Agincourt adults and other Southern African populations are subject to extensive temporary labor migration, with consequent high mobility, making the provision of chronic, ongoing care especially challenging.

While a full account of health system limitations is beyond the scope of this paper, current understanding of the health transition in Agincourt does highlight particular areas that require strengthening. Although fiscal constraints may put achievement of all aspects beyond the short-term reach of South African health services, and certainly those of other sub-Saharan African countries, much can be achieved through better use and some reallocation of existing resources.

Three key issues are considered. While based on experience of the South African rural health care system, general principles are of relevance to other developing settings.

Building Clinical Management Capacity

Staffing of health facilities in a district should include an appropriate mix of skills at different levels of care (clinic, health center, district hospital) based on the morbidity and mortality patterns prevalent in the area. While of variable quality and accessibility, EPI (Expanded Programme on Immunisation) and nutrition programs have long been provided in many developing country settings, IMCI (Integrated Management of Childhood Illnesses) services have been introduced more recently, and VCT (HIV Voluntary Counselling and Testing) services are becoming available in some. Nurses competent to manage adult health conditions at the clinic level are now required, and the Integrated Management of Adolescent and Adult Illness (IMAI) is being developed by the World Health Organization to support this (IMAI has a focus on acute illness as well as on chronic disease and HIV/AIDS). A "step-up" in care between different levels of the health service, such as clinic, health center, and district hospital, needs to be planned, and staff with the requisite skills employed at each level. An understanding of the evolving patterns of illness also needs to influence curriculum development for basic health worker training programs and priorities for continuing professional development. Screening programs should be introduced for conditions in which diagnosis and treatment can be sustained. Greater emphasis needs to be placed on noncommunicable disease diagnosis and management and on the detection of complications. An understanding of risk factors, including hypertension, obesity, and such lifestyle factors as smoking and alcohol consumption, as well as methods of reducing them, is needed.

Two strategies to improve the clinical care of patients are clinical protocols and patient-retained records. Clinical protocols, or structured treatment guidelines, are tools designed to promote standardized, cost-effective, high-quality treatment of particular conditions. Staff tend not to follow these guidelines if passively disseminated, however (Daniels et al., 2000; Goodman et al., 1996), and their introduction and continued use needs to be maintained by in-service training programs. Particular strategies for promoting the use of guidelines can have additional advantages; an example is inclusion of the guidelines in a structured clinical record. This can become a useful tool for audit and evaluation of the quality of care, providing opportunity for discussions regarding patient care, thereby improving both education and teamwork (Daniels et al., 2000).

A patient-retained record can also serve to improve patient care. Advantages include better compliance through an implied partnership with the health service and decreased waiting time at the clinic through elimination of queuing for clinic records (Daniels et al., 2000). This removes one disincentive for patients to return for follow-up visits. In regions with high levels of circular migration, such as much of Southern Africa, patients may attend different facilities depending on whether they are at their temporary place of work or at their permanent residence at the time of the follow-up visit. A patient-retained record ensures that full clinical, laboratory, and treatment information is available to all health providers, while clinical guidelines together with medication from an essential drugs list enable continuity of appropriate care.

Improving Access to Care

While a health service should respond to the needs and demands of its catchment population, these are not necessarily the same. Whereas needs are largely determined by the health status of a community, demand depends also on the community's perceptions of illness, which may result in excessive or inappropriately low use of services (Bobadilla and Possas, 1993). Understanding how people perceive the cause of illness is critical in understanding patterns of health care used. In settings in which people tend to access plural health care, encouraging earlier consultation and regular follow-up at Western primary care services may be an important part of developing patient literacy around noncommunicable diseases and their management.

Treatment of hypertension in sub-Saharan Africa, despite the cost and difficulties, is a priority. Yet investment in a better organized health care system is needed in order to realize the gains in adult health (Cooper, Rotimi, Kaufman, Muna, and Mensah, 1998). With regular follow-up care a critical component of chronic disease management, addressing common barriers is imperative to ensuring patient return. These include ineffective drug distribution systems, malfunctioning equipment, inadequate staff training, and poor staff attitudes.

A less rigid approach to the provision of chronic disease services will go some way to improving quality and addressing the needs of patients. Scheduling of clinic hours and patient waiting times will need attention to facilitate attendance of working adults. Clinics must be equipped with functioning blood pressure cuffs, adult weight scales, and glucometers, and a regular drug supply must be ensured to prevent patients from bypassing the primary care level or failing to attend for follow-up at all. A comprehensive approach that seeks synergy between different chronic care programs will produce benefits for each. This will be particularly the case in settings in which antiretroviral therapy is offered, as these require high-quality services, an uninterrupted drug supply, and access to laboratory facilities.

Controlling Escalating Costs

The high costs of many interventions for noncommunicable diseases are of concern in considering sustainable programs for resource-constrained health systems (Bobadilla and Possas, 1993; Burdon, 1998; Cooper et al., 1998). Interventions with low cost-effectiveness should certainly be limited, and appropriate use of allocated resources needs to be monitored. The goal for adult health programs should be early detection of common chronic conditions (those that can reasonably occur at the primary care level), thus saving resources by delaying progress to complications and advanced stages of disease that require hospitalization (Bobadilla and Possas, 1993). Improvements in quality at the primary care level, discussed above, are essential if screening, diagnostic procedures, and cost-effective ambulatory care are to be successfully devolved to this level.

CONCLUSION

Evidence from the Agincourt study site in rural South Africa, drawn from multiple sources, highlights limitations of classical epidemiological transition theory and reinforces the need for a less rigid, more flexible notion of "complex, multi-sided processes of change in particular societies" (Chen, Kleinman and Ware, 1994). Data from Agincourt demonstrate a counter transition in which mortality is increasing rather than declining as epidemiological transition theory would predict. Sequential passage through Omran's stages—from the era of pestilence and famine, through receding pandemics, to degenerative and manmade diseases—is too linear a model and does not fit the complex interplay of social, economic, behavioral, and environmental factors that act on populations. Instead, the transition under way in rural South Africa better fits the more contemporary framework used to describe transition in other middle-income countries (Frenk et al., 1989). In Agincourt, we have a protracted or prolonged transition in which change is incomplete and different stages are spanned simultaneously. The population is experiencing coexistence of the unfinished agenda of diseases of poverty (persisting infection and malnutrition), together with emerging noncommunicable diseases and escalating HIV/AIDS (Kahn et al., 1999). The HIV/AIDS epidemic provides stark evidence that infectious diseases are not likely to be conquered and replaced with manmade and degenerative diseases. Rather, societies will have to contend with new infectious diseases concurrent with emerging noncommunicable diseases.

As shown elsewhere, noncommunicable diseases are the leading causes of death in adults (Phillips et al., 1993), with the burden falling more on women than on men in Agincourt. Evidence on stroke and cardiovascular risk factors, particularly hypertension, indicates that this population is in the early stage of health transition and is an "early adopter" community within the sub-Saharan African context (Thorogood et al., 2005). The South African experience may well anticipate that of other countries in the region.

The coexistence of communicable and noncommunicable diseases poses multiple challenges for households, policy makers, and health system planners and managers. Efforts to project the prevalence of chronic diseases for purposes of health budgeting and planning need to take into account the impact of HIV/AIDS; fewer infected people will survive to middle and older ages at which noncommunicable diseases reach their peak age-specific prevalence, resulting in lower chronic disease prevalence rates (Panz and Joffe, 1999). Developing health systems—to cater to the chronic, ongoing requirements of adult noncommunicable disease prevention and control while at the same time preserving the acute, short-term care of maternal and child health services—calls for calculated reorientation on the part of policy makers and planners. Scarce public-sector resources will have to be creatively managed to contend with multiple and divergent health problems. A comprehensive approach should ensure that health-sector human resources and organizational and management improvements benefit both HIV/AIDS and noncommunicable disease programs.

While there are calls for further theoretical development of the health transition framework (Beaglehole and Bonita, 2004; Frenk et al., 1994), building an understanding of actual transition experience through empirical research is critical for the formulation of effective public health and social policy (Bell and Chen, 1994).

REFERENCES

Barnett, T., and Whiteside, A. (2002). *AIDS in the twenty-first century: Disease and globalization.* New York: Palgrave Macmillan.

Beaglehole, R., and Bonita, R. (2004). *Public health at the crossroads: Achievements and prospects, second edition.* Cambridge, England: Cambridge University Press.

Bell, D.E., and Chen, L.C. (1994). Responding to health transitions: From research to action. In L.C. Chen, A. Kleinman, and N.C. Ware (Eds.), *Health and social change in international perspective* (pp. 491-501). Cambridge, MA: Harvard University Press.

Bobadilla, J.L., and Possas, C. de A. (1993). Health policy issues in three Latin American countries: Implications of the epidemiological transition. In National Research Council, *The epidemiological transition: Policy and planning implications for developing countries* (pp. 145-169). Committee on Population, J.N. Gribble and S.H. Preston (Eds.). Washington, DC: National Academy Press.

Bonita, R., Solomon, N., and Broad, J.B. (1997). Prevalence of stroke and stroke-related disability: Estimates from the Auckland Stroke Studies. *Stroke, 28,* 1898-1902.

Burdon, J. (1998). Figure of $1,800 per life saved seems optimistic (letter). *British Medical Journal, 317,* 76.

Caldwell, J.C. (2001). Population health in transition. *Bulletin of the World Health Organization, 79*(2), 159-160.

Cappuccio, F.P. (2004). Commentary: Epidemiological transition, migration, and cardiovascular disease. *International Journal of Epidemiology, 33,* 387-388.

Chen, L.C., Kleinman, A., and Ware, N.C. (1994). Overview. In L.C. Chen, A. Kleinman, and N.C. Ware (Eds.), *Health and social change in international perspective* (p. xiv). Cambridge, MA: Harvard University Press.

Collinson, M., Mokoena, O., Mgiba, N., Kahn, K., Tollman, S., Garenne, M., Herbst, K., Malomane, E., and Shackleton, S. (2002). Agincourt DSS, South Africa. In *INDEPTH network, population, and health in developing countries, volume 1. Population, health, and survival at INDEPTH sites* (pp. 197-205). Ottawa, Canada: International Development Research Centre.

Commission on Health Research for Development. (1990). *Health research: Essential link to equity in development.* New York: Oxford University Press.

Cooper, R.S., Rotimi, C.N., Kaufman, J.S., Muna, W.F.T., and Mensah, G.A. (1998). Hypertension treatment and control in sub-Saharan Africa: The epidemiological basis for policy. *British Medical Journal, 316,* 614-617.

Daniels, A.R., Patel, M., Biesma, R., Otten, J., Levitt, N.S., Steyn, K., Martell, R., and Dick, J. (2000). A structured record to implement the national guidelines for diabetes and hypertension care. *South African Medical Journal, 90*(1), 53-56.

Dolan, C., Tollman, S., Nkuna, V., and Gear, J. (1997). The links between legal status and environmental health: A case study of Mozambican refugees and their hosts in the Mpumalanga (eastern Transvaal) Lowveld, South Africa. *International Journal of Health and Human Rights, 2*(2), 62-84.

Dorrington, R., Bourne, D., Bradshaw, D., Laubsher, R., and Timaeus, I.M. (2001) *The impact of HIV/AIDS on adult mortality in South Africa.* Report. Cape Town: South African Medical Research Council.

Feachem R.G.A., Phillips M.A., and Bulatao R.A. (1992). Introducing adult health. In R.G.A. Feacham, T. Kjellstrom, C.J.L. Murray, M. Over, and M.A. Phillips (Eds.), *The health of adults in the developing world* (pp. 1-22). New York: Oxford University Press.

Frenk, J., Bobadilla, J.L., Sepulveda, J., and Cervantes, M.L. (1989). Health transition in middle-income countries: New challenges for health care. *Health Policy and Planning, 4*(1), 29-39.

Frenk, J., Bobadilla, J-L., Stern, C., Frejka, T., and Lozano, R. (1994). Elements for a theory of the health transition. In L.C. Chen, A. Kleinman, and N.C. Ware (Eds.), *Health and social change in international perspective* (pp. 25-49). Cambridge, MA: Harvard University Press.

Garenne, M., Tollman, S., and Kahn, K. (2000). Premarital fertility in rural South Africa: A challenge to existing population policy. *Studies in Family Planning, 31*(1), 47-54.

Gaylin, D.S., and Kates, J. (1997). Refocusing the lens: Epidemiologic transition theory, mortality differentials, and the AIDS pandemic. *Social Science and Medicine, 44*(5), 609-621.

Goodman, G.R., Zwarenstein, M.F., Robinson, I.I., and Levitt, N.S. (1996). Staff knowledge, attitudes, and practices in public sector primary care of diabetes in Cape Town. *South African Medical Journal, 87*(3), 305-309.

Gregson, S. (1994). Will HIV become a major determinant of fertility in sub-Saharan Africa? *Journal of Development Studies, 30*(3), 650-679.

Gregson, S., Zaba, B., and Garnett, G.P. (1999). Low fertility in women with HIV and the impact of the epidemic on orphanhood and early childhood mortality in sub-Saharan Africa. *AIDS, 13*(Suppl A), S249-S257.

Gwatkin, D.R. and Guillot, M. (2000). *The burden of disease among the global poor: Current situation, future trends, and implications for strategy.* (Human Development Network. Health, Nutrition and Population). Washington, DC: The World Bank.

Gwatkin, D.R., Guillot, M., and Heuveline, P. (1999). The burden of disease among the global poor. *The Lancet, 354,* 586-589.

Hargreaves, J.R., Collinson, M.A., Kahn, K., Clark, C., and Tollman, S.M. (2004). Childhood mortality among Mozambican refugees and their hosts in rural South Africa. *International Journal of Epidemiology, 33,* 1271-1278.

Heligman, L., Chen, N., and Babkol, O. (1993). Shifts in the structure of population and deaths in less developed regions. In National Research Council, *The epidemiological transition: Policy and planning implications for developing countries* (pp. 9-41). Committee on Population, J.N. Gribble and S.H. Preston (Eds.). Washington, DC: National Academy Press.

Joint United Nations Programme on HIV/AIDS. (2002, July). *Report on the global HIV/AIDS pandemic.* Geneva, Switzerland: Author.

Kahn, K., and Tollman, S.M. (1999). Stroke in rural South Africa: Contributing to the little known about a big problem. *South African Medical Journal, 89*(1), 63-65.

Kahn, K., Tollman, S.M., Garenne, M., and Gear, J.S.S. (1999). Who dies from what? Determining cause of death in South Africa's rural northeast. *Tropical Medicine and International Health, 4,* 433-441.

Kahn, K., Tollman, S.M., Garenne, M., and Gear, J.S.S. (2000). Validation and application of verbal autopsies in a rural area of South Africa. *Tropical Medicine and International Health, 5*(11), 824-831.

Kahn, K., Garenne, M., Tollman S, and Collinson, M. (in press). Mortality trends in a new South Africa (Agincourt 1992-2003): Hard to make a fresh start. *Scandinavian Journal of Public Health.*

Levitt, N.S., Zwarenstein, M.F., Doepfmer, S., Bawa, A.A., Katzenellenbogen, J., and Bradshaw, D. (1996). Public sector primary care of diabetics: A record review of quality of care in Cape Town. *South African Medical Journal, 86*(8), 1013-1017.

Lewando Hundt, G., Stuttaford, M., and Ngoma, B. (2004). The social diagnostics of stroke like symptoms: Healers, doctors and prophets in Agincourt, Limpopo Province, South Africa. *Journal of Biosocial Sciences, 36*, 433-443.

Mosely, W.H., and Gray, R. (1993). Childhood precursors of adult morbidity and mortality in developing countries: Implications for health programs. In National Research Council, *The epidemiological transition: Policy and planning implications for developing countries* (pp. 69-100). Committee on Population, J.N. Gribble and S.H. Preston (Eds.). Washington, DC: National Academy Press.

National Research Council. (1993). *The epidemiological transition: Policy and planning implications for developing countries. Report of a Workshop.* Committee on Population, J.N. Gribble and S.H. Preston (Eds.). Washington, DC: National Academy Press.

Olshansky, S.J, and Ault, E.B. (1986). The fourth stage of the epidemiologic transition: The age of delayed degenerative diseases. *Milbank Memorial Fund Quarterly, 64*, 355-391.

Omran, A.R. (1971). The epidemiologic transition. *Milbank Memorial Fund Quarterly, 49*(4), 509-538.

Omran, A.R. (1982). Epidemiologic transition. In J.A. Ross (Ed.), *International encyclopaedia of population* (pp. 172-183). London, England: Free Press.

Panz, V.R., and Joffe, B.I. (1999). Impact of HIV infection and AIDS on prevalence of type 2 diabetes in South Africa in 2010 (letter). *British Medical Journal, 318*, 1351-1352.

Pearson, T.A. (1999). Cardiovascular disease in developing countries: Myths, realities, and opportunities. *Cardiovascular Drugs and Therapy, 13*, 95-104.

Phillips, M., Feachem, R.G.A., Murray, C.J.L., Over, M., and Kjellstrom, T. (1993). Adult health: A legitimate concern for developing countries. *American Journal of Public Health, 83*(11), 1527-1530.

Reddy, K.S. (1999). The burden of disease among the global poor (letter). *The Lancet, 354*, 1477.

SASPI Project Team. (2003). *Workshop of the Southern Africa stroke prevention initiative.* (Report. 2-4 November). Division of Health in the Community, University of Warwick and School of Public Health, University of the Witwatersrand.

SASPI Project Team. (2004a). Prevalence of stroke survivors in rural South Africa: Results from the Southern Africa stroke prevention initiative (SASPI), Agincourt field site. *Stroke, March*, 627-632.

SASPI Project Team. (2004b). Secondary prevention of stroke: Results from the Southern Africa stroke prevention initiative (SASPI), Agincourt field site. *Bulletin of the World Health Organization, 82*(7), 503-508.

Thorogood, M., Connor, M., Tollman, S., Lewando-Hundt, G., and Marsh, J. (2005). *The prevalence of cardiovascular risk factors in a rural South African population: Evidence of the impending cardiovascular epidemic from the Southern Africa stroke prevention initiative (SASPI).* Unpublished manuscript, Warwick Medical School, Coventry, England.

Timaeus, I.M. (1998). Impact of the HIV epidemic on mortality in sub-Saharan Africa: Evidence from national surveys and censuses. *AIDS, 12*(Suppl. 1), S15-S27.

Tollman, S., Herbst, K., and Garenne, M. (1995). *The Agincourt demographic and health study: Phase 1*. Johannesburg, South Africa: Health Systems Development Unit, Department of Community Health, University of the Witwatersrand.

Tollman, S.M., Kahn, K., Garenne, M., and Gear, J.S.S. (1999). Reversal in mortality trends: Evidence from the Agincourt field site, South Africa, 1992-1995. *AIDS, 13*, 1091-1097.

United Nations, Population Division, Department of Economic and Social Affairs. (1999). *Population ageing 1999*. (UN Publication ST/ESA/SER.A/179). New York: Author.

Unwin, N., Setel, P., Rashid, S., Mugusi, F., Mbanya, J., Kitange, H., Hayes, L., Edwards, R., Aspray, T., and Alberti, K.G.M.M. (2001). Noncommunicable diseases in sub-Saharan Africa: Where do they feature in the health research agenda? *Bulletin of the World Health Organization, 79*(10), 947-953.

Walker, R.W., McLarty, D.G., Masuku, G., Kitange, H.M., Whiting, D., Moshi, A.F., Massawe, G., Amaro, R., Mhina, A., and Alberti, K.G.M.M. (2000). Age specific prevalence of impairment and disability relating to hemiplegic stroke in the Hai district of northern Tanzania. *Journal of Neurology and Neurosurgery Psychiatry, 68*, 749.

Yusuf, S., Reddy, S., Ounpuu, S., and Anand, S. (2001). Global burden of cardiovascular diseases Part I: General considerations, the epidemiologic transitions, risk factors, and the impact of urbanization. *Circulation, 104*, 2746-2753.

6

The Situation of Older People in Poor Urban Settings: The Case of Nairobi, Kenya

Alex C. Ezeh, Gloria Chepngeno,
Abdhalah Ziraba Kasiira, and Zewdu Woubalem

INTRODUCTION

Urban growth in sub-Saharan Africa continues to be fueled by rural-urban migration, especially of youths and young adults under 30 years of age. For many African countries, this trend dates back to the early 1960s with the attainment of independence in some of the countries. Drawn largely by the expanding urban economies and social amenities in the 1960s and 1970s, which offered opportunities for cash or wage employment and trade, city-ward migration soon became associated with social and economic mobility (Anderson, 2001; Barber and Milne, 1988; Bigsten, 1996; Johnnie, 1988; Nigeria Institute of Social and Economic Research, 1997). Residence in cities quickly became a status symbol for at least the rural residents in many parts of Africa, and this, among other reasons, has continued to propel this pattern of migration and rapid urbanization in the region.

Africa's rapid urbanization has occurred amidst stagnating economies and poor governance, which have created massive and abject poverty in overcrowded slum settlements across major cities in the region. Recent studies have highlighted huge inequities in social indicators and in health and reproductive health outcomes between the urban poor and other subgroups, including residents of rural areas, with the urban poor recording the worst outcomes (African Population and Health Research Center, 2002; Dodoo, Zulu, and Ezeh, forthcoming; Gulis, Mulumba, Juma, and Kakosova, 2003; Magadi, Zulu, and Brockerhoff, 2003; Zulu, Dodoo, and Ezeh, 2003). Despite the poor outcomes observed among the urban poor in sub-Saharan Africa, cities continue to attract a large influx of migrants from rural areas, causing urban growth to remain high across sub-Saharan Africa (Government of Kenya, 2000; Oucho, 1998).

Migration to urban areas has generally been thought of as a temporary phenomenon, with migrants maintaining strong ties with their rural origins (Grant, 1995; Gugler, 1991; Trager, 1998). The assumption has also been that they will return to their rural homes upon retirement. However, the presence and the growing numbers of older people in urban areas call for a better understanding of the context of aging in sub-Saharan Africa as well as the situation of older people living in urban areas in the region. These urban areas are characterized by worsening economic and social conditions, especially in the sprawling, informal settlements of cities across sub-Saharan Africa.

Even though sub-Saharan Africa has the lowest proportion of people age 60 and older, at about 5 percent compared with 10 percent globally, the region has one of the highest rates of growth for this age group, with projections reaching as high as 12 percent of the region's total population by 2050 (Population Reference Bureau, 2005; World Health Organization, 2002). Recent comparative analysis of Demographic and Health Survey data conducted in the early to mid-1990s in 20 sub-Saharan African countries noted that, on average, people 60 years and over accounted for about 6 percent of the population, with the average for Southern African countries reaching 7 percent (Ayad and Otto, 1997). In Kenya, various estimates put the proportion age 60 and over at about 4 percent (Thumbi, 2005). The 1999 Kenyan census puts the proportion 60 and over at 4.7 percent, significantly lower compared with the 6.1 percent recorded in the 1989 census (Republic of Kenya, 2001). These differences may result from age misreporting in censuses and surveys, especially for older ages, since interviewers generally rely on physical features to estimate age.

Little research has focused on older people in sub-Saharan Africa. The limited work that has been done has focused mostly on rural areas, and attention to older people living in urban areas is almost nonexistent. This paper aims to reduce this dearth of knowledge by exploring the living arrangements, economic activities, and health status of older people living in two informal settlements in Nairobi, Kenya.

The Study Setting

Nairobi typifies the current urban population boom and its associated health and poverty problems, characteristic of many sub-Saharan African cities. During the colonial era, restrictive settlement policies on migration to the city maintained the growth within certain limits, with a population of 120,000 in 1948 (Muwonge, 1980). With the elimination of the "pass" system, in which migrants were required to obtain a permit to reside in Nairobi, and the relaxation of other migration rules following Kenya's independence in 1963, Nairobi's growth entered its second phase; its population reached 350,000 in 1962 and 500,000 in 1971, with an estimated one-third living in unauthorized housing (Muwonge, 1980). The 1999 Kenyan Population Census enumerated the population of Nairobi at 2.3 million (Republic of Kenya, 2001). With economic declines since the 1980s, 60 to 70 percent of the Nairobi population is currently estimated to be living in informal settlements that occupy only 5 percent of the residential land area of the city (Matrix Development Consultants, 1993; UN-Habitat, 2003).

This study covers 2 of the more than 40 informal settlements in Nairobi: Viwandani and Korogocho. Although the two communities are similar in many respects, they also have some key differences. Viwandani, which is located very close to the city's industrial area, is home to many low-income industrial workers, as reflected in the relatively high proportion of men of working age (15-49). In line with its strategic location near the major source of employment in the city (the industrial area), Viwandani attracts somewhat more educated residents than Korogocho. However, this means that the population is also more transient, with residents on average having lived there only six years, whereas Korogocho residents have spent an average of 11.5 years in the community. Also, while Viwandani has more than 53 percent of the total population of the two settlements, it has less than a quarter of the population age 60 and over.

The two communities also share a number of features characteristic of informal settlements in Nairobi. Most households live in one-room houses that serve multiple purposes, including sleeping, sitting, and cooking and eating. Over 95 percent of the households cook in the same room they use for sleeping. Over 90 percent of the households do not have any organized mechanism for garbage disposal, while fewer than 5 percent have their own toilets. Similar patterns are observed for water supply: over 90 percent of households depend on poor-quality water distributed by vendors or kiosks for which they pay three or more times the tariff charged by the Nairobi City Council to pipe water to middle or upper income households (African Population and Health Research Center, 2002; Matrix Development Consultants, 1993; UNICEF, 2002). The social, economic, and environmental conditions prevailing in informal settlements provide a challenge to the well-being of older people living in this setting, given their increased vulnerability due to declining physical and health status and reduced economic productivity. It is against this background that this paper seeks to explore the living conditions of the elderly in the informal settlements in Nairobi.

Data and Methods

The quantitative data are drawn from the Nairobi Urban Health and Demographic Surveillance System (NUHDSS) that the African Population and Health Research Centre set up in 2002. The NUHDSS covers a population of about 60,000 living in about 23,000 households in the two informal settlements. The NUHDSS involves visits to all the households once every four months to continuously update information on pregnancies and pregnancy outcomes, migration, episodes of morbidity, health-seeking behavior, mortality and causes of death, livelihood activities, vaccination coverage, marital status, and school attendance. Data on 791 persons age 60 and older present at the end of the three waves of observation in 2003 are used in this analysis.

Qualitative data are also used to examine the meanings attached to being old by older people themselves and other residents of the communities under study and also to provide a snapshot of older people through the use of case studies. The qualitative research involved focus group discussions and in-depth interviews with older persons, as well as focus group discussions with other members of the two communities. The focus group data were collected to provide an overview of the communities' attitudes and opinions toward older people and aging. They addressed a number of issues relating to community perceptions and definitions of an older person, roles older people play in the community and how these might vary between men and women, support networks available, and general problems older people encounter in urban informal settlements. The focus group participants were randomly selected and stratified according to age. In the in-depth interviews, different categories of older people (those living alone, those living only with children under age 15, those with physical disabilities or chronic conditions, those who recently lost an adult child, etc.) were purposively selected for interview. The interviews focused on obtaining case histories of their lives and experiences, support networks, and reasons why they continue to reside where they do. Although these qualitative data are rich and deserve fuller exploration beyond the scope of this paper, we have made only limited use of them, generally to underscore the results emerging from the quantitative data and to highlight the lives of specific older people in the form of case studies.

Who Are Regarded as Older People in Poor Urban Communities?

Although old age is defined differently by various cultures and societies, age 60 is widely used as the cutoff age to define older people. Chronological age, physical features, and social attributes are widely used as characteristics that define old age. The concept of defining old age by chronological age in sub-Saharan Africa has severely been criticized (Bledsoe and Fatoumatta, 2002; HelpAge International, 2002; Kimuna and Adamchak, 1999; United Nations, 1991). Social definitions that see old age as both a process and a stage have been recommended instead, as this comes much closer to local perceptions and notions regarding old age. The qualitative study explored the meanings attached to being old among the study population. Analysis of the data shows clearly that being an older person is perceived both as a process and a stage that a person enters after attaining a certain age or reproductive and other life experiences.

Most of the discussants define an older person according to their physical characteristics, their marital or childbearing experiences, their dress, or the sort of lifestyle they lead. In 15 of the 24 focus group discussions, physical attributes, such as having grey hair and wrinkles, using a walking stick, or having a stooped back, were mentioned in defining an older person. Reproductive experience, especially having grandchildren, and personal character, especially manner of dressing, were also said to define an older person. The degree of contribution to community-wide programs or the ability to command respect in the community are other common descriptions of older people, often made without much regard to chronological age. These nonphysical notions of who an older person is were mentioned in about two-thirds of the focus group discussions. For some discussants, being an older person is equated with importance in men, the onset of menopause for women, and loss of interest in sex for both sexes. Declining physical strength and health status and increased physical and financial dependence and vulnerability were also mentioned as characterizing older people.

Apart from physical features and reproductive experiences, the roles that older people play in their community, especially in arbitrating disputes and providing guidance and local leadership, are also seen as their defining characteristics. Older people were said to play an important role in the community, for example in settling disputes both at the domestic or family level and at the community level. In about 21 of the 24 focus groups, older people were said to be nonpartisan when settling disputes because of their wealth of experience and knowledge, hence their ability to give valuable advice on various issues. They were also said to play a major role in security matters in the community and to participate and provide leadership in community development initiatives, such as the construction of schools, bridges, and toilets, the provision of water, and ensuring that the community is clean. During calamities or disasters such as fires, older people are said to play a lead role in mobilizing the community. The excerpts below provide examples of the views on older people mentioned above.

> You may identify an old person by looking at his age and especially for men you may also see their grey hair. Women normally wear head scarves so you

may not see the hair. He may also use a walking stick, have impaired vision and may occasionally need assistance from another person (women ages 15-24, Korogocho).

Res6: It means being unable to do things for themselves. There is no work you can do. Even in employment you cannot work. It is like being a child. It is like sickness.

Res9: An older person is someone who is sickly, has no one to help them. They wake up and stare through the window and pray to God and leave everything to God. I am old and I have nothing. I have nobody to help me. I am sick and I have nobody to give me water or to do anything for me. I am old.

Res6: Like me, the way I was last year is not the same this year. I am now incapacitated. I feel I cannot walk. I have aches in the limbs and the back. I feel my whole body paining now.

Res1: It is when your body is incapacitated. It does not concern money but when you can no longer work or do things for yourself then you are old (women age 60 and older, Korogocho).

Res6: An older person cannot walk and his life is almost over. You will shake while walking. Others have no food and this food we are given by our children while others go without food. That is one of the problems the older people face because you are old and you cannot fend for yourself. When you are sick there is nobody to give you health care. Perhaps you have children but they are poor and they wander around because you never gave them proper upbringing due to your poverty status (men age 60 and older, Viwandani).

Res3: They are involved in the administration of the community. Most of them act as chairmen in the community leadership. They attend to community problems like fire outbreaks, shortage of water and village cleanliness, and so on (men ages 25-49, Viwandani).

Those who use chronological age in defining older people often mentioned ages ranging from 35 to 65 and over as the cutoff. Specific ages were given in 13 of the 24 focus groups. Each age group appears to consider anyone in the age groups above theirs as an old person. Discussants in the age group 15-24 were more likely to report age 35 or 40 as the cutoff age. Those ages 25-49 were more likely to mention age 50 or 55 as the cutoff, while most discussants ages 50-59 gave the cutoff as 65. It is interesting that, except for those age 60 and older who feel incapacitated, people do not regard themselves as older. It is unclear the extent to which the negative images often used in describing older people in the slum communities contribute to this view.

The defining characteristics ascribed to older people as noted above suggest that being an older person is not only a function of having attained a certain age, but also reflects certain physical attributes, reproductive experiences, and roles performed in the community. This gives a different perspective on who is an older person as seen through the eyes of members of these communities. The different meanings attached to being an older person call for caution in conducting studies that look at older people in such settings. The discussion below, however, focuses on persons age 60 and above in line with the international definition of older persons.

STUDY RESULTS

Sociodemographic Characteristics of Study Participants

Table 6-1 shows the sociodemographic characteristics of older people resident in the two informal settlements. There is a variation in the sex distribution across and within each slum community. There are generally more men than women in the overall population, and this is also reflected in the population age 60 and over. It may reflect historical migration patterns in many parts of sub-Saharan Africa, which are largely dominated by male migration. As noted earlier, Viwandani tends to attract more men: 58 percent of the total male population in the two communities resides in Viwandani (statistics not shown in table). A slightly larger proportion (57 percent) of the total population of the two slum communities also resides in Viwandani. However, only 23 percent of the population age 60 and over resides here. This can be attributed to the fact that Viwandani attracts a more youthful population, who work in the adjoining industries. The imbalance in the older population between Viwandani and Korogocho is also reflected in the gender distribution. Whereas only 56 percent of the total older population is male, this proportion rises to 74 percent in Viwandani, whereas the proportion in Korogocho is the same as that of older women.

Almost one-third of the total population consists of people from the Kikuyu ethnic group, and the proportion rises to more than one half (54 percent) among the population age 60 and older. Across the sexes, more than two-thirds of older women in the two slum communities are Kikuyu compared with only 43 percent of the older men. The overrepresentation of Kikuyu older women in the two slum communities may reflect a combination of factors, including the fact that Nairobi is almost surrounded by Central Province, which is largely dominated by the Kikuyu ethnic group. It may also be the case that older women from other ethnic groups may be more likely to return to their rural origins in old age or less likely to have migrated to Nairobi in the past. With growing poverty, it is also possible that poor women from Kikuyu-dominated districts surrounding Nairobi may decide to move to Nairobi to beg or carry out petty business and there-

TABLE 6-1 Sociodemographic Characteristics of the Overall Population and Older People Age 60 and Above, Nairobi Demographic Surveillance System, 2003

	Total Population			Population 60+		
	Women	Men	Total	Women	Men	Total
Ethnic Group						
Kamba	20.2	27.2	24.2	8.9	15.4	12.5
Kikuyu	33.6	29.1	31.1	67.4	43.3	54.0
Luhya	13.9	13.2	13.5	2.9	10.9	7.3
Luo	18.3	16.1	17.1	2.6	8.6	5.9
Other	13.9	14.3	14.1	18.3	21.8	20.2
Education						
No education	9.8	5.1	7.1	69.1	38.2	51.9
Primary	67.7	59.8	63.1	30.0	55.6	44.3
Secondary+	22.4	35.1	29.8	0.9	6.3	3.9
Marital Status						
Currently married	51.4	57.7	55.2	20.1	76.5	50.8
Formerly married	13.4	4.4	8.1	75.5	21.5	46.1
Never married	35.2	37.9	36.8	4.5	2.0	3.1
Residing with Spouse						
Yes	96.7	65.6	77.6	70.2	52.8	56.0
No	3.3	34.4	22.4	29.9	47.2	44.1
Number of Cases	23,021	30,525	53,546	350	441	791
Percent	43.0	57.0		44.2	55.8	

SOURCE: African Population and Health Research Center (2002-2003).

fore more likely to reside in the slums. The large disparity between older men and women from the Kikuyu ethnic group is not reflected in the overall ethnic distribution of the total population in the two slum communities. Kikuyu women account for only 34 percent of the total female population, similar to Kikuyu men, who account for 29 percent of the total male population. Across other ethnic groups, older men are more predominant than women in both slum communities.

Slightly more than half of the older population have no education, and less than 5 percent have attained secondary or higher education. The disparity between the sexes in terms of level of education is very wide: more than two-thirds of the older women have no formal education compared with only 38 percent of the older men. Older men are almost eight times more likely than older women to have secondary or higher education.

Korogocho Population 60+			Viwandani Population 60+		
Women	Men	Total	Women	Men	Total
6.3	7.6	6.9	25.0	32.9	30.8
67.9	45.7	56.8	64.6	38.0	44.9
3.0	10.9	6.9	2.1	11.0	8.7
3.0	10.9	6.9	0.0	3.7	2.7
19.9	25.0	22.4	8.3	14.6	13.0
69.6	42.3	55.9	66.0	28.8	38.6
29.7	51.7	40.8	31.9	64.4	55.9
0.7	6.0	3.4	2.1	6.8	5.6
18.6	71.2	44.8	29.6	90.2	73.1
77.9	26.7	52.4	59.1	8.0	22.4
3.5	2.1	2.8	11.4	1.8	4.5
77.8	64.2	67.1	38.5	29.3	30.4
22.2	35.8	33.0	61.5	70.7	69.6
302	304	606	48	137	185
49.8	50.2		25.9	74.1	

Among older women, about one in five is currently married compared with 77 percent of older men. An overwhelming majority of the women (76 percent) are formerly married, the majority of these being widowed, and 5 percent have never been married. For the older men, only 21 percent are formerly married, reflecting the higher propensity of widowed and divorced men to remarry, often to much younger women. Widowed or divorced older women, in contrast, rarely remarry and may end up living alone or with their children or other adult relatives.

Among the currently married, older women are more likely to reside with their spouse than are men, and this is true of residents of Korogocho more often than Viwandani. While almost two-thirds of the currently married older men in Korogocho live with their wives, only 29 percent of those living in Viwandani do so. Also, while more than three-quarters of currently married older women in Korogocho live with their spouses, fewer than 40 percent of their counterparts in Viwandani do so. These patterns of gender and slum location differentials in coresidence also exist in the general population, with 96 to 98 percent of currently married women in the two communities coresiding with their husbands compared with only 71 and 61 percent (not shown) of the currently married men in Viwandani and Korogocho, respectively. One plausible explanation for these gender differentials may be differences in reasons for rural-urban migration between men and women: married men may migrate to the city in search of jobs, leaving their families behind, while the women may migrate to join their husbands in the city.

The sociodemographic profile of older people living in urban informal settlements as described above may have implications for their well-being. For example, older women who are largely uneducated and unmarried may face more severe forms of poverty, isolation, and vulnerability than men, and they may be more likely to be excluded from formal employment in the past and social support systems in the present, such as the country's contributory pension scheme. We use the case study of an in-depth interview with an 82-year-old woman to highlight the vulnerability women face in the urban informal settlements (Box 6-1).

Living Arrangements

The living arrangements of older people greatly affect their social, economic, and health status and overall well-being. Older people who live alone may lack the necessary social capital and networks to survive in urban informal settlements. Table 6-2 shows the living arrangements of the study group. Overall, 47 and 38 percent of older men and women, respectively, live alone in one-person dwelling units in the two slum communities. In both Korogocho and Viwandani, 7 and 10 percent of the older women, respectively, live only with children under age 15 compared with about 1 percent of the men in each of the slum communities. This finding supports earlier reports suggesting that older women, who may be more vulnerable economically and socially, are often more likely to shoulder the burden of caring for orphaned grandchildren or relatives (Ntozi and Zirimenya, 1999). Among older people who reported being currently married, older men are about 2.5 times more likely than older women to live with only a spouse or with a spouse and children under age 15. The greater proportion of older men living with a spouse may reflect the higher likelihood of widowed or divorced men remarrying, often to much younger women, compared with widowed or divorced women. Overall, close to one-half of older women live with at least one other adult (other than the spouse) who is age 15 or older compared with only a third of the men.

Across the two slum communities, there are substantial variations in

---

BOX 6-1
Case Study 1: Female Living Alone, Viwandani

She is 82 years old and has been living alone for the past year after her two adopted children were admitted to a boarding school, which also serves as a rehabilitation center. She ran away from her matrimonial home 20 years ago to escape physical abuse from the husband who had married two other wives after she could not bear children. She settled in this community and did various casual jobs until she decided to become self-employed as a hawker of secondhand clothes in the streets of Nairobi. She stopped the business after hawkers were banned from operating in the streets, and she has not been employed since. She was also finding it difficult to continue hawking after she was hit by a vehicle and her leg was seriously injured. She owns the house she currently occupies but the house has burned down a couple of times.

About 10 years ago she decided to adopt a set of twins from a woman who had planned to abandon the children after delivery. Her adopted children got into bad company and became delinquent, refusing to go to school. To salvage the situation, she took the children to a rehabilitation center, where all their expenses and upkeep are taken care of by a religious group running the center. The children do not come home to visit her even during holidays, but she does visit them once in a long while.

She relies on well-wishers, including neighbors and relief organizations, to provide her with food and water. A religious organization also provides her with free health care. She is able to do household chores with little difficulty. One disadvantage of living alone, according to her, is that there is no one to assist her at times of difficulty. Living alone, however, also has its advantages because she is catering only to her own needs. According to her, "If you feel hungry, you feel the hunger alone. If you cook food, you cook your own which you know it is enough for two days or one only."

---

living arrangements. More than half of older people in Viwandani (54 percent) live alone compared with only 40 percent in Korogocho. In Viwandani, 60 percent of older men live alone in one-person dwelling units, compared with only 36 percent of the women in the same community. While 12 percent of the older men in Korogocho live with only a spouse, less than 4 percent of those in Viwandani reported living with only their spouse. Compared with estimates for Nairobi from the 1999 census in which only 16.8 percent of the older people live alone, those in the two informal settlements (43 percent) are 2.5 times more likely to live alone. This suggests that older

TABLE 6-2 Living Arrangements of Older People, Nairobi Demographic Surveillance System, 2003 (in percentage)

Living Arrangements	Total Population 60+		Korogocho Population 60+		Viwandani Population 60+	
	Women	Men	Women	Men	Women	Men
Person Living with:						
Lives alone	37.6	47.0	37.9	41.2	36.0	59.9
Lives with child(ren) < 15 years	7.3	1.1	6.9	1.3	10.0	0.7
Lives with spouse only	4.8	9.5	4.6	12.1	6.0	3.7
Lives with spouse and children < 15	1.4	5.2	1.6	6.9	0.0	1.5
Lives with at least 1 adult (not spouse)	48.9	37.3	49.0	38.6	48.0	34.3
Relationship to Household Head:						
Head	77.8	92.6	78.4	92.5	74.0	92.7
Spouse	9.6	1.6	10.1	2.0	6.0	1.0
Other relative	12.6	5.6	11.4	5.2	20.0	6.6
Number of Cases	356	442	306	305	50	137

SOURCE: African Population and Health Research Center (2002-2003).

people in poor urban settings may experience much higher levels of isolation. A recent analysis of Demographic and Health Survey data from several African countries suggests that only 6.5 and 5.1 percent of older people age 65 and above in the urban and rural areas, respectively, live alone (Bongaarts and Zimmer, 2005). Most of the older people are heads of their households. This can be attributed to the fact that a large proportion of them live alone and are hence heads of their single-member households. Older women are more likely to report being a spouse or other relative to the head of households compared with men.

The living arrangement categories highlighted above may not adequately capture the range of vulnerabilities that older people face in urban informal settlements. Even when an older person lives with a spouse or other adults, their situation may not necessarily improve, especially if they have primary responsibility for the upkeep of the household. The experiences of two case studies may help highlight this point clearly (Box 6-2). Although these older persons do not live alone, their situations are as bad as those of many other older people who do live alone.

Economic Status

Table 6-3 shows the labor force participation of the study population, the type of activity they are engaged in, and reasons for not working for those not engaged in any type of income-generating activity. Although the retirement age in Kenya is 55, more than half and close to two-thirds of older women and men, respectively, living in the two slum communities were engaged in an income-generating activity at the time of the study. Nearly three-quarters of the older women and half of the older men who are currently working are engaged in businesses—mainly petty trading, such as selling vegetables along walkways in the community. More than one in five of both men and women are still working in formal employment, whereas 27 percent of the men and only 7 percent of the women are engaged in informal employment—mainly casual labor. There are few variations in the proportions working or type of work across the two communities: older men in Viwandani (39 percent) are more than twice as likely as older men in Korogocho to be working in formal employment. These are largely employed in the industries around Viwandani slum, often as security guards.

For those not working, 63 percent of the women and 55 percent of the men reported they are too old or have retired, while 19 percent of the women and 15 percent of the men reported being sick or too ill to work. A total of 30 percent of households headed by an older woman and 15 percent of those headed by a man receive transfers or remittances; nearly half of the transfers come from children and other relatives for both men and

BOX 6-2
Two Case Studies
Case Study #2: Man with a Disability Living with a Spouse, Korogocho

The subject is a 90-year-old man whose leg was crippled by injuries he sustained following a bicycle accident five years ago. Although he lives with his wife, he seems totally helpless, with no one to provide any assistance since his wife has a mental illness. He claims to have been among the first people to settle in this slum almost 30 years ago. Compared with other people in his neighborhood, his house seems to be in a very poor state, with the roof leaking almost from all sides. The house gets flooded with water even with the lightest rainfall. His other health problem is insomnia.

His life took a complete turn after he was involved in the bicycle accident. He seems very lonely and rarely gets any visitors who are interested in his situation. He was very happy to talk to the interviewer and broke down in tears on several occasions during the interview, especially when recalling some of the hardships he has had to undergo due to his disability. He and his wife mainly depend on well-wishers for their survival.

Case Study #3: Woman with a Disability and Living with Grandchildren, Viwandani

The subject is a 59-year-old widow living with her younger sister, who is ill, and seven of her orphaned grandchildren in the same house-

women. Older women (34 percent) are more likely than men (26 percent) to receive support from religious organizations, nongovernmental organizations, or the government, probably because they are more likely to reside with younger children, unlike the men. Only 2 percent of older women and 10 percent of men participate in some form of welfare program, mainly the National Social Security Fund. Since it is a contributory scheme, this disparity may reflect traditional gender inequities in employment, with men being much more likely to be in formal employment and therefore to contribute to the program. Indeed, the difference between the two slum communities also points to this fact. In Viwandani, where about 40 percent of the older men report having formal employment, almost one in four reported receiving social security support compared with only 2 to 4 percent of older men in Korogocho and women in both slum communities who receive social security support.

hold. She has been married twice and came to live in Nairobi from the rural areas after separating from her first husband in 1989. Her only surviving child lives in the same community with his family. She worked as a domestic servant after moving to Nairobi and stopped only after she developed difficulty walking due to pain in her legs. The pain has limited her movements, including performing daily activities such as bathing and using the toilet, which she does with great difficulty and requires assistance during days when the pain is most severe. She cannot afford to follow up on treatment for her legs and the little money she gets goes toward buying food for her household.

For her livelihood, she sells water on behalf of someone and is paid in kind. She also doubles up as an herbalist selling traditional medicine meant to treat eye infections. The grandchildren also contribute to the household income, especially during school vacation, when they do manual labor, including working as domestic servants. Her household also relies on handouts from well-wishers in the community. The interviewer found her contemplating her next move because of a notice issued to her and her neighbors to vacate their dwelling units, which were to be demolished due to being too close to electricity main grid lines.

Her wish is to start up a business selling vegetables outside her doorstep and joining a welfare group that would advance her credit to expand on the business. She longs for the day when her grandchildren have finished school and will be able to take care of her.

One of the biggest challenges to the economic well-being of older people in the urban informal settlements is the informality of their economic activities. A majority of the residents work in the informal sector, and even those who have formal employment often lack job security despite working in high-risk jobs. The case in Box 6-3 highlights the complex linkages between economic activity, health status, and aging among the urban poor.

Health Status

Table 6-4 shows 30 percent of older women and 18 percent of the men reported being sick during a two-week period preceding a visit to their households between January and April 2003. A look at the main illnesses reported by these older people show few differences by gender and slum location. Overall, musculoskeletal illnesses account for 57 percent of the

TABLE 6-3 Working Status, Reasons for Not Working, and Other Economic Indicators, Nairobi Demographic Surveillance System, 2003 (in percentage)

	Total Population 60+		Korogocho Population 60+		Viwandani Population 60+	
	Women	Men	Women	Men	Women	Men
Percentage Currently Working	51.5	62.1	52.3	63.1	46.9	59.9
Type of Work:						
Petty trading	72.7	50.2	71.9	57.0	78.3	34.2
Formal employment	20.8	22.9	21.3	16.1	17.4	39.0
Informal employment	6.6	26.9	6.9	26.9	4.4	26.8
Reason for Not Working:						
Too old/retired	62.7	54.5	62.5	52.7	64.3	63.6
Sick/ill	19.1	15.2	18.8	16.4	21.4	9.1
Other reasons	18.2	30.3	18.8	30.9	13.3	27.3
Household Receives Remittances	30.1	15.2	29.7	17.8	32.4	9.4
Receives Social Security (e.g., NSSF)	2.2	10.2	2.3	4.3	2	23.4
Number of Cases	356	442	306	305	50	137

SOURCE: African Population and Health Research Center (2002-2003).

BOX 6-3
Case Study #4: Man with a Disability (Blindness), Viwandani

The subject is a 61-year-old man living with his wife and two school-age children. He moved to Nairobi during the preindependence period and has lived in this particular slum community for close to 25 years. He was employed as a plant operator in one of the neighboring industries. His eyesight started deteriorating after an industrial accident at work that exposed his eyes to dangerous chemicals. His employment was terminated on health grounds when it became apparent that he was almost totally blind. He has been unemployed for about 10 years. He made several attempts to save his eyesight, including undergoing about five eye operations. The hospital expenses of these surgeries cost him all his savings and put him in debt.

After exhausting his savings and losing his job at the factory, he was resigned to fate. He has undergone rehabilitation and training on the use of the white cane and is now able to move around his neighborhood unaided and is even able to walk to the main road and take public transport. He is also able to perform most household chores, such as washing clothes, lighting the stove, cooking, and washing utensils. He likes to be independent and does not want to stay idle, so he prefers to do most of the household chores, even though his wife and children are always eager to assist.

He owns the structure that his household currently occupies in addition to two others in the community that have been rented out. Most of his income comes from the rental structures. His wife also runs a business selling vegetables in the market. He prefers life in the city, which he believes is better than in the rural areas, since his parents left a piece of land too small to farm, and the brothers he left behind have already taken it over and refused to share it with him.

---

illnesses reported by the women in both slum communities but for only 35 to 47 percent of the illnesses reported by men. Men are more likely to report respiratory illnesses, with one in four in Viwandani reporting this compared with only 15 percent of the women in Korogocho and Viwandani. Equal proportions of men and women in Korogocho reported gastrointestinal illnesses, reflecting the common environmental conditions affecting health in this particular slum community. In contrast to Korogocho, no woman in Viwandani reported gastrointestinal illness, although 10 percent of the men in the community reported it.

Between 10 and 18 percent of the men and women reported illnesses associated with the central nervous system. Although there are indications

TABLE 6-4 Health Status and Treatment-Seeking Behavior Among Older People, Nairobi Demographic Surveillance System, 2003 (in percentage)

Health Status and Care Seeking	Total Population 60+		Korogocho Population 60+		Viwandani Population 60+	
	Women	Men	Women	Men	Women	Men
Sick (past two weeks)	29.6	18.1	28.8	19.6	34.7	14.6
Type of Illness:						
Musculoskeletal	57.1	43.8	56.8	46.7	58.8	35.0
Respiratory	15.2	22.5	14.8	21.7	17.7	25.0
Gastrointestinal	5.7	7.5	6.8	6.7	0.0	10.0
Central nervous	13.3	16.3	12.5	18.3	17.7	10.0
Other	8.6	10.0	9.1	6.7	5.9	20.0
Sought Care for Illness	44.8	47.5	42.0	45.0	58.8	55.0
Number of Cases	356	442	306	305	50	137

SOURCE: African Population and Health Research Center (2002-2003).

that depression and dementia are less common in Africa, there might be gross underreporting given the fact that the occurrence of neurovascular disorders, dementia, and depression increases with age. Again, since the reports are generally obtained from the household respondent, who may not necessarily be the older person, such proxy reports on such illnesses as depression may be poor (Alverado-Esquivel et al., 2004; Heun and Hein, 2005; Prince, Acosta, Chiu, Scazufca, and Varghese, 2003). Although older women are more than 1.5 times as likely as older men to be sick, they are not any more likely to have sought care during an illness episode. In general, treatment seeking is quite low among older people, with less than one-half of the sick receiving treatment.

A major health challenge faced by older people is the increasing prevalence of noncommunicable diseases often requiring constant long-term care. These illnesses have the potential of affecting every aspect of their lives, including their families, as some spend all household resources on medication, often at the expense of other basic needs. The case in Box 6-4, a diabetic octogenarian, highlights the situation of older people in dealing with chronic illnesses.

Interaction of Living Arrangements, Health, and Economic Status

Table 6-5 looks at the health and working status of older people in the two slum communities by their living arrangements. In Korogocho where the sample is large enough, older women and men living alone are more likely to report being sick than those who live with a spouse or children (or both) or those living with other adults. While 37 percent of older women living alone reported being sick, only 23 percent of those living with other adults reported an illness. Similar patterns are also observed for men, with those living alone being more than two times as likely to report an illness as those living with at least one other adult.

Data on treatment-seeking behavior by living arrangement suggests that older women and men living alone may have less access to treatment when ill compared with those living with at least one other adult. Among older women and those in Korogocho, those who live with at least one other adult (other than the spouse) reported higher levels of seeking treatment during an illness episode compared with those who live alone. The number of cases is too small to explore treatment-seeking behavior in other forms of living arrangements. From the qualitative data, lack of transport fare and absence of health personnel at the health facilities were often cited as major hindrances to seeking health care in hospitals. This may partly explain why older people living alone are less likely to seek care even though they are sicker.

In addition, the table shows that in both slum communities and for

BOX 6-4
Case Study #5: Man Living Alone, Korogocho

The subject is almost 90 years old and has been living alone for the past 5 years. His three children moved out of Nairobi to different parts of the country, and his wife moved in with their son to help look after her son's children. The wife visits him in the city frequently. He pays someone to come twice a week to do household chores for him, such as cleaning and cooking. He used to run businesses that were able to sustain him and his entire family. He had even employed a number of people to help him manage the businesses, including all his children. However, after he was diagnosed to be diabetic, a lot of funds were diverted to treating his ailment, forcing all his businesses to collapse. This also contributed to his children leaving the community to earn a living elsewhere. He owns the structure that he now occupies, including six other dwelling units (rentable rooms) that are rented out; some of these units were unoccupied during the time of the interview.

He is currently under medication and has to buy all the drugs himself, sometimes assisted by his children. His ailment has depleted his resources and assets and he is on a special diet according to doctor's advice. He says "I may want medication but it is expensive at these private clinics, so I wonder what to do. This is what finishes our money. Medicine is expensive. The amount you pay for government hospital wards and the health services is as much as you pay to private clinics for one or two pills. Especially for us diabetics, one tablet costs twenty shillings. To get a packet of ten tablets is two hundred shillings. Yet you must buy the medicine, you have no choice." The diabetic condition has affected his eyesight and he has undergone an operation to remove cataract from his eyes.

His view is that without money one cannot access health care. He prefers to seek treatment in government-run facilities as opposed to private clinics or hospitals. He argued that health facilities should have special services for older people to treat particular ailments and also special diets if they are admitted as inpatients. Older people should also be cared for by the government by providing them with food, shelter, or a monthly allowance. He considers an older person to be someone with disability who requires constant care. On special services for older people, he said "I think old people should be separated from the rest. They should have their own hospital. It should be based on a certain cutoff age. If the old have their own ward in a hospital, it would be good because they will be fed as old people. As it is now, when patients are being fed on bones, even the old people are given the bones to eat."

When asked what his greatest wish was, he says he wished to be reunited with his children and that the children would come back to live with him. He acknowledges that this is not possible because the children have settled down wherever they are, and there will be nothing to keep them going should they decide to move back.

TABLE 6-5 Health and Economic Status by Living Arrangement, Nairobi Demographic Surveillance System, 2003

	Lives Alone	(N)	Lives with Spouse/ Children	(N)	Lives with at Least 1 Other Adult	(N)
Those Who Reported Sick						
Korogocho						
Women	37.1	(116)	25.0	(40)	23.3	(150)
Men	27.8	(126)	16.1	(62)	12.7	(118)
Viwandani						
Women	41.2	(17)	—	(2/5)	33.3	(24)
Men	13.4	(82)	0.0	0	19.1	(47)
Sought Treatment by Gender:						
Women	40.0	(50)	—	(6/12)	48.8	(43)
Men	47.8	(46)	—	(4/10)	50.0	(24)
Sought Treatment by Slum:						
Korogocho	41.0	(78)	40.0	(20)	48.0	(50)
Viwandani	—	(10/18)	—	(2/2)	—	(9/17)
Currently Working:						
Korogocho						
Women	73.2	(97)	63.2	(19)	55.0	(140)
Men	80.6	(98)	90.9	(22)	73.4	(128)
Viwandani						
Women	78.6	(11/14)	—	(1/3)	55.0	(20)
Men	94.0	(50)	—	(3/3)	80.0	(40)

both men and women, older people who live alone are more likely to continue working to support themselves than those who live with at least one other adult. This is further evidence that older people who live alone may face greater vulnerability than those who live with other adults. Compared with their female counterparts, older men are more likely to be currently working irrespective of their living arrangement.

CONCLUSION

Differences do exist between the two slum communities, Viwandani and Korogocho, both in terms of the share of older people living in the particular slum and also in the sociodemographic characteristics of the older population. Older people are more likely to reside in the Korogocho community, although Viwandani has a larger share of the total population of the two communities. This may result from the fact that Viwandani tends to attract a more youthful population seeking employment because of its proximity to the city's industrial zone. With regard to the currently married, more than two-thirds of those in Viwandani do not reside with their spouses compared with only one-third in Korogocho.

A large proportion of older people living in the informal settings live alone contrary to findings from other studies (for example, Bongaarts and Zimmer, 2001) in which most older people, especially those in rural areas, live in large households. Older men are more likely to live alone compared with women, who were more likely to reside only with children under age 15. Coresidence of older women with young children normally referred to as skipped-generation households could reflect the high incidence of mortality in the middle age groups due to HIV/AIDS. Women were more likely to report not being currently married, whereas the majority were formerly married, with a few having never married. This may reflect the combined effect of higher life expectancy for women, higher remarriage among men, and age differences between spouses (African men usually marrying younger women). Older women living in informal settlements are more likely to be vulnerable to poverty as a result of their low participation in employment, which is worsened by their low educational attainment.

The informal sector is the major employer to the majority of residents in the slums of Nairobi, hence they are left out of the contributory pension program, which is accessible only to those employed in the formal sector. Less than 10 percent of older people in the two slums were receiving any form of pension. Lack of social security in old age could be a reason for the continued participation of a high percentage of older people in employment coupled with the cash economy of urban settings. The declining health and physical status of older people together with a competitive employment market that discriminates on age reduces the chances of older people finding well-paying jobs, as reflected in the nature of their employment, which is mainly petty trading. Although old age signifies an increase in the need for health care, there is low utilization of health care services among older people living in the two slum communities. Less than half of those who reported an illness in the two weeks preceding the visit to their households sought care for their ailment. Older people living alone were also more likely to report being sick compared with those living with a spouse or other adults, but they are less likely to seek treatment in a health facility.

This paper has provided an overview of the sociodemographic characteristics, living arrangements, health, and economic status of older people living in two slum communities of Nairobi. The paper has highlighted a number of vulnerabilities older people in urban informal settlements may face. Unlike other older people, those in urban informal settlements are more likely to live alone in single-person households. Consequently, they are unlikely to benefit from the type of support and care traditionally provided to older people by extended family. The majority of them, despite being old and fragile, continue to be engaged in one form of economic activity or the other, especially for those living alone. The small sample, however, could not permit a fuller assessment of how the living arrangements of older people affect other aspects of their well-being. Given the unique challenges faced by older people in the urban informal settlements, a more detailed analysis of their situation across various cities in sub-Saharan Africa is needed to facilitate the development of comprehensive policy and action to improve the well-being of older people living in urban informal settlements.

ACKNOWLEDGMENTS

The authors acknowledge support for the Nairobi Urban Health and Demographic Surveillance System from the Rockefeller Foundation (Grant no. 2004AR037) and the Hewlett Foundation (Grant no. 2004-9699). This analysis and the qualitative data collection were supported in part by the National Institute on Aging (Grant no. P30 A9017248-0351) through the University of Colorado's Population Aging Center (Subaward no. 0000047604) in collaboration with Jane Menken.

REFERENCES

African Population and Health Research Center. (2002). *Population and health dynamics in Nairobi informal settlements*. Nairobi, Kenya: Author.

African Population and Health Research Center. (2002-2003). *Nairobi urban health and demographic surveillance system*. Nairobi: Author.

Alvarado-Esquivel, C., Hernandez-Alvarado, A.B., Tapia-Rodriguez, R.O., Guerrero-Iturbe, A., Rodriguez-Corral, K., and Martinez, S.E. (2004). Prevalence of dementia and Alzheimer's disease in elders of nursing homes and a senior center of Durango City, Mexico. *BMC Psychiatry, 18*(4), 3.

Anderson, J.A. (2001). Mobile workers, urban employment and "rural" identities: Rural-urban networks of Buhera migrants, Zimbabwe. In M. Dedruijn, R. Van Dijk, and R Foeken (Eds.), *Mobile Africa: Changing patterns of movement in Africa and beyond*. Lieden, The Netherlands: Brill.

Ayad, M.B., and Otto, B.J. (1997). *Demographic and health surveys comparative studies: Demographic and socio-economic characteristics of households*. Calverton, MD: Macro International.

Barber, G.M., and Milne, W.J. (1988). Modeling internal migration in Kenya: An econometric analysis with limited data. *Environment and Planning A, 20*(9), 1185-1196.

Bigsten, A. (1996). The circular migration of smallholders in Kenya. *Journal of African Economics, 5*(1), 1-20.

Bledsoe, C.H., and Fatoumatta, B. (2002). *Contingent lives: Fertility, time, and aging in West Africa*. Chicago, IL: University of Chicago Press.

Bongaarts, J., and Zimmer, Z. (2001). *Living arrangements of older adults in the developing world: An analysis of DHS household surveys*. (Policy Research Division Working Paper No. 148). Available: http://www.popcouncil.org/pdfs/wp/148.pdf [accessed October 2005].

Dodoo, F.N., Zulu, E.M., and Ezeh. A.C. (Forthcoming). Urban-rural differences in the socio-economic deprivation: The sexual behavior link. *Social Science and Medicine*.

Government of Kenya. (2000). *Second report on poverty in Kenya. Volume I: Incidence and depth of poverty.* Nairobi: Central Bureau of Statistics, Ministry of Planning and National Development. Available: http://www4.worldbank.org/afr/poverty/pdf/docnav/02880.pdf.

Grant, M. (1995). Movement patterns and the medium sized city: Tenants on the move in Gweru, Zimbabwe. *Habitat International, 19*(3), 357-369.

Gugler, J. (1991). Life in a dual system revisited: Urban-rural ties in Enugu, Nigeria, 1961-1987. *World Development, 19*(5), 399-409.

Gulis, G., Mulumba, J.A.A., Juma, O., and Kakosova, B. (2003). Health status of people of slums in Nairobi, Kenya. *Environmental Research, 96*(2), 219-227.

HelpAge International. (2002). *State of the world's older people 2002.* London, England: Author.

Heun, R., and Hein, S. (2005). Risk factors of major depression in the elderly. *European Psychiatry, 20*(3), 199-204.

Johnnie, P.B. (1988). Rural-urban migration in Nigeria: Consequences on housing, health-care and employment. *Migration World Magazine, 16*(3), 22-29.

Kimuna, S.R., and Adamchak, D.J. (1999). Population ageing and elderly support: A Kenya profile. *Quarterly Journal of INIA (International Institute on Ageing), 10*(1), 6-16.

Magadi, M.A., Zulu, E.M., and Brockerhoff, M. (2003). The inequality of maternal health care in urban sub-Saharan Africa in the 1990s. *Population Studies, 57*(3), 347-366.

Matrix Development Consultants. (1993). *Nairobi's informal settlements: An inventory.* (A report prepared for USAID/REDSO/ESA.) Nairobi, Kenya: U.S. Agency for International Development.

Muwonge, J.W. (1980). Urban policy and patterns of low-income settlement in Nairobi, Kenya. *Population and Development Review, 6,* 595-613.

Nigeria Institute of Social and Economic Research. (1997). *Nigeria migration and urbanization survey, 1993.* Ibadan, Nigeria: Author.

Ntozi, J.P.M., and Zirimenya, S. (1999). Changes in household composition and family structure during the AIDS epidemic in Uganda. In J.C. Caldwell, I.O. Orubuloye, and J.P.M. Ntozi (Eds.), *The continuing African HIV/AIDS epidemic* (pp. 193-209). Canberra: Health Transition Centre, National Centre for Epidemiology and Population Health, Australian National University.

Oucho, J.O. (1998). Recent internal migration processes in sub-Saharan Africa; determinants, consequences, and data adequacy issues. In R.E. Bilsborrow (Ed.), *Migration, urbanization and development: New directions and issues.* New York: UNPF/Kluwer Academic.

Population Reference Bureau. (2005). *World population data sheet 2005.* Washington, DC: Author.

Prince, M., Acosta, D., Chiu, H., Scazufca, M., and Varghese, M. (2003). Dementia diagnosis in developing countries: A cross-cultural validation study. *The Lancet, 361*(9361), 909-917.

Republic of Kenya. (2001). *The 1999 population and housing census, volume 1: Population distribution by administrative areas and urban centers.* Nairobi: Government Press.

Thumbi, P.W. (2005). *Kenya country report on reproductive health and reproductive rights.* National Council for Population and Development, Kenya. Available: http://www.uneca.org/eca_resources/Major_ECA_Websites/icpd/fourth/Kenya.htm [accessed October 2005].

Trager, L. (1998). Home town linkages and local development in South Western Nigeria: Whose agenda, what impact? *Africa, 68*(3), 360-382.

UN-Habitat (United Nations Human Settlement Programme). (2003). *Slums of the world: The face of urban poverty in the new millennium?* Nairobi, Kenya: Global Urban Observatory.

UNICEF. (2002). *Poverty and exclusion among urban children*. (Innocent Digest No. 10). UNICEF Innocent Research Centre. Available: www.unicef-isdc.org.

United Nations. (1991). *The world ageing situation*. New York: Author.

World Health Organization. (2002, April). *Active ageing: A policy framework*. WHO contribution to the Second United Nations World Assembly on Ageing, April 8-12, Madrid.

Zulu, E.M., Dodoo, F.M., and Ezeh, A.C. (2003). Urbanization, poverty and sex: Roots of risky sexual behaviors in slum settlements in Nairobi, Kenya. In E. Kalipeni, J. Oppong, S. Craddock, and J. Ghosh (Eds.), *HIV/AIDS in Africa: Beyond technology* (pp. 167-174). Malden, MA: Blackwell.

7

Labor Force Withdrawal of the Elderly in South Africa

David Lam, Murray Leibbrandt, and Vimal Ranchhod

INTRODUCTION

The elderly in South Africa face a complex set of challenges. South Africans over age 50 have spent most of their lives under the system of apartheid. Levels of inequality in education between races and within races are far greater among these older cohorts than they are for younger South Africans. Elderly black South Africans have lived their most productive years under the restrictions on employment, residence, and other opportunities that apartheid imposed. As they now enter retirement, they face new pressures caused by the impact of HIV/AIDS and high unemployment on the next generation. At the same time, South Africa's elderly have access to an old age pension system that is among the most generous in the developing world. The old age pension helps lift many older South Africans out of the most extreme forms of poverty, putting many of them in a position to support their children and grandchildren.

Decisions of the elderly about work and retirement are made in this complex set of circumstances. Older workers face an increasingly competitive labor market characterized by high unemployment, with limited opportunities for those with poor education and training. They often live in large extended households in which their own resources may be an important source of economic support. The pension provides such a source without necessarily competing with work.

The state old age pension program has spawned a considerable body of research. This research is reviewed in the next section of the paper. The review shows that the state old age pension is the key plank of South Africa's social safety net, that these pensions are well targeted to the poor, and, because of the large number of three-generation and skipped-generation households in South Africa, they reach many poor children. In addition, it seems that many of the unemployed survive through their links to related pensioners. More recent research has begun to explore the impact of these pensions on labor participation behavior.

Given all of the above, the dearth of research on the elderly themselves is surprising. We know very little about the circumstances of the elderly, their health, and how they cope with the pressures placed on them by the importance of their pension income to their extended families. Two recent studies have begun to address these issues (Møller and Devey, 2003; Møller and Ferreira, 2003). The first of these studies compares older and younger households on the basis of data from 1995 and 1998 national surveys, defining older households as those that include at least one member age 60 or older. The second study is based on a 2002 survey of the living conditions and financial and health situations of 1,111 older nonwhite households in Cape Town and the rural Eastern Cape. Here, older was defined as households containing 1 person age 55 or older.

The first study confirms that older households are larger and include larger numbers of dependents and unemployed members than younger households. In both 1995 and 1998, roughly half of older black households included three or more generations. Such households tend to be concentrated in rural areas. The Møller and Ferreira (2003) study shows that among black older households, the percentage of household members under age 25 was 58 percent in rural areas and 51 percent in urban areas. In contrast, less than a quarter of these household members were actually age 55 or older. Less than 10 percent of older people lived alone.

Møller and Devey (2003) show that many older black households are poor. However, access to state old age pensions strongly decreases the probability that such households fall into the lowest expenditure quintile. Pensioner households have better access to services and express significantly higher levels of satisfaction with their living conditions than nonpensioner older households.

Møller and Ferreira (2003) confirm the dominance of the state old age pension as the primary income source in older households. They found that pension income is often the sole income in these households, especially in rural areas. They describe three elements of a "gradient of disadvantage" that makes older rural households worse off than older urban households. First, household well-being as measured by income or expenditure per capita is lower in the rural households. Second, the drain on the resources of the rural elderly through expenditures on other members of the household is higher in rural areas. Third, urban households are far more successful at accessing other government grants, such as the child support grants and disability grants for which the members of their household may be eligible. All in all this leads to a situation in which the elderly in urban areas are better placed to use their pensions for their own support.

Aside from work on the old age pension, the magnitude of South Africa's unemployment problem has spawned a growing body of work on labor force participation in the country. This work shows that South African participation rates are low by international standards, especially for women (Winter, 1998). However, participation rates, and female participation rates in particular, rose sharply in the 1990s, despite the fact that many of these new participants did not move into employment but joined the ranks of the unemployed (Casale and Posel, 2002; Klasen and Woolard, 2000). Research by Mlatsheni and Leibbrandt (2001) and Leibbrandt and Bhorat (2001) highlights the importance of education as a factor affecting female participation rates.

However, this literature on participation has given very little specific attention to the labor market behavior of the elderly. Given the considerable focus on the impact of the old age pension on the work activity of the nonelderly, it is surprising that the labor force behavior of those who actually receive these pensions has received so little attention. The fact that it is the elderly who are facing a retirement decision as part of this participation behavior would seem to make their labor force behavior especially interesting.

This paper provides a broad overview of the labor force activity of older workers in South Africa. We begin the paper with a discussion of important features of the social and economic environment that provide a background for the analysis. Drawing on excellent microdata, we then analyze the age profile of participation, focusing in particular on the possible effects of the old age pension on retirement. We look at several important variables that may affect the economic activity of the elderly, including marital status, living arrangements, the pension system, and education. We estimate probit regressions in order to look at key determinants of labor force activity.

SOCIAL AND ECONOMIC BACKGROUND

A number of features of South African society and economy are important to keep in mind in analyzing the economic activity of the elderly. In this section of the paper we discuss some of these important features, with particular focus on the old age pension system and patterns of household structure.

South Africa's Old Age Pension

No analysis of the elderly in South Africa would be complete without a discussion of the country's old age pension system. Social assistance in South Africa consists of three main programs: pensions for the elderly, grants for the disabled, and grants for the support of poor children. Old age and disability pensions are set at generous levels. The 2005 level is R780 per month, about $120. Relative to this amount, the child support grant is set at a meager R180 or about $28 per month and is payable for children up to and including the age of 14. All three grants are supposedly means-tested, but in practice the means test is rarely administered for applicants who appear poor. A total of between 4 and 5 million people (or 10 percent of the total population) receive one or the other grant. South Africa's public welfare system is exceptional among developing countries and is a major pillar in its highly redistributive social policies (Seekings, 2002; Van der Berg, 2001; Van der Berg and Bredenkamp, 2002).

The state old age pension system is unique and the most important aspect of the South Africa social assistance system. It has an interesting history, as it evolved from a grant that was paid exclusively to white South Africans to one that was paid to all South Africans regardless of racial categorization. The grant was first introduced in 1928 as a form of income support for poor elderly whites (Sagner, 2000). Only in 1944 did the preapartheid state extend the social pension to include members of other race groups, and, even then, pension payment size was legally determined by race at a ratio of 4:2:1 for whites, Indians/coloreds, and blacks/Africans, respectively. Beginning in the late 1970s, the racial gap in pensions was significantly reduced through the allocation of large additional funds to this scheme by the apartheid state. During the 1980s, the size of pensions more than doubled for Africans, while it declined by 40 percent (in real terms) for whites (Ferreira, 1999). By 1985, white pensions were only 2.5 times higher than those of blacks and 1.5 times higher than those for those categorized as coloreds and Indians (Schlemmer and Møller, 1997). Take-up rates, particularly among elderly black South Africans, increased markedly during this time. The Social Assistance Act of 1992 provided steps to deracialize pensions and achieve pension parity, which was finally achieved in 1993, just one year prior to the first democratic elections. By 1993, the take-up rate among eligible black South African men and women stood at 80 percent.

Case and Deaton (1998) provide a comprehensive analysis of the workings of the South African pension system. The key features of the system are that it is paid to women age 60 and over and men age 65 and over, with a means test that allows 80 percent of age-eligible black South Africans to receive the pension. Most receive the maximum benefit. The benefit was about 2.5 times the median per capita income by 2000. The 2005 pension of R780 per month can be compared to the minimum wage for domestic workers, which was set at R754 in rural areas in 2005.

The means test for the pension in 2004, if enforced, would have applied at annual income levels of about R18,000 for single individuals and about R34,000 for married couples. This implies that many elderly could receive the full value of the pension while continuing to work full time, even with the means test (below we show that some elderly do in fact work while receiving the pension, although the percentages are low). Given the weak enforcement of the means test, the receipt of the pension does not have a direct negative incentive on work for many low-income elderly. The impact of the pension on labor supply is thus primarily an income effect.

Considerable research has been done on the impact of the old age pension. Duflo (2003) found a positive effect of the pension on the health outcomes of young girls in the household. Jensen (2004) found that the pension tends to "crowd out" private transfers from family members living away from home. Looking at the impact of the pension on labor supply, Bertrand, Mullainathan, and Miller (2003) found that the pension tends to reduce the labor supply of working-age adults. Posel, Fairburn, and Lund (2004) found a more complex effect of the pension on labor supply, with the pension increasing the probability that prime-age adults migrate for work. Edmonds (2005) found a negative effect of the pension on the work activity of children. Given the attention focused on the pension's impact on the labor supply and other outcomes of prime-age adults and children, it is surprising that little attention has been given to the pension's impact on the labor supply of the elderly themselves. This is an issue we analyze in detail below.

Household Structure

As noted above, another dimension of South African society that is important in analyzing the economic activity of the elderly is the complex extended household structure that is common among black South African households. As noted by Case and Deaton (1998), one of the reasons the pension system is so effective in reducing poverty in South Africa is that the elderly recipients of the pension often live in households with young children. While these complex extended household patterns have long historical roots in South Africa, they have taken on new importance as HIV/AIDS and high unemployment have weakened the ability of prime-age adults to support their families. Edmonds, Mammen, and Miller (2005) remind us how unusual this situation is when they note that the standard literature on old age pensions focuses on how pensions enable the elderly to maintain their independence. They conclude that the arrival of a state old age pension into a black South African household leads to the departure of prime-age working women and the arrival of children under age 5 and women of childbearing age. They see this behavior as evidence of the household's making use of the pension to reshape itself according to the comparative advantage for work inside and outside the household. In line with this behavior, we would expect that the labor supply decisions of the elderly are therefore often being made simultaneously with decisions about living arrangements. We look at the links between household structure and the labor force activity of the elderly in some detail. Although we do not identify the causal links between household structure and the work activity of the elderly, we show that there appear to be important links between these variables.

DATA

We use two main data sets for our analysis, each with strengths and weaknesses. We use the 10 percent sample of the 2001 census for many of our estimates, taking advantage of the large sample size. With roughly 4 million total observations, the census gives us thousands of observations at single years of age, even at ages from 60 to 70. For example, the number of individuals in the 70-74 age group in the census sample is over 12,800 black South African men, 25,000 black South African women, 4,500 white men, and 6,000 white women. The census provides standard information on employment status, along with information on schooling, household structure, and marital status. For comparative purposes we also use the 10 percent sample of the 1996 census.

The other important data set used in our analysis is the South Africa Labor Force Survey (LFS), a nationally representative household survey of about 30,000 households collected by Statistics South Africa. We use the September 2000 LFS for some of our analysis because it has greater detail than the census for such variables as work activity and pension receipt. The drawback of the LFS is the smaller sample size. For example, in the 50-79 age group there are roughly 4,000 black South African men and 6,000 black South African women, making it difficult to look at fine age detail and making it almost impossible to look at any population group other than black South Africans. For certain parts of our analysis, we pool the LFS data for September 2000 and September 2001, giving us a larger sample size. Although the LFS is designed with a rotating panel structure, a new sample was introduced in September 2001. There is therefore no overlap in the two waves that we pool. We also merge the September LFS with the 2000 Income and Expenditure Survey (IES), allowing us to look at the impact of pension income on total household income.

AGE PROFILES OF LABOR FORCE PARTICIPATION

Figure 7-1 shows the age profile of labor force participation and employment for men and women ages 45-75 who identify themselves as black/African in the 1996 and 2001 census.[1] The ages of eligibility for the state old age pension (65 for men and 60 for women) are indicated on the figure for reference. The measure of labor force participation used in Figure 7-1 follows standard international definitions, counting labor force participants as those who were either working, on vacation or sick leave from work, or looking for work. The "working" series includes those who were working and those who were on vacation or sick leave during the week before the census. Work is defined broadly, including any work for pay, profit, or family gain.[2] One of the stark features of Figure 7-1 is the large gap between the "in labor force" and "working" series, confirming the high rates of unemployment for both men and women in South Africa. The unemployment rate at age 50 in 2001, for example, is 34 percent for men and 40 percent for women.[3]

Figure 7-1 shows a relatively rapid rate of withdrawal from the labor force for both men and women after age 50. In the 2001 census, male participation rates fall from around 75 percent at age 50 to 47 percent at age 60 and 10 percent at age 70. Participation rates for women in 2001 fall from around 55 percent at age 55 to about 20 percent at age 60 and below 5 percent at age 70. The percentage who are actually working is well below the participation rate for both men and women around age 50, but, like the participation rate, it falls steadily with age. The percentage of men working in 2001 is about 50 percent at age 50, falls to 30 percent at age 60, and is below 10 percent at age 70. Put another way, if we could interpret this cross-sectional relationship as the life-cycle work profile of a cohort of men, it would imply that over half of the men who were working at age 50

---

[1] The census asked the following question for each household member: "How would (the person) describe him/herself in terms of population group?" The possible responses and proportions giving each response were "Black/African" (79%), "Colored" (9%), "Indian or Asian" (3%), and "White" (9%). Henceforth we refer to the black/African group, which is our main focus, as African.

[2] The wording of the census questionnaire is the following: "Does (the person) work (for pay, profit, or family gain)? Answer yes for formal work for a salary or wage. Also answer yes for informal work such as making things for sale or selling things or rendering a service. Also answer yes for work on a farm or the land, whether for a wage or as part of the household's farming activities. Otherwise answer no."

[3] The standard definition of the unemployment rate is the number of unemployed (actively searching) divided by the number in the labor force. In Figure 7-1 this is the difference between the "in labor force" and "working" values divided by the "in labor force" value. For men age 50 this is 0.25/0.74 = 0.34.

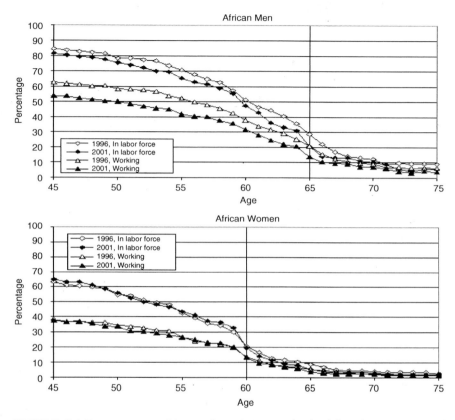

FIGURE 7-1 Percentage working and participating in the labor force, 1996 and 2001 censuses.

stopped working several years before they reached the age of eligibility for the state old age pension.

Comparisons between 1996 and 2001 census data are interesting for a number of reasons. First, it helps to disentangle age and cohort effects that would be impossible to separate in a single cross-section. In this paper we often interpret the age patterns in labor force activity as indicating changes over the life cycle. But it is important to remember that the age patterns we observe may be affected by differences in the behavior of different cohorts. For example, as we document below, younger cohorts are considerably better educated than older cohorts, especially among Africans. This may lead to differences in life-cycle labor force behavior that will show up in the age profile of participation at any given point in time. By looking at two censuses five years apart, we can be clearer about age and cohort effects and more certain about whether we are seeing life-cycle labor force behavior. The age profiles from the 1996 census shown in Figure 7-1 suggest that the basic shape of the age profile in work and labor force participation did not change much between 1996 and 2001, although both rates for men dropped at all ages. Looking at the figure for women, the 1996 and 2001 lines are almost indistinguishable for both labor force participation and work.

Figure 7-1 shows that there are sharp drop-offs in labor force participation and work for both men and women around the age of eligibility for the old age pension (age 60 for women and age 65 for men). These declines around the pension age are larger in 2001 than they are in 1996. The decline in labor force participation rate for men between ages 64 and 66 is 13.6 percentage points in 1996 and 16.9 percentage points in 2001. This implies that 54.5 percent of those still in the labor force at age 64 have left it by age 66 in 2001. Exit from work is at a similar rate, with the percentage of men working at age 66 roughly half of the percentage working at age 64. The figure for women shows a similar discontinuity around the pension age in rates of labor force participation and employment. The decline in labor force participation rates for women between ages 59 and 61 is 18.4 percentage points, or 57 percent of the age 59 rate. The decline in the percentage working is 10.3 percentage points, or 52 percent of the age 59 rate.

Figure 7-2 shows participation rates for all four of the major population groups. As this figure shows, there are relatively small racial differences in participation rates for men at all ages. Participation rates are somewhat lower for African and colored men from ages 45 to 55, with similar rates of decline in participation for all groups from ages 55 to 65. Participation rates for women are considerably lower at all ages, falling from around 60 percent at age 45 to 20 percent at age 60 and under 5 percent at age 70. Racial differences in participation rates are larger for women than for men, with Indian women having the lowest rates. Participation rates for African and white women are almost identical up to age 59, with the participation of African women showing a larger drop in participation at age 60. Participation rates above age 65 are between 10 and 20 percent for men, rates that are much lower than the 65 percent participation rate reported for Southern Africa in a cross-national analysis of 1980 data (Clark and Anker, 1993). Participation rates of older men in South Africa are somewhat higher than those for most European countries, however. As shown in the cross-national study of retirement in Organisation for Economic Co-operation and Development (OECD) countries coordinated by the National Bureau of Economic Research (NBER), participation rates for men ages 60-64 were below 20 percent in France, Belgium, and the Netherlands around 1995 (Gruber and Wise, 1999). We discuss comparisons to OECD countries in more detail below.

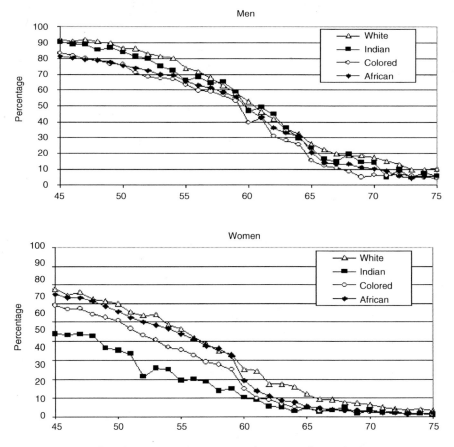

FIGURE 7-2 Labor force participation rates by age and population group, 2001 South Africa census.

COMPONENTS OF LABOR FORCE ACTIVITY

Figure 7-3 shows the 2001 distribution of labor force activity in more detail for African men, white men, African women, and white women. Four categories of activity are shown. The two components of labor force participation—working and unemployed—are shown separately. In the 2001 census, respondents were asked to give the reason for not working for all those who were not working in the previous seven days. Two of these categories are included in Figure 7-3: the percentage reported as being a "pensioner or retired person/too old to work" and the percentage reported as "unable to work due to illness or disability." Additional possible reasons

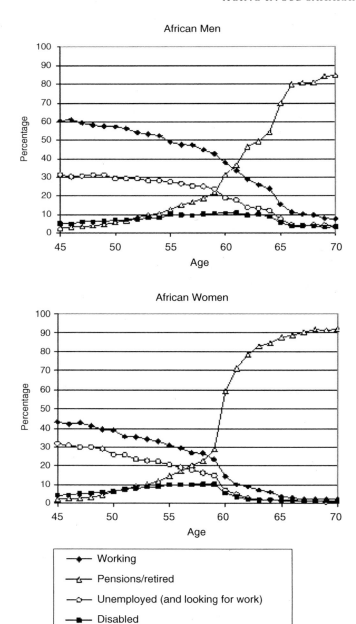

FIGURE 7-3 Distribution of labor force activity by age, African and white men and women, South Africa, 2001 census.

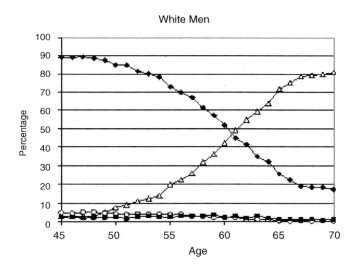

White Men

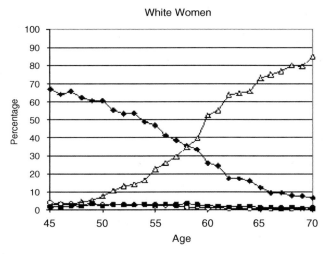

White Women

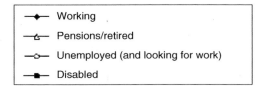

- Working
- Pensions/retired
- Unemployed (and looking for work)
- Disabled

for not working that are not included in the figure include student, house-wife/homemaker, and "does not choose to work." Figure 7-3 once again shows the high rate of unemployment for African men and women, even in what would usually be considered prime working years. Over 20 percent of both African men and African women ages 45-55 reported that they were unemployed and looking for work in 2001. These high rates of unemployment are an important characteristic of the South African labor market that must be kept in mind throughout our analysis.

The percentage of African men and women who are unemployed declines steadily with age, with many of these individuals presumably reclassifying themselves as retired as they get older. The percentage of men who are reported as "pensioner or retired/too old to work" climbs steeply after age 65, reaching about 80 percent by age 66. Women show an even sharper jump in the percentage reported as being retired around age 60, with the percentage jumping from 30 to 70 percent between ages 59 and 61. The age profiles for white men and women show steady declines in participation and steady increases in the percentage retired with increasing age, but the changes around age 60 and age 65 are less sharp than the changes for Africans.

The percentage of men and women of either racial group reported as disabled is relatively low, reaching highs of around 10 percent for African men and women approaching retirement age. It is interesting to compare this to the significantly higher rates of disability reported for many OECD countries in the NBER study (Gruber and Wise, 1999). For example, in the Netherlands, a country with generous disability insurance, well over 20 percent of men ages 60-64 were reported as being disabled in 1994 (Kapteyn and de Vos, 1999). Disability rates for Africans drop at the retirement ages, as men and women presumably reclassify themselves from disabled to retired.

Further detail on the economic activity of older workers is provided in the LFS, which asks a series of separate questions about specific types of economic activity. In addition to providing greater detail than the census, these questions may elicit higher levels of economic activity than the single question used in the census. Table 7-1 shows detailed breakdowns of work activity for African men and women in 5-year age groups using the merged September 2000 and September 2001 LFS. Due to small cell sizes, we do not attempt this breakdown for other population groups. Column 2 shows the percentage engaged in work for pay, excluding domestic workers. About 54 percent of men are in this category in the merged 2000-2001 LFS data. This percentage drops to 41 percent in the 55-59 age group, then drops sharply to 26 percent in the 60-64 age group and 11 percent in the 65-69 age group. Column 3 shows the percentage employed as domestic workers, an occupation that is, not surprisingly, concentrated among women. Combining the first two columns for women, about 37 percent are engaged in work for pay in the age group 45-49. There is a sharp drop from 29 percent to under 10 percent between the 55-59 and 60-64 age groups.

Column 5 in Table 7-1 shows the percentage reporting that they work on a family plot or farm.[4] This is an activity that is counted as economically active in many surveys, including the LFS and the census. While under 4 percent of men report that they work on a family plot in the 45-49 age group, this rises to about 10 percent among 65-69-year-olds and remains at about that level through the 75-79 age group. Column 7 shows the percentage working in any of the categories in Columns 2-6. Although the categories in Columns 2-6 are not mutually exclusive, the total percentage working in Column 7 is calculated to eliminate double counting. Comparing the estimates of the percentage working from the LFS in Table 7-1 with the estimates from the census in Figure 7-3, it appears that the specific questions about work on a family plot in the LFS lead to higher estimates of work activity for older workers than the census, even though the census question should theoretically include the same components as those included in Table 7-1. For example, the total percentage of men working in the 65-69 age group is 25 percent in the LFS figures in Table 7-1, while the percentage is under 20 percent for the census in Figure 7-3. We suspect that the difference is the result of higher response to the specific question directed at work on a family plot in the LFS.

Hazard Rates for Withdrawal from Labor Force

A useful way of focusing on withdrawal from the labor force is to calculate hazard rates for exit from the labor force. Figure 7-4 shows hazard rates of leaving the labor force for African men and women. These are calculated using the proportions who are economically active (those working and those unemployed by the narrow definition) at each age shown in Figure 7-1. The hazard rate can be thought of as an estimate of the probability of leaving the labor force at a given age, conditional on being in the labor force in the previous year. It is important to keep in mind that it is being estimated from cross-sectional rather than longitudinal data, and therefore it does not show the actual retirement experience of individuals. In our data it is simply the percentage decline in the proportion who are economically active between age x and age $x + 1$.

---

[4]Specifically, the LFS asks whether in the past seven days a person "did any work on his/her own or the family's plot, garden, cattle post or kraal, or help in growing produce or in looking after animals for the household."

TABLE 7-1 Percentage in Various Categories of Labor Market Status, African Men and Women, 2000-2001 South Africa Labor Force Survey

Age Group (1)	Percentage Working by Category of Work					
	For Pay (not domestic) (2)	Domestic Worker (3)	Own Business (4)	Family Plot (5)	Unpaid Family Business (6)	Total (7)
Men						
45-49	53.9	2.1	10.6	3.7	0.5	68.6
50-54	47.6	2.8	10.0	5.5	0.3	63.6
55-59	41.3	2.9	10.9	6.5	0.1	59.3
60-64	26.1	3.5	10.6	7.1	0.4	45.8
65-69	10.6	0.4	5.9	9.9	0.1	25.3
70-74	3.5	1.3	5.2	8.9	0.5	18.2
75-79	2.0	0.4	3.3	9.5	0.0	15.2
Women						
45-49	22.5	15.1	11.4	5.3	0.7	52.7
50-54	20.5	14.2	11.7	5.3	0.5	49.9
55-59	15.6	12.8	9.5	5.4	0.3	14.7
60-64	5.2	4.2	5.4	7.3	0.4	21.9
65-69	1.8	1.8	4.1	6.7	0.3	13.7
70-74	0.8	0.4	2.7	5.5	0.2	9.5
75-79	0.4	0.1	1.1	6.0	0.0	7.4

NOTES: Columns 2-6 are not mutually exclusive. Column 7 is based on answers to questions shown in columns 2-6 but avoids double counting; column 10 is the sum of 7 + 8; column 11 is the sum of 7 + 9.

Figure 7-4 shows the annual hazard rate of retirement for African men and women in the 2001 census. For African women the hazard rate has a very sharp peak of about 40 percent at age 60, the age at which women become eligible for the old age pension. If we estimated this hazard rate for women between ages 59 and 61, the rate would be 57 percent. That is, the labor force participation rate for women at age 61 is 57 percent smaller than the rate at age 60. The hazard rate for women remains at over 20 percent at ages 61-63, drops to 10 percent at age 64, then rises again to a second peak of around 30 percent at age 65.

For African men the hazard rate for leaving the labor force is below 5 percent until age 60, reaches 10 to 15 percent between ages 60 and 64, then jumps to over 30 percent at ages 65 and 66. Calculated between ages 64 and 66—one year before the pension age to one year after—the probability of retiring, conditional on being in the labor force at age 64, is 55 percent. As Figure 7-1 shows, these hazard rates would be very similar if estimated

Percentage Unemployed		Percentage in Labor Force	
Narrow (8)	Broad (9)	Narrow (10)	Broad (11)
14.4	22.1	83.3	91.0
11.9	20.9	75.8	84.8
10.5	17.8	70.4	77.7
5.1	10.6	51.4	56.8
1.5	5.0	27.2	30.7
0.7	2.2	19.0	20.5
0.6	1.5	16.1	16.9
13.1	27.4	66.2	80.5
8.4	19.7	58.7	70.0
5.7	14.5	47.8	56.6
1.6	4.1	23.8	26.4
0.7	2.4	14.5	16.2
0.1	0.8	9.8	10.5
0.3	0.6	7.9	8.2

for employment rather than labor force participation. The proportion of men working and the proportion of men in the labor force both fall by over 50 percent between ages 64 and 66.

These hazard rates can be compared with the rates estimated in NBER's cross-national comparative study of OECD countries (Gruber and Wise, 1999). One of the striking results in that study is the very high hazard rates of labor force exit at particular ages in many countries. These high hazard rates are typically observed at ages associated with strong incentives to retire due to features of the retirement system. For example, they estimate hazard rates of over 60 percent at age 60 in France and hazard rates of almost 70 percent at age 65 in Spain and the United Kingdom. The South African hazard rates at the age of eligibility for the old age pension are not quite as high as those observed at key pension policy age thresholds in France, Spain, and the United Kingdom. The South African spikes in retirement at age 60 for women and 65 for men are very high, however, in spite

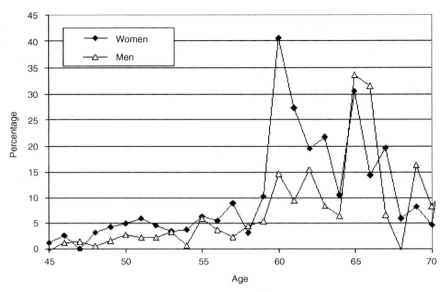

FIGURE 7-4 Hazard rate for leaving employment by age, African men and women, South Africa, 2001 census.

of the fact that the direct incentive to retire (or tax on continuing to work) associated with South Africa's old age pension is much lower than in the OECD countries. The sharp increases in retirement for both men and women around the age of pension eligibility suggest that South Africa's elderly do adjust their labor market behavior in response to the old age pension.

Comparative Estimates of Unused Productive Capacity

A useful summary measure of the labor force participation rates of older workers is the measure of unused productive capacity used in the Gruber and Wise (1999) NBER study. Figure 7-5 plots this measure for 11 OECD countries included in the NBER study, along with two measures for South Africa. The measure is calculated by summing the proportions out of the labor force between ages 55 and 65 and dividing by 11. The measure of 60 for France in Figure 7-5, for example, can be interpreted as meaning that a cohort experiencing the participation rates of France would work only 40 percent of the potential number of person-years available for work between ages 55 and 65. As emphasized in the Gruber and Wise volume, this measure of unused capacity varies substantially across OECD countries, from a low of 22 percent in Japan to a high of 67 percent in Belgium. A major

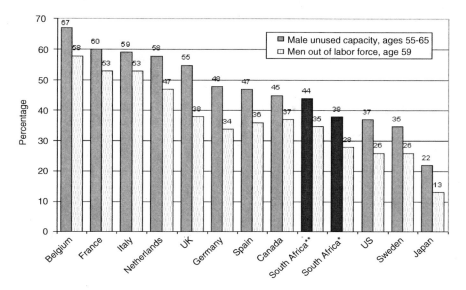

FIGURE 7-5 Measures of unused productive capacity for OECD countries and South Africa.
NOTES: OECD estimates taken from Gruber and Wise (1999); South Africa estimates are based on the 2000-2001 Labor Force Survey.
*Narrow measure of participation.
**Broad measure of participation.

focus of the NBER project is to document a strong positive relationship between this measure of unused capacity and a measure of the implicit tax on working built into each country's pension system.

Above we document very high unemployment rates for South Africans in this age range. In the South African case, it is therefore not correct to assume that all retirees would have been productively employed if they had continued their participation in the labor market. This makes the notion of unused capacity more problematic in the South African context than it is in the OECD countries. While we need to bear this caution in mind, it remains a useful comparative exercise to calculate these measures of formal retirement from the labor market in South Africa. Two measures of participation for South Africa are used to compare with the OECD countries. The narrow measure of participation is a standard measure that should be similar to that used in the OECD countries. It corresponds to the measure used in Figure 7-1, counting labor force participants as those who report that they are employed or unemployed and looking for work. The broader measure of participation also includes those who report that they would be willing to work, even though they are not actively looking for work. Using either of these measures, South Africa compares favorably to Canada and the United States, two countries on the lower end of unused capacity in the NBER study, with between 38 and 44 percent of men ages 55-65 out of the labor force.

A second simple measure of labor force withdrawal shown in Figure 7-5 is the percentage of men who are out of the labor force at age 59. This measure gives a fairly similar picture to that of the unused labor capacity measure. South Africa is once again between Canada and the United States, with less than 40 percent of men having withdrawn from the labor force by age 59 by either the broad or the narrow measures of participation. South Africa would presumably fare worse in these comparisons if we use the proportion working rather the proportion in the labor force. The high unemployment rates shown in Figure 7-3 imply that the percentage of unused capacity between ages 55 and 65 would be much higher if the unemployed were included in unused capacity. We do not attempt to address this issue here, in part because many OECD countries also have fairly high unemployment rates, and in part because we want to maintain comparability with the estimates in the Gruber and Wise study. While any estimate of unused capacity will have limitations, we present these comparisons here simply to demonstrate that the age profile of withdrawal from the labor force observed in South Africa is not unusual in its shape or in the level of participation observed in the 55-65 age group.

DETERMINANTS OF THE ELDERLY LABOR SUPPLY

We now look at some of the important variables that are likely to be related to the economic activity of the elderly. These include household structure, marital status, public and private pensions, and education. After discussing these variables in isolation, we estimate probit regressions to estimate the relationship between these variables and the work activity of the elderly. It is important to keep in mind that a number of these variables may be endogenous outcomes of joint decisions about living arrangements and residential location. The point of our analysis is not necessarily to identify causal determinants of the elderly labor supply, but to identify the important patterns that are associated with the economic activity of elderly South Africans.

Household Structure and Marital Status

One of the important differences between the elderly in South Africa and the elderly living in the United States or Europe is that South Africa's elderly often live in large extended households. Table 7-2 presents details on household living arrangements and marital status for African and white men and women using the 2001 census. The table documents large differences in living arrangements for Africans and whites. African women ages 60-64, for example, live in households with 5.5 household members, compared with 2.6 household members for white women of the same ages. Especially striking is the number of children living with elderly Africans. African women age 60-64 have an average of 2.3 coresident household members under age 18, compared with an average of 0.25 such members living with white women ages 60-64. This tendency to live in extended households is further demonstrated in the proportions living alone or with only a spouse. For African women the percentage living alone stays at around 6-7 percent in all age groups from ages 30-34 to ages 70-74. White women, by contrast, show the kinds of large increases in the probability of living alone that are observed in the United States. The percentage of white women living alone stays around 5 percent or less until the age group 50-54, then rises steadily with age, reaching over 30 percent for the 70-74 age group.

The last three columns of Table 7-2 show the distribution of marital status. Marriage is defined broadly, including any kind of formal or informal cohabiting partnership. African men and women are less likely to be married than whites at all ages. The combined effect of higher male mortality and the age gap between husbands and wives is evident in the proportions married and widowed at older ages. Men of both races who are still alive in the older age groups are very likely to be married. Only about 14 percent of African men and 10 percent of white men ages 70-74 are widowed, while 55 percent of African women and 45 percent of white women ages 70-74 are widowed.

Looking at age groups around the age when many men and women leave the labor market, Table 7-2 indicates that the great majority of men still have living partners at these ages. About 80 percent of African men and 85 percent of white men are still married in the 60-64 and 60-65 age groups. The situation for women is considerably different. Only 45 percent of African women are married at age 60-64, with 36 percent widowed and 5 percent divorced or separated (the remainder were never married). Among white women ages 60-64, 67 percent are married, 20 percent widowed, and 9 percent divorced or separated.

Public and Private Pensions

As noted above, South Africa's state old age pension program plays an important role in the lives of elderly South Africans. Figure 7-6 shows the percentage of African and white men and women who report in the Septem-

TABLE 7-2 Household Living Arrangements and Marital Status,
2001 Census

Age Group	Number (N)	Number Living in Household		
		Total	Under 18	Age 18-59
African Women				
30-34	111,649	5.22	2.40	2.57
35-39	104,057	5.20	2.49	2.49
40-44	85,041	5.24	2.31	2.73
45-49	69,747	5.23	2.13	2.92
50-54	51,689	5.33	2.10	2.99
55-59	37,598	5.40	2.13	2.94
60-64	38,096	5.51	2.29	1.88
65-69	30,209	5.52	2.33	1.89
70-74	25,055	5.50	2.36	1.89
African Men				
30-34	94,925	4.40	1.45	2.70
35-39	84,697	4.38	1.67	2.48
40-44	70,770	4.51	1.80	2.52
45-49	56,565	4.68	1.80	2.73
50-54	43.290	4.86	1.77	2.95
55-59	29,538	5.03	1.80	3.08
60-64	24,179	5.28	1.95	20.6
65-69	16,413	5.46	2.06	1.94
70-74	12,759	5.57	2.14	1.88
White Women				
30-34	13,063	3.76	1.43	2.18
35-39	12,946	3.98	1.62	2.19
40-44	13,068	3.90	1.26	2.47
45-49	12,144	3.47	0.66	2.65
50-54	11,373	3.04	0.33	2.49
55-59	9,884	2.68	0.22	1.99
60-64	8,442	2.57	0.25	0.64
65-69	6,714	2.42	0.23	0.56
70-74	5,815	2.30	0.20	0.58
White Men				
30-34	12,218	3.50	1.11	2.25
35-39	11,767	3.84	1.49	2.18
40-44	12,061	3.94	1.42	2.36
45-49	10,948	3.77	0.95	2.67
50-54	10,558	3.33	0.50	2.69
55-59	9,156	2.96	0.29	2.51
60-64	7,602	2.71	0.22	1.07
65-69	5,726	2.58	0.20	0.66
70-74	4,521	2.46	0.16	0.49

Marital Status

Pension Eligible	Percentage Living Alone	Percentage Living Only with Spouse	Percentage Married	Percentage Widowed	Percentage Divorced
0.23	5.9	7.3	52.0	1.9	2.5
0.20	5.9	6.9	58.5	3.8	4.5
0.18	5.9	6.8	59.1	6.9	6.4
0.15	6.4	6.9	58.5	11.1	7.4
0.16	6.7	6.3	55.5	17.4	7.3
0.20	6.6	5.9	51.2	24.8	6.3
1.26	5.9	4.9	44.8	35.5	4.7
1.27	5.8	4.1	38.6	46.1	3.5
1.23	5.9	3.5	32.7	55.2	2.4
0.22	15.6	9.7	47.7	0.4	1.2
0.20	15.2	9.9	63.6	0.8	2.4
0.18	15.0	9.8	71.1	1.3	3.7
0.14	14.5	10.1	75.7	1.9	4.5
0.13	13.8	10.0	77.7	3.1	4.6
0.14	13.0	9.8	78.7	4.6	4.4
0.26	11.4	9.5	78.5	7.2	3.8
1.45	9.3	9.0	77.8	10.2	3.6
1.54	8.6	8.4	75.7	13.7	3.0
0.11	4.4	11.7	79.2	0.9	7.3
0.14	3.9	7.7	80.9	1.5	9.5
0.15	3.8	8.7	80.4	2.6	11.2
0.14	5.1	17.3	79.4	4.3	11.5
0.14	7.3	30.4	77.6	7.4	11.2
0.19	11.1	43.3	74.8	11.7	9.8
1.41	16.2	44.8	67.0	20.2	9.2
1.58	22.7	43.8	59.4	31.0	6.4
1.50	30.9	36.5	47.1	45.1	4.8
0.11	6.5	16.6	76.8	0.2	4.5
0.14	5.7	9.7	82.7	0.4	6.0
0.15	5.1	8.6	85.7	0.6	6.9
0.14	4.6	12.8	86.2	0.8	7.9
0.13	5.5	25.4	87.0	1.6	7.0
0.15	5.9	40.6	87.9	2.2	6.2
0.41	6.3	52.9	87.8	3.6	5.2
1.72	8.2	58.9	85.9	6.7	4.6
1.80	9.7	62.5	84.3	9.4	3.6

ber 2000 LFS that they were receiving the state old age pension. The top panel shows the high prevalence of the pension among elderly Africans, with over 80 percent of men and women age 70 and above receiving it. The age eligibility rules appear to be fairly strictly enforced for women, with sharp increases in the percentage receiving the pension at ages 60 and 61. Something over 5 percent of women in the 55-59 age group report receiving the pension, in spite of not having reached the official age of eligibility of 60. Possible explanations for these anomalies, as noted by Case and Deaton (1998), are age misreporting in the census or exercise of local discretion in eligibility criteria. The percentage of African women receiving the pension

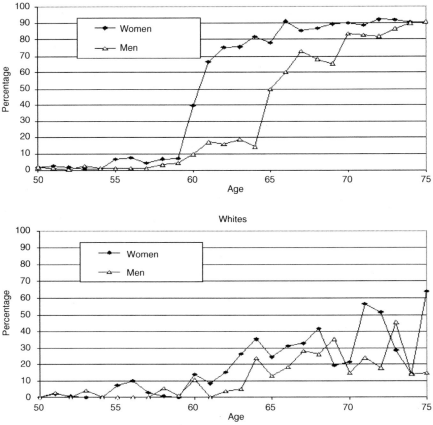

FIGURE 7-6 Percentage receiving old age pension, September 2000, South Africa LFS.

increases to 40 percent at age 60 and 70 percent at age 61, rising to about 90 percent from age 66 and higher. An even larger discrepancy between the technical age eligibility rules and the report of pension receipt is observed for African men. About 15 percent of men are reported as receiving the pension between ages 60 and 64, in spite of not having reached the official age of eligibility of 65. The proportion of men receiving the pension jumps to 50 percent at age 65, then continues rising until it reaches a peak of 90 percent at age 75.

The bottom panel of Figure 7-6 shows the percentage of whites receiving the state old age pension. These percentages are much smaller than those for Africans, although they are not inconsequential. Small cell sizes make these estimates at single years of age for whites somewhat erratic, but about 30 percent of women and 25 percent of men report receiving the pension above age 64.

Figure 7-7 documents the importance of pensions in the economic situation of African households. The figure shows the proportion of total household income attributable to the old age pension for individuals at every age from 50 to 80. It is derived by merging the September 2000 LFS with income data for the same households from the October 2000 IES. The pension income of all household members is included in the calculation. The figure shows that pension income accounts for more than 50 percent of household income for both men and women beginning around age 70. There is a sharp increase for women beginning at age 60, the age at which they

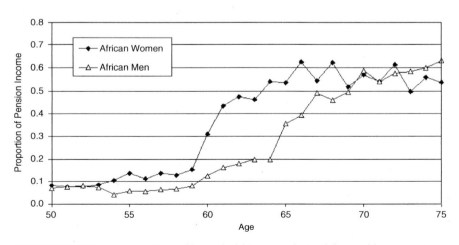

FIGURE 7-7 Mean proportion of household income derived from old age pension, South Africa LFS/IES, September 2000.

themselves begin receiving the pension. Similarly, we see a sharp increase in the proportion of household income attributable to pension income for men beginning at age 65, the age at which they begin receiving the pension. Recalling from Figure 7-6 that at least 10 percent of African men and women do not receive the pension, the levels in Figure 7-7 suggest that pension income accounts for an even higher fraction of household income in those households that do receive the pension.

Figure 7-8 shows the percentage of African and white men and women receiving employer-provided pensions. The top panel shows that employer-provided pensions are very uncommon for Africans, with fewer than 10 percent of men and 5 percent of women receiving them at most ages. The bottom panel shows that private pensions are much more important for whites. The percentage of white men receiving private pensions rises from around 10 percent at age 54 to well over 50 percent above age 64. The percentage of women receiving private pensions (presumably in the form of spouse benefits in many cases) is also high, reaching levels of around 40 percent above age 65. The most pronounced age spike in receipt of private pensions for white men occurs at age 64, where there is an increase from about 20 to 50 percent receiving pensions.

An important feature of the South African old age pension system is that receiving the pension is not necessarily incompatible with working. This is true both because the means test does not preclude work and because the rules of the system may be somewhat flexibly applied. Table 7-3 analyzes the extent to which African individuals work and receive the pension at the same time, as reported in the September 2000 LFS. Two definitions of work are used in Table 7-3. One is a broad definition that includes the family plot category used in Column 5 of Table 7-1. The second is a narrower definition that excludes those working only on a family plot.

Looking at men ages 65-69, a group in which all men have reached pension age, Table 7-3 shows that the employment rate among men who are not receiving the pension is 47 percent by the broad definition and 41 percent by the narrower definition. The employment rate among men ages 65-69 who *are* receiving the pension is considerably lower, 22 percent by the broad measure and 7 percent by the narrow measure. At older ages almost 20 percent of men receiving pensions are reported as working by the broad measure, but these men are almost all working only on a family plot. A similar result is observed for women. Although 21 percent of women receiving the pension in the 60-64 age group are working by the broad definition, only 7 percent are working by the narrow definition.

These results suggest that while we do observe individuals working and receiving the pension at the same time, employment rates are much lower among pension recipients than among nonrecipients. Using the narrow em-

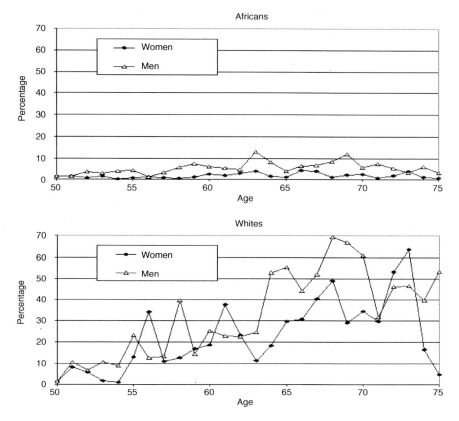

FIGURE 7-8 Percentage receiving employer-provided pension, September 2000 South Africa LFS.

ployment measure, we estimate employment rates of less than 10 percent for pension recipients.

Schooling

Schooling is an important determinant of employment at all ages, affecting both labor demand and labor supply. In many countries it is observed that better educated workers have later ages of retirement (Peracchi and Welch, 1994). There is a strong effect of schooling on both wages and the probability of employment for prime age workers in South Africa (Anderson, Case, and Lam, 2001; Mwabu and Schultz, 1996). It is there-

TABLE 7-3 Percentage Working by Pension Status, African Men and Women, September 2000, South Africa LFS

Age Group	Number	Percentage Receiving Pension	Not Receiving Pension			Receiving Pension		
			Number	Percentage Working		Number	Percentage Working	
				Broad	Narrow		Broad	Narrow
Men								
50-54	1,253	1.6	1,233	67.2	62.3	20	13.6	7.1
55-59	884	2.4	857	66.7	61.0	27	20.8	9.1
60-64	776	14.6	653	53.8	47.1	123	13.0	6.8
65-69	548	63.8	201	46.6	41.0	347	21.9	6.6
70-74	415	84.4	66	26.3	17.0	349	18.7	7.9
75-79	228	86.9	31	20.2	20.2	197	17.6	3.3
Total	4,104	24.9	3,041	61.9	56.4	1,063	18.9	6.5
Women								
50-54	1,520	1.8	1,487	55.3	49.5	33	28.2	13.1
55-59	1,136	6.8	1,064	46.4	40.7	72	14.0	4.3
60-64	1,253	62.9	459	43.1	33.7	794	20.7	7.5
65-69	859	85.2	127	27.4	22.5	732	16.7	5.5
70-74	768	90.4	75	11.3	7.7	693	11.8	3.0
75-79	380	93.1	25	21.3	2.0	355	9.1	1.4
Total	5,916	43.6	3,237	48.5	42.2	2,679	15.5	4.9

NOTE: Broad measure of work includes work on family plot; narrow measure does not.

fore natural to look at the impact of schooling on the work activity of the elderly.

Table 7-4 shows summary statistics for the distribution of schooling for African men and women by 5-year age groups. As the table clearly shows, levels of schooling among the elderly in South Africa are very low. Over 45 percent of men and over 50 percent of women age 60 and above in the 2001 census had 0 years of schooling. The percentage completing 7th grade is under 30 percent for those age 60 and older, and the percentage completing secondary school is below 5 percent for all age groups age 55 and older. Although men have more schooling than women in older age groups, the gender gap is relatively small compared with many African countries and narrows substantially at younger ages. As shown by Anderson and colleagues (2001), a female advantage in schooling has clearly emerged among younger cohorts. Table 7-4 shows the substantial improvements in schooling that have taken place in South Africa over time, with mean years of schooling more than doubling from the 60-64 to the 30-34 age group.

Figure 7-9 shows the age profile of employment for African men and women, dividing the sample into those with less than 7 years of schooling and those with at least 7 years of schooling. The better educated group has higher rates of employment at all ages for both men and women. Less educated men begin to withdraw from employment at a faster rate in their late 50s, dropping to employment rates below 30 percent by age 60. The gap in employment between the schooling groups is much larger for African women, for whom there is about a 20 percentage point difference in employment rates between the education groups at ages up to 60. The better educated women appear to have a steeper rate of decline in employment beginning at age 60, with both groups falling to employment rates of below 10 percent by age 65. The combination of large improvements in schooling over time and the strong positive relationship between schooling and employment should create a tendency for increasing employment rates for older South Africans over time. This may be especially true for women, for whom the impact of schooling on employment is particularly large.

PROBIT REGRESSIONS

In order to get a clearer picture of the variables affecting the work activity of the elderly in South Africa, we use the 2001 census data to estimate probit regressions of the probability of employment. The dependent variable is one if the individual was working in the week prior to the census and zero for everyone else, whether or not they are in the labor force. The regressions are estimated for the sample of Africans ages 50-75, with separate regressions estimated for men and women. Two specifications are used in the regressions. The first includes years of schooling,

TABLE 7-4 Schooling Attainment of African Men and Women by Age Group, 2001 Census

	Mean Years of Schooling		Percentage Completing Zero Schooling	
Age Group	Women	Men	Women	Men
30-34	8.20	8.33	14.4	11.9
35-39	7.03	7.38	20.1	15.9
40-44	6.06	6.54	25.7	20.2
45-49	5.18	5.70	30.9	25.2
50-54	4.42	4.86	37.2	31.9
55-59	3.97	4.29	41.7	37.0
60-64	3.04	3.56	53.1	45.8
65-69	2.66	3.16	58.0	51.5
70-74	2.12	2.64	65.4	57.9

dummy variables for marital status, a flexible parameterization of age, and dummy variables for province and urban residence. The second regression adds measures of household composition. As noted above, living arrangements are likely to be endogenous, determined jointly with decisions about labor supply, so these variables are included simply to indicate the association between living arrangements and the elderly labor supply and not as indicators of causation.

Table 7-5 presents the estimates of these probit regressions. Regressions 1 and 2 present estimates of the first specification for women and men, respectively. As suggested by Figure 7-9, the coefficient on years of schooling is positive and highly significant for both men and women. The marginal effects (dF/dx) column indicates that 1 year of additional schooling is associated with about a 1 percentage point increase in the probability of working for both men and women, evaluated at the sample means of the independent variables. This translates into a similar percentage point increase in schooling for men and women, although it is a smaller proportional change for men given their higher levels of employment.

The marital status dummies, with married as the omitted category, indicate that unmarried women are significantly more likely to work, controlling for all of the other variables in the regression, with the largest effect for divorced women. Evaluated at sample means, the percentage increase in the probability of work compared with married women is 0.5 percentage points for widows, 8 percentage points for divorced women, and 4 percentage points for women who have never married. The effects of marriage for men go in the opposite direction, with married men having significantly higher probabilities of employment than widowed, divorced, or never married men. Married men have probabilities of employment at least 10 percentage points

At Least 4 Years		At Least 7 Years		At Least 12 Years	
Women	Men	Women	Men	Women	Men
82.0	83.7	70.8	71.1	30.5	31.4
74.7	78.5	60.0	62.7	20.6	22.4
67.7	72.5	50.6	54.6	14.7	16.6
61.1	66.1	42.8	46.9	9.8	12.0
54.1	58.5	35.5	39.0	6.6	8.2
49.6	52.8	31.7	33.9	5.1	6.3
38.6	44.0	23.0	27.1	3.5	4.9
33.8	39.0	19.9	24.0	2.9	4.5
27.0	32.4	15.2	19.3	2.2	3.8

higher than men in any of the other categories of marital status, even with very flexible controls for age.

We use a cubic function of age to permit a flexible shape for the age-employment profile. We also include two dummy variables, permitting shifts in the age profile at ages 60 and 65. The age 60 dummy is equal to one for age 60 and above; the age 65 dummy is equal to one for age 65 and above. For women we estimate a decline of 3.4 percentage points in employment probabilities at age 60, the age at which women become eligible for the state old age pension. We also estimate a positive effect of the age 65 dummy for women, with a decline in the probability of employment of 2.9 percentage points. For men the coefficient on the age 60 dummy is not statistically significant, but we estimate a significant negative effect of the age 65 dummy. This suggests that men speed up their withdrawal from employment when they reach the age of pension eligibility, with a predicted drop of 7.2 percentage points in the probability of employment at age 65.

The coefficient on the urban dummy indicates that both men and women are significantly more likely to work in urban areas, with a larger coefficient for women. We observe substantial differences in employment across provinces with significantly lower probabilities of employment for both women and men in Eastern Cape, Northern Cape, KwaZulu-Natal, and Northern Province when compared with Western Cape. Gauteng has higher rates of employment than Western Cape for women, but differences between Gauteng and Western Cape are not statistically significant for men. We caution that none of the locational variables can be considered exogenous, since the decision about where to live may be made jointly with the decision about whether to retire.

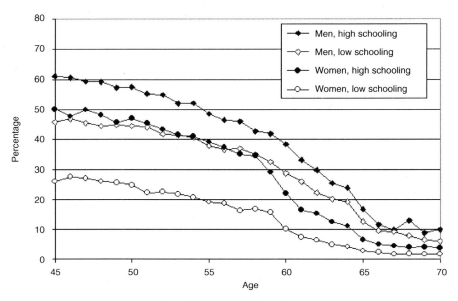

FIGURE 7-9 Percentage working by years of schooling, 2001 census.
NOTE: High schooling is 7 or more years of schooling; low schooling is under 7 years.

Regressions 3 and 4 add three household composition variables to the regression—the number of household members under the age of 18, the number of men ages 18-59, and the number of women ages 18-59. The number of household members under age 18 is negatively associated with the employment of both men and women, with a larger coefficient for women. This may reflect a trade-off between labor market work and caring for grandchildren, especially for women. The number of adult men in the household is negatively associated with the employment of women but positively associated with the employment of men, although both effects are extremely small. The effect of the number of adult women in the household is slightly positive on the employment of women and statistically insignificant in its effect on the employment of men. Since we have controlled for the presence of children, the positive effect of women ages 18-59 on the employment of women may indicate that older women are less needed for child care responsibilities if the children's mother is in the household.

As with the locational variables, we caution again that household living arrangements are likely to be endogenous with respect to the labor supply decisions of potential household members. Unobserved variables, such as the health of elderly household members, are likely to affect both living arrangements and work activity. Since the living arrangements of the elderly are likely to be influenced by many of the same unobservable variables that affect labor supply, the coefficients on these household composition variables should not be given a causal interpretation.

CONCLUSIONS

We have referred to the large literature showing the importance of the noncontributory old age pension for poor households in South Africa. Those elderly who do not have pension income are among the poorest South Africans. Many of those with a pension live in three-generation or skipped-generation households. Indeed, we have made reference to a literature arguing that this extended household structure may in part be a response to the pension. Leaving aside these difficult issues of endogenous household structure, the fact remains that the African elderly are usually in the minority in their own households, and their pension income is available to support large numbers of children and working-age adults. This makes the state old age pension a key element in South Africa's social safety net and a central plank in overall social welfare policy. It also implies that an unusual burden is placed on South Africa's elderly. Given this, it strikes us as an omission that the existing literature has devoted so much attention to the impact of the pension on labor supply and other outcomes of the nonelderly without interrogating the impact on the elderly themselves. This paper has sought to fill in this gap by examining the labor supply behavior of the elderly.

Our analysis of South African census and survey data indicates that withdrawal from the labor force occurs at a fairly rapid rate above age 45. According to the 2001 census, male participation rates fall from around 80 percent at age 45 to 50 percent at age 60 and 10 percent at age 70, with only modest differences across the four main population groups. Participation rates for women are lower at all ages, with participation rates for African women falling from around 60 percent at age 45 to 20 percent at age 60 and 5 percent at age 70. Using the metric of unused productive capacity developed by Gruber and Wise (1999) this pattern of labor force withdrawal leads to somewhat less unused capacity than most European countries and slightly more unused capacity than the United States.

For black South Africans, the noncontributory old age pension system is triggered almost entirely by simple age eligibility rules, with women becoming eligible at age 60 and men becoming eligible at age 65. The fraction of women receiving the pension jumps from under 10 percent at age 59 to almost 70 percent at age 61, with the pension becoming almost 50 percent of household income for women age 61. Although the pension does not necessarily imply a tax on work, especially for low-wage workers, we find that the age of pension eligibility is associated with increased rates of retire-

TABLE 7-5 Probit Regressions for Employment, Africans Ages 50-75, 2001 Census

| | Probit Regression Coefficients and Robust Standard Errors | | | | | |
| | Female Regression 1 | | | Male Regression 2 | | |
Variable	b	SE	dF/dX	b	SE	dF/dX
Years of schooling	0.064	(0.001)***	0.010	0.032	(0.001)***	0.011
Widowed	0.030	(0.010)***	0.005	−0.329	(0.019)***	−0.098
Divorced	0.388	(0.021)***	0.080	−0.426	(0.031)***	−0.120
Never Married	0.203	(0.011)***	0.036	−0.655	(0.015)***	−0.178
Age ≥ 60	−0.207	(0.023)***	−0.034	−0.017	(0.022)	−0.005
Age ≥ 65	−0.185	(0.030)***	−0.029	−0.228	(0.027)***	−0.072
Age-50	0.023	(0.008)***	0.004	0.001	(0.008)	0.000
(Age 50) squared	−0.008	(0.001)***	−0.001	−0.005	(0.001)***	−0.002
(Age 50) cubed	0.000	(0.000)***	0.000	0.000	(0.000)***	0.000
Urban	0.265	(0.011)***	0.045	0.038	(0.011)***	0.012
Eastern Cape	−0.355	(0.028)***	−0.050	−0.650	(0.026)***	−0.186
Northern Cape	−0.258	(0.050)***	−0.035	−0.080	(0.043)*	−0.026
Free State	−0.035	(0.029)	−0.006	−0.117	(0.027)***	−0.037
KwaZulu-Natal	−0.204	(0.027)***	−0.031	−0.402	(0.026)***	−0.121
Northwest	−0.161	(0.028)***	−0.024	−0.144	(0.026)***	−0.046
Gauteng	0.115	(0.026)***	0.020	0.023	(0.024)	0.008
Mpumulanga	0.049	(0.029)*	0.008	0.024	(0.027)	0.008
Northern Province	−0.096	(0.029)***	−0.015	−0.144	(0.027)***	−0.104
Number < 18						
Men 18-59						
Women 18-59						
Constant	−0.943	(0.031)***		0.108	(0.029)***	
Sample size		172,241			118,858	
Pseudo R-squared		0.208			0.156	
Log likelihood		−56986			−62038	

NOTES: Robust standard errors in parentheses. Significance levels: *** = 0.01, ** = 0.05, * = 0.1. Omitted categories: Married, Western Cape.

ment. Reaching the age of pension eligibility leads to an increase in the hazard rate of leaving employment for women from 5 percent at age 58 to over 40 percent at age 60. Men also retire at a faster rate when they reach the pension-eligibility age of 65, with the hazard rate rising to over 30 percent at ages 65 and 66. While this is a sharp jump in retirement, it is not as large as observed in many European countries, where hazard rates can be as high as 60 percent at key program eligibility ages.

We found large effects of schooling on employment of the elderly. Our probit regressions imply about a 1 percentage point increase in the probability of employment for each year of schooling for both men and women. Since schooling levels rise rapidly from older to younger ages, especially for

Female Regression 3			Male Regression 4		
b	SE	dF/dX	b	SE	dF/dX
0.062	(0.001)***	0.010	0.031	(0.001)***	0.010
0.030	(0.011)***	0.005	−0.345	(0.019)***	−0.102
0.370	(0.021)***	0.074	−0.463	(0.031)***	−0.129
0.181	(0.012)***	0.032	−0.678	(0.015)***	−0.182
−0.206	(0.023)***	−0.034	−0.011	(0.022)	−0.004
−0.188	(0.030)***	−0.029	−0.228	(0.027)***	−0.072
0.021	(0.008)***	0.003	0.001	(0.008)	0.000
−0.008	(0.001)***	−0.001	−0.005	(0.001)***	−0.002
0.000	(0.000)***	0.000	0.000	(0.000)***	0.000
0.244	(0.011)***	0.041	0.025	(0.011)**	0.008
−0.344	(0.028)***	−0.048	−0.647	(0.026)***	−0.182
−0.256	(0.050)***	−0.035	−0.079	(0.043)*	−0.025
−0.035	(0.029)	−0.005	−0.117	(0.027)***	−0.037
−0.170	(0.027)***	−0.026	−0.377	(0.026)***	−0.114
−0.158	(0.028)***	−0.023	−0.156	(0.026)***	−0.049
0.104	(0.026)***	0.017	0.012	(0.025)	0.004
0.064	(0.030)**	0.011	0.031	(0.027)	0.010
−0.083	(0.029)***	−0.013	−0.325	(0.027)***	−0.098
−0.058	(0.007)***	−0.009	−0.037	(0.004)***	−0.012
−0.009	(0.005)*	−0.002	0.003	(0.000)***	0.000
0.004	(0.001)***	0.001	0.000	(0.003)	0.001
−0.807	(0.036)***		0.174	(0.030)***	
	172,241			118,858	
	0.214			0.160	
	−56569			−61759	

Africans, this implies that employment rates at older ages may increase in the future. Employment rates at older ages may also be pushed upward by the fact that younger cohorts are more likely to live in urban areas, since we estimate a substantial positive effect of urban residence on employment.

It is beyond the scope of this paper to fully explain the patterns in labor force withdrawal that we have documented. While some factors, such as the age eligibility for the old age pension, appear to play an important role, many questions remain. For example, even if the pension helps explain sharp drops in labor force participation immediately around the pension age, it presumably cannot explain the steady declines in participation that begin around age 45. Health may be important in these declines, but existing data sources provide limited information on health and disability. The lack of panel data also complicates interpretation of our results, especially as they relate to the high level of unemployment. Does the decline in participation result from individuals retiring from their jobs, or from individuals losing their jobs and deciding not to search for a new one? Further research on the labor supply of the elderly in South Africa would clearly benefit from longitudinal data that includes data on health and disability.

REFERENCES

Anderson, K., Case, A., and Lam, D. (2001). Causes and consequences of schooling outcomes in South Africa: Evidence from survey data. *Social Dynamics, 27*(1), 1-23.

Bertrand, M., Mullainathan, S., and Miller, D. (2003). Public policy and extended families: Evidence from pensions in South Africa. *World Bank Economic Review, 17*(1), 27-50.

Casale, D.M., and Posel, D.R. (2002). The continued feminization of the labor force in South Africa: An analysis of recent data and trends. *South African Journal of Economics, 70*(1), 156-184.

Case, A., and Deaton, A. (1998). Large cash transfers to the elderly in South Africa. *Economic Journal, 108,* 1330-1361.

Clark, R.L., and Anker, R. (1993). Cross-national analysis of labor force participation of older men and women. *Economic Development and Cultural Change, 41*(3), 489-512.

Duflo, E. (2003). Grandmothers and granddaughters: Old age pension and intra-household allocation in South Africa. *World Bank Economic Review, 17*(1), 1-25.

Edmonds, E. (2005). Child labor and schooling responses to anticipated income in South Africa. *Journal of Development Economics.* Available: http://72.14.209.104/search?q= cache:I0wPhNpkmh4J:www.dartmouth.edu/~eedmonds/liquidity.pdf+child+labor+and+ schooling+responses+to+anticipated+income+in+South+Africa&hl=en&gl=us&ct=clnk&cd=1 [accessed September 2006].

Edmonds, E., Mammen, K., and Miller, D. (2005). Rearranging the family? Household composition responses to large pension receipts. *Journal of Human Resources, 40*(1), 186-207.

Ferreira, M. (1999). The generosity and universality of South Africa's pension system. *The EU Courier, 176.*

Gruber, J., and Wise, D.A. (1999). *Social security and retirement around the world.* Chicago, IL: University of Chicago Press.

Kapteyn, A., and de Vos, K. (1999). Social security and retirement in the Netherlands. In J. Gruber and D.A. Wise (Eds.), *Social security and retirement around the world.* Chicago, IL: University of Chicago Press.

Klasen, S., and Woolard, I. (2000). *Unemployment and employment in South Africa, 1995-1997.* Report to the Department of Finance, South Africa.

Jensen, R.T. (2004). Do private transfers displace the benefits of public transfers? Evidence from South Africa. *Journal of Public Economics, 88*(1-2), 89-112.

Leibbrandt, M., and Bhorat, H. (2001). Modeling vulnerability in the South African labor market. In B. Haroon, M. Leibbrandt, M. Maziya, S. van der Bberg, and I. Woolard (Eds.), *Fighting poverty: Labor markets and inequality in South Africa.* Cape Town, South Africa: University of Cape Town Press.

Mlatsheni, C., and Leibbrandt, M. (2001, September). *The role of education and fertility in the participation and employment of African women in South Africa.* (DPRU Working Paper No 01/54). Cape Town, South Africa: School of Economics, University of Cape Town.

Møller, V., and Devey, R. (2003). Trends in the living conditions and satisfaction among poorer older South Africans: Objective and subjective indicators of quality of life in the October Household Survey. *Development Southern Africa, 20*(4), 457-476.

Møller, V., and Ferreira, M. (2003). *Getting by . . . benefits of noncontributory pension income for older South African households.* Cape Town, South Africa: Institute of Ageing in Africa, University of Cape Town.

Mwabu, G., and Schultz, P.T. (1996, May). Education returns across quantiles of the wage function: Alternative explanations for returns to education by race in South Africa. *American Economic Review, 86*(2), 335-339.

Peracchi, F., and Welch, F. (1994). Trends in labor force transitions of older men and women. *Journal of Labor Economics, 12*(2), 210-242.

Posel, D., Fairburn, J., and Lund, F. (2004, July). *Labor migration and households: A reconsideration of the effects of the social pension on labor supply in South Africa.* Paper presented at the National Research Council Conference on Aging in Africa, Johannesburg.

Sagner, A. (2000). Ageing and social policy in South Africa: Historical perspectives with particular reference to the Eastern Cape. *Journal of Southern African Studies, 26*(3), 523-553.

Schlemmer, L., and Møller, V. (1997). The shape of South African society and its challenges. *Social Indicators Research, 41*(1-3), 15-50.

Seekings, J. (2002). The broader importance of welfare reform in South Africa. *Social Dynamics, 28*(2), 1-38.

Van der Berg, S. (2001). Redistribution through the budget: Public expenditure incidence in South Africa, 1993-1997. *Social Dynamics, 27*(1), 140-164.

Van der Berg, S., and Bredenkamp, C. (2002). Devising social security interventions for maximum policy impact. *Social Dynamics, 28*(2), 39-68.

Winter, C. (1998). *Women workers in South Africa: Participation, pay and prejudice in the formal labor market.* Unpublished manuscript, World Bank, Washington, DC.

8

HIV/AIDS and Older People in South Africa

Victoria Hosegood and Ian M. Timaeus

INTRODUCTION

South Africa is experiencing a rapidly growing and severe HIV/AIDS epidemic. National antenatal clinic data show a rise in seroprevalence from 1 percent in 1990 to 25 percent in 2000 (Karim and Karim, 1999; South Africa Department of Health, 2005). By 2000, 40 percent of adult deaths at ages 15-49 were due to HIV/AIDS (Dorrington, Bourne, Bradshaw, Laubscher, and Timaeus, 2001). This disastrous epidemic has enormous implications for older people. They are at risk of HIV infection and AIDS mortality themselves. In addition, many more older people face the consequences of AIDS-related illness and deaths among their own children and other relatives and of the wider social and economic changes wrought by the epidemic. The rising burden of morbidity and mortality among younger adults is likely to increase the importance of the practical contributions made by older people to their households. In South Africa, these include the contribution the monthly old age pension makes to family incomes as well as older people's role in caring for grandchildren and other children whose parents are absent (HelpAge International, 2003).

In their international review of AIDS and older people, Knodel, Watkins, and VanLandingham (2003) extensively consider the evidence concerning the sociodemographic impact of AIDS on older people in Africa (Knodel et al., 2003). This paper complements their review by focusing on South Africa. The survival of the apartheid system in South Africa long after decolonization of the rest of the continent and the economic advantages of the country mean that older South Africans live in a very different social, political, and economic environment from older people in other African countries. These distinctions, coupled with a very severe HIV epidemic, suggest that the impact of HIV/AIDS on older people in South Africa may be very different from that in other countries with generalized HIV epidemics.

We begin by describing some of the more important social, demographic, and economic aspects of older people's lives in South Africa and then discuss the direct and indirect consequences of the HIV epidemic for them. The last section of the paper presents data on the living arrangements of older people in rural KwaZulu-Natal in South Africa and examines their households' experience of adult mortality, in particular AIDS mortality.

OLDER PEOPLE IN SOUTH AFRICA

The impact of the HIV epidemic on older people is shaped by the social, political, demographic, and economic circumstances in which they live. This section highlights some of the relevant characteristics of South African society.

South Africa Has the Highest Proportion of Older People in Africa

Population aging has commenced in most African countries as a consequence of the transition to lower levels of fertility and mortality. The population age 60 or more is projected to increase sixfold by 2050 (HelpAge International, 2000). The degree of population aging has been exceptionally large in South Africa primarily because of the early onset of fertility transition. Fertility has been falling since the 1960s, when total fertility was nearly seven births per woman, with the rate of decline accelerating in the early 1980s to reach total fertility of around 3.5 in 1996. South Africa's total fertility is currently the lowest in mainland sub-Saharan Africa (Moultrie and Timaeus, 2002, 2003).

South Africa has a higher proportion of older people in its population than any other mainland sub-Saharan African country. In 1997, 7 percent of the population were age 60 or older (Kinsella and Ferreira, 1997). The demographic profiles of the different racial groups in South Africa are markedly different.[1] In the African population, 6 percent were age 60 or older in

---

[1]We regard race as a social reality produced by racism, not a biological characteristic. This paper follows South African practice and uses the term "African" to refer to the majority racial group. In South Africa, "black" has the connotation "nonwhite." Statistical sources on South Africa usually distinguish four population groups: Africans, whites, coloreds, and Asians.

1997 in contrast to 14 percent in the white population, whose population structure closely resembles that of European countries (Kinsella and Ferreira, 1997). By 2030 the proportion of older people in South Africa is projected to increase to 11 percent (U.S. Census Bureau, 2005).

The Sex Ratio in South Africa's Older Population Is Exceptionally Low

In all African countries, women constitute the majority of the older population, reflecting the higher mortality of men. However, the excess in men's mortality in South Africa has always been exceptionally large (Timaeus, 1999). In 1985, the probability of dying between ages 15 and 60 in South Africa was 24 percent for women but 37 percent for men. By 2001 it was 34 percent for women and 51 percent for men (Dorrington, Moultrie, and Timaeus, 2004). Much of the excess in men's mortality in this age range is due to the high death rate from accidents and homicides (Dorrington et al., 2001; Hosegood, Vanneste, and Timaeus, 2004). Thus, according to the 2001 census, the sex ratio at age 60 or more in South Africa was only 62 men per 100 women, compared with 85 in sub-Saharan Africa as a whole (U.S. Census Bureau, 2005).

South Africa's Political History Has Shaped Older People's Lives

South Africa's history of apartheid and labor migration profoundly influences contemporary life there. The Apartheid Group Areas Act and the labor migration system systematically divided African families by recruiting younger men and women to the centers of employment, including mining, farming, and urban areas. Restrictions on the movement and settlement of those not employed meant that most children, unemployed younger adults, and older people were required to live in rural or periurban areas (Leliveld, 1997; Mazur, 1998; Spiegel, 1987). Older people facilitated the economic migration of younger adults by caring for their grandchildren and safeguarding the family land and assets. This became essential to both maintaining the labor migration system and ensuring the long-term survival of households (Izzard, 1985; Leliveld, 1997; Mazur, 1998; Murray, 1980). Consequently, in South Africa the role of older people, particularly grandmothers, in caring for children affected by HIV, builds on a long-established set of social structures related to child care (Madhavan, 2004; Van der Waal, 1996).

In traditional African societies, older men were the principal authority figures both in their households and in the wider community. In South Africa, rapid social change and the transition to democratic government are transforming family relations. Studies have highlighted increasing intergenerational tensions and adaptations of the patriarchal structures in family and community life (Campbell, 1994; Nhongo, 2004). In most countries, fertility decline and economic development are leading to an evolution of household structures away from large, extended households toward smaller households based around the conjugal unit (Bongaarts and Zimmer, 2002). In this transition, increasing numbers of older people will live alone or with a partner. Such changes in household structure do not appear to be occurring readily in South Africa. The reasons for this include very low marriage rates, low rates of cohabitation in nonmarital relationships, the dependence of children and younger adults on the economic and material support of older people, and the limited availability of land for and cost of housing. Thus, in 1996, only 6 percent of Africans were living alone (Noumbissi, Bawah, and Zuberi, 2005). In contrast, other phenomena, such as matrifocal and other women-headed households,[2] have emerged and become a common household arrangement in both rural and urban areas (Preston-Whyte, 1988).

Older Africans Have Worse Health than Older People from Other Racial Groups

The massive social and economic inequalities that the apartheid system served to maintain are mirrored in enormous inequalities in health status among the different racial groups in South Africa. In 1997, life expectancy at birth was 77 years for white women, compared with 55 years for African women (Kinsella and Ferreira, 1997). The 1990-1991 Multidimensional Survey of Elderly South Africans found that older Africans living in rural areas experienced greater health and financial problems than other older people. This can be attributed to isolation, poor housing, lack of income, poor access to health care facilities, and the political and economic marginalization that resulted from apartheid policies (Ferreira, Møller, Prinsloo, and Gillis, 1992). Other studies have found high levels of self-reported depression and ill health among Africans living in urban areas (Ferreira, 2000; Gillis, Welman, Koch, and Joyi, 1991).

The cause-specific mortality profile in South Africa also differs among

---

[2]Several types of households headed by women have been described in South Africa, including those headed by women following the death or separation of their spouse and matrifocal or female-linked households. These are households formed by younger, never married women and their children. In such households the dominant relationships are between mother and daughters and, to a lesser extent, sisters. Husbands and other male partners are not necessarily absent, but the unions may be temporary or not socially recognized (Preston-Whyte, 1978, 1988).

racial groups. Prior to the HIV epidemic, an epidemiological transition had been occurring in all racial groups. Thus, in 2000 in an almost exclusively African population in rural KwaZulu-Natal, noncommunicable diseases accounted for 76 and 71 percent of deaths of women and men, respectively, in the age group 60 or more (Hosegood et al., 2004). The proportion of deaths from heart disease is lower among Africans than other racial groups, but they suffer higher death rates from hypertension, stroke, infectious diseases, accidents, and violence (Bradshaw, Bourne, Schneider, and Sayed, 1995).

The Majority of Older People in South Africa Receive a State Pension

In South Africa, a means-tested, noncontributory state old age pension is paid in cash to women age 60 or more and men age 65 or more. This pension is relatively large—R780 a month in 2005—and had a purchasing power equivalent to about U.S. $280. Thus, in 1998 the pension was about twice the median income per head in African households (Case, 2001; Case and Deaton, 1998; Case, Hosegood, and Lund, 2005; Mohatle and de Graft Agyarko, 1999; Møller and Ferreira, 2003). The existence of a noncontributory pension scheme is a product of South Africa's political past and its ability and political will to currently finance large-scale, public welfare schemes. The means-tested state pension was introduced in 1928 to provide for poor whites with inadequate occupational pensions. Although African workers were generally excluded from occupation pension schemes, the state pension was extended to Africans in 1944 and the value equalized for all population groups after the democratic elections in 1994 (Sagner, 2000).

Older People Use Their Income to Support Other Members of Their Household

In South Africa, older people's pensions do not provide only for their own needs. Many older people also use this income to support the basic needs of their family, including food, clothing, and school fees for children. For many rural African households, the state pension and, to a lesser extent, other government grants are the main source of income. For example, in the Western and Eastern Cape provinces, Møller and Ferreira (2003) found that the old age pension competed with wage earnings as the most important source of income in the households they surveyed, in terms of both access and amount. In one-third of households interviewed in a study in KwaZulu-Natal, a pension was the only source of household income (Møller and Sotshongaye, 1996).

A study examining the role of pensions in poverty alleviation in South

Africa found that both older men and older women spend 30-40 percent of their income on school expenses for dependents. This was in addition to other expenditures on food and household utilities (Mohatle and de Graft Agyarko, 1999). In another study in the Western Cape province, Case (2001) demonstrated that the pension had a measurable protective effect on indicators of health and self-reported well-being. In households whose members pool their income, the presence of an older recipient of a state old age pension in the household had a significant, protective effect on the health of not only the older person themselves, but also all household members. Most studies indicate that the majority of African pensioners share their income with other members of their household. As fewer than 5 percent of pensioners live alone in South Africa (Kinsella and Ferreira, 1997), pension income is a substantial source of financial support for many younger adults and children.

There are several additional social welfare grants for which older people may apply on behalf of someone else (Hunter and Rushby, 2002; Women's Budget Initiative, 2003). In 2001 approximately 10 percent of child support grants in a rural area of KwaZulu-Natal were held by grandmothers (Case, Hosegood, and Lund, 2003, 2005).

The Support That Older People Provide Others Affects Their Own Welfare

The state pension policy has had a profound influence on social arrangements, particularly in rural areas. It has influenced the way in which communities perceive and relate to older people, as well as the social and economic role that older people feel obliged to fulfill as income providers (Burman, 1995). Sagner (2000) argues that, even though the African pension prior to 1994 was an inadequate amount to live on, it served to ensure that many households survived economically (Sagner, 2000). While the contribution made by pensions to poorer households may increase the self-respect and social status of old age pensioners, it also makes younger people dependent on them. Several studies and government inquiries have highlighted the problem of financial and physical abuse of older household members. Both younger and older respondents report that younger people pressuring older people for money is common (Mohatle and de Graft Agyarko, 1999; South Africa Department of Social Development, 2001). However, the old age pension may have slowed the loss of social status and increasing marginalization of older people relative to younger generations that has been described in other countries undergoing substantial social change and economic development (Du Toit, 1994; Johnson, 1989).

Poverty and Older People in South Africa

The take-up of the old age pension is high, particularly in the poorest groups and at the oldest ages. Using data from the 1998 and 1999 October Household Surveys, May (2003a, 2003b) reports that 84 percent of people age 64 or older in households that were on or below a consumption-based poverty line were receiving a government pension. However, the pension is often insufficient to support the number of household members who are dependent on it. Indeed, evidence exists that the pension may attract dependents to the household, thereby reducing the value of the pension per household member (Møller and Sotshongaye, 1996). Thus, despite the state pension, many older people live in severe poverty. In 1998-1999, 25 percent of older people were living in households whose income fell below half the poverty line, compared with 28 percent of the population as a whole (May, 2003a).

DIRECT AND INDIRECT CONSEQUENCES OF HIV/AIDS FOR OLDER PEOPLE IN SOUTH AFRICA

This section considers the impact of the HIV epidemic on older people in South Africa. The rapid development of a severe epidemic has resulted in substantial increases in adult mortality since the mid-1990s, which have reversed improvements in health and survival made in the 1970s and 1980s. The mortality of women ages 25-29 in 1999-2000 was 3.5 times higher than in 1985, while the mortality of men ages 30-39 doubled in the same period (Dorrington et al., 2001).

HIV Infection and AIDS Mortality in Older People

In the United States and Europe, attention has been given to both HIV prevention and the treatment and care of HIV-positive older people (Levy, Ory, and Crystal, 2003). In Africa, however, HIV/AIDS health education programs and the health services largely ignore the risk of HIV infection and AIDS in older people (Wilson and Adamchak, 2001). One of the factors contributing to this neglect is that the available data on HIV infection are restricted largely to women of reproductive age. Most of the seroprevalence data on South Africa have been collected from pregnant women seen at government antenatal clinics. However, the national HIV prevalence survey conducted by the Human Sciences Research Council collected HIV data on a small number of people age 55 or more (Human Sciences Research Council, 2002). Their report presents a graph indicating that approximately 7 percent (95 percent confidence interval, CI, approximately 4-10) of women age 55 or more and 7 percent (95 percent CI approximately 3-15) of men in the same age group were HIV positive. These data probably suffer from a number of biases. In particular, they probably overrepresent younger members of this age group. However, they do suggest that appreciable numbers of older South Africans are HIV positive. Moreover, as people may not develop AIDS until many years after they were infected with HIV, significant numbers of AIDS cases and deaths are likely to occur in this age group. A study in rural KwaZulu-Natal in 2000 found that 2 percent of people dying of AIDS with or without tuberculosis were age 60 or more, representing 5 percent of all deaths in this age group (Hosegood et al., 2004).

Older People as Members of Households Affected by HIV/AIDS

Although they are at risk of being infected with HIV themselves, the major impact of the HIV epidemic on older people is indirect. Knodel and colleagues (2003) identify seven pathways though which older people experience the impact of the AIDS epidemic at the family or household level: caregiving, coresidence with an ill adult child, loss of the child, providing financial or material support during the time the adult child is ill, paying for the funeral of the deceased child, fostering grandchildren, and negative community reaction. Both in South Africa and elsewhere in the African region, most studies examining the indirect impact of HIV/AIDS on older people have focused on the role of older people in caring for people with AIDS or their orphaned children, rather than on outcomes for the older people themselves, such as effects on their physical and mental health, economic status, or living arrangements.

The role of older people in the care of relatives with AIDS has been relatively well documented. Many of the empirical studies have been in the United States (Berk, Schur, Dunbar, Bozette, and Shapiro, 2003; Ellis and Muschkin, 1996) and Thailand (Knodel and VanLandingham, 2001; Knodel, Saengtienchai, Im-em, and VanLandingham, 2001a, 2001b). Qualitative studies in Tanzania, Zimbabwe, and South Africa have also shown the important role that older people play in caring for those of their children who develop AIDS (Ferreira, Keikelame, and Mosaval, 2001; Foster et al., 1995; World Health Organization, 2002). In Uganda, 48 percent of people with AIDS were cared for by a parent for at least for some time during their illness (Ntozi and Nakayiwa, 1999). Although the focus of caring has often been on women, men are also involved in supporting ill and bereaved people. In Tanzania, older men and women were equally likely to care for sick household members, although women spent twice as much time as men on caregiving activities (Dayton and Ainsworth, 2002).

In rural South Africa, many of those needing care will have been migrants, often labor migrants, prior to their illness. Their living arrangements at their place of work often fail to provide them with the level of physical, emotional, and financial support that they can receive from their parents and others in their natal household. Therefore, they often return to their parents' households when they become chronically sick. As many as 14 percent of the people dying in one area of rural KwaZulu-Natal in 2001-2002 had arrived in the area less than 6 months before they died (Gafos, 2003).

Widespread awareness exists in the media, research, and program arenas of the role of older people in fostering children orphaned by parental deaths due to AIDS. Studies in Zimbabwe, Uganda, and Kenya show that grandmothers, in particular, care voluntarily not only for their orphaned grandchildren but also for other closely related children (Drew, Makufa, and Foster, 1998; Guest, 2001; Nyambedha, Wandibba, and Aagaard-Hansen, 2003).

Few studies in Africa have examined the impact of HIV/AIDS on caregivers' own health and well-being. AIDS illness and death have short-term and long-term economic consequences for households and their surviving members, including reduced economic status (Rugalema, 1999; Yamano and Jayne, 2004). Since many older people in developing countries are dependent on financial and material assistance from their children and grandchildren, increased mortality of working-age adults will weaken their support networks (Adamchak, Wilson, Nyanguru, and Hampson, 1991).

A qualitative study of grandmothers caring for a child with HIV/AIDS as well as their grandchildren in townships in the Western Cape province of South Africa found that the cost of caring for the sick person (transport, medical bills), as well as taking on more of the costs of childrearing (school fees, food), drove these older women and their households into poverty. In addition, the women reported that their health had worsened as a result of the experience due to the physical demands involved in caregiving and the emotional trauma that they had suffered (Ferreira et al., 2001).

In one of the few longitudinal studies in Africa to investigate the impact of adult deaths on older household members, Dayton and Ainsworth (2002) found that, controlling for poverty, the body mass index of older people decreased significantly in the period immediately following the death of an adult member of their household. In Zimbabwe, elevated levels of emotional and psychological stress have been reported among older caregivers (World Health Organization, 2002).

Older People Living in HIV/AIDS-Affected Communities

The macro-level economic and social impact of the HIV epidemic in Africa is also likely to have implications for older people, for example, by increasing demands on or worsening the quality of health and welfare services, reducing opportunities for paid work, and adversely affecting the supply of adequate foodstuffs (Barnett and Whiteside, 1999, 2000). Water supply, sanitation, and clinic-based and hospital care are particularly important for older people and public health expenditures in South Africa fell from 8.2 percent of the gross domestic product in 1994 to 4.1 percent in 2000 (Walker, 2001).

Even in remote rural areas, older people in South Africa experience a high burden of chronic diseases due to noncommunicable diseases and disorders, principally obesity in women, hypertension, diabetes, stroke, and cancer (Bradshaw et al., 1995; Kahn and Tollman, 1999; Walker, 2001). Almost three-quarters of older people report having at least one chronic illness or ongoing health problem, and more than half of them report a physical disability (Ferreira, 2000). Government health services, particularly in rural areas, are inadequately equipped to provide long-term support for people with chronic diseases, and this is unlikely to improve in the context of the overwhelming pressure on them resulting from the tuberculosis and HIV/AIDS epidemics.

OLDER PEOPLE'S LIVING ARRANGEMENTS AND MORTALITY IN RURAL KWAZULU-NATAL

Demographic surveillance systems (DSS) with longitudinal observations on individuals and households provide opportunities to measure the sociodemographic impact of the HIV epidemic. In this section, we describe the demographic and socioeconomic characteristics, composition, and experience of adult deaths of the households of older people using data from a DSS site in rural KwaZulu-Natal. The results presented are from an analysis of a subset of longitudinal data from the Africa Centre Demographic Information System (ACDIS) (Hosegood and Timaeus, 2005).

Study Area

The study area is part of the rural district of Umkhanyakude in northern KwaZulu-Natal. It is situated about 250 km north of the provincial capital of Durban. The area includes both land under tribal authority that was designated as a Zulu "homeland" under South Africa's former apartheid policy and a township under municipal authority. Infrastructure is poor. In 2001 only 13 percent of households had access to either their own piped water supply or a communal tap. Although this is a rural area, there is little subsistence agriculture. Most households rely on wage income and pensions. Unemployment is high: 67 percent of women and 56 percent of men ages 16-59 were unemployed in 2001 (Case and Ardington, 2004). Few local employment opportunities exist, and consequently labor migration is high. Approximately 40 percent of the men and 35 percent of women age 18 years or more who report that they are members of households in the study area also report that they reside outside the area most of the time (Hosegood and Timaeus, 2005).

KwaZulu-Natal is the province of South Africa with the highest prevalence of HIV infection among those attending antenatal clinics (South Africa Department of Health, 2005). An antenatal survey conducted in the study area in 1998 found that 41 percent (95 percent CI: 34.7-47.9) of pregnant women were infected with HIV (Wilkinson, Connolly, and Rotchford, 1999). Preliminary results from a population-based HIV surveillance study in the same area in 2003 found HIV seroprevalence to be 22.2 (95 percent CI: 20.4-24.1) in women ages 15-49 and 12.1 (95 percent CI: 10.4-14.1) in men ages 15-54 (Weltz and Hosegood, 2003). HIV prevalence was highest among men ages 30-34 (42.5, 95 percent CI: 31.0-54.6) and women ages 25-29 (43.2, 95 percent CI: 35.7-51.1).

Data Source

ACDIS started data collection on January 1, 2000. The demographic study area was mapped and all households were registered. The study population includes all members of households living in a dwelling in the study area. ACDIS collects data on both the resident members of a household who sleep at the dwelling most of the time and nonresident members who acknowledge the authority of the household head and visit the household at least once a year. The initial round of fieldwork registered 79,354 individuals as members of 10,612 households. Demographic and health information is collected two or three times a year from all registered households and individuals. It includes reports of all births and deaths and moves between households and in and out of the area. The causes of all notified deaths (of both resident and nonresident household members) are established by clinicians on the basis of a verbal autopsy interview conducted by nurses with the family or caregivers of the deceased (Hosegood et al., 2004). The conceptual and operational design of ACDIS has been described in more detail elsewhere (Hosegood and Timaeus, 2005).

Because of the importance of the old-age pension in South Africa for both pensioners and other members of their household, our analysis of older people's living arrangements focuses on those of pensionable age. We present information on the individual and household characteristics of the 3,657 women age 60 or more and men age 65 or more who were resident in the study area on January 1, 2000. We also examine changes in the structure of their households by January 1, 2002, together with the structure of the households of the 528 additional people of pensionable age residing in the study area by then. The methods used to generate the data on individual and household relationships are described elsewhere and are available from the authors on request.

Characterizing Household Structure

In ACDIS, the relationship of each member of the household to its head is collected at each round, but establishing the nature of the relationship between two members when neither is the head of the household is more difficult. It is complicated by high levels of extramarital fertility and the frequent presence in households in this area of distantly related or unrelated individuals. In addition, respondents often report socially as well as biologically related individuals as kin or report kin to be more closely related than they are. This is particularly a problem with foster parents and half-siblings (Noumbissi and Zuberi, 2001; Townsend, 1997).

In contrast, ages are available for all household members and provide an unambiguous way of comparing households in the study area. Instead of classifying household structures on the basis of the relationship of other members to the older person, such as coresidence with a grandchild under age 15 (Zimmer and Dayton, 2003), we distinguish four groups of households defined on the basis of the ages of younger household members irrespective of whether the household includes any older people other than the index individual. These are: (a) households in which the older person of pensionable age is the only member or that has other older members only, (b) households with younger adult members but with no members under age 18, (c) households whose membership includes both younger adults and children under age 18, and (d) households with members under age 18 but no adult members below pensionable age. Older people are included in the analysis only as an index individual in the household in which they are resident, but we analyze the composition both of the other residents and of everyone recognized as a member of the household.

One of the primary hypotheses of both researchers and policy makers has been that the deaths of younger adults due to HIV/AIDS in Southern Africa will result in an increase in what are termed "skipped-generation households." This concept has been defined in various ways. It is generally applied to households made up of coresident grandparents and grandchildren. However, some authors use the term for households that include younger adults, providing that they are not a child of an older household member (Knodel et al., 2003). This analysis equates skipped-generation households with our final group of households, those in which one or more older persons live in a household whose membership includes at least one child but no younger adults.

Living Arrangements of Older People in Rural KwaZulu-Natal

On January 1, 2000, 5 percent of the resident population of the study area were of pensionable age. Some 29 percent of the households in the study area had at least one resident member of pensionable age. Table 8-1 presents individual and household characteristics of these older men and women. Older men and women differ significantly (p < 0.01) in their individual characteristics. Older men are more likely than older women to be married, to be the head of the household, to live in households with more assets, and to live alone.

The majority of people of pensionable age (87 percent) live in households with both younger adult and child members. Most of these households would be classified as "extended households" by other authors (Noumbissi and Zuberi, 2001), although our classification does not specify the kinship relationships among the members. Table 8-2 looks jointly at the composition of all members and the other residents in older people's households. It shows that, while about 15 percent of older people live in households without any younger adult residents, less than half of those living alone or only with other older people, and less than a third of those residing only with other older people and children, live in households than have no younger adult members. Thus, few older people (2 percent) live in households consisting of only other older people and children.

Noumbissi and Zuberi (2001) present estimates of the living arrangements of older people in South Africa based on census and Demographic and Health Survey data. The 1996 Census of South Africa suggests that 79 percent of Africans age 60 or more lived in extended or nuclear households, while 6 percent lived alone and 16 percent lived with both family members and nonrelatives (Noumbissi and Zuberi, 2001). While they do not specifically identify skipped-generation households, modeling by Merli and Palloni (this volume, Chapter 4) based on several sources of data suggests that by 1998 some 15 percent of older people in KwaZulu-Natal were living with a grandchild under age 15 but none of their adult children. This percentage is higher than in the data from Umkhanyakude (in the northeastern part of the Kwazulu-Natal province). Their figures also suggest that less than 2 percent of older people were living alone with one or more grandchildren, both of whose parents had died.

The differences between these three sets of estimates undoubtedly result to a considerable degree from differing definitions in the various inquiries of what "living with" someone means. The 1991 and 1996 South African censuses enumerated only the de facto population. Any household member who resided elsewhere (e.g., adult labor migrants) was excluded from the household schedule. Given the extent of labor migration in such provinces as KwaZulu-Natal, de facto data on households mask the distinction be-

TABLE 8-1 Characteristics of Older People and Their Households, Persons of Pensionable Age[a] Resident in the Demographic Surveillance Area on January 1, 2000

Characteristic	All	Women	Men
Mean Age in Years (SD)	70.4 (7.7)	69.6 (7.9)	72.8 (6.4)
Marital Status Distribution (%)			
Currently married	1,362 (37)	722 (26)	640 (71)
Widowed/divorced/separated	1,858 (51)	1,761 (64)	97 (11)
Never married	425 (12)	267 (10)	158 (18)
Unknown	12 (<1)	10 (<1)	2 (<1)
Education Status Distribution (%)			
None	2,310 (63)	1,763 (64)	547 (61)
Primary	743 (20)	587 (21)	156 (17)
Secondary and higher	205 (6)	143 (5)	62 (7)
Unknown	399 (11)	267 (10)	132 (15)
Mean household assets[b]	7.4	7.2	7.6
Percentage of households owning a luxury item[b]	49	48	51
Mean number of household members (SD)	9.9 (5.4)	9.9 (5.3)	9.8 (5.6)
Mean number of resident members (SD)	7.0 (4.1)	7.0 (4.0)	7.0 (4.3)
Percentage living alone	2	1	3
Distribution by composition of household members (%)			
Lives alone or other older people only	113 (3)	65 (2)	48 (5)
Younger adults but no children	271 (7)	199 (7)	72 (8)
Younger adults and children	3,189 (87)	2,433 (88)	756 (84)
Children but no younger adults	84 (2)	63 (2)	21 (2)
Distribution by composition of resident members (%)			
Lives alone or older people only	233 (6)	148 (5)	85 (9)
Younger adults but no children	303 (8)	221 (8)	82 (9)
Younger adults and children	2,798 (77)	2,133 (77)	665 (74)
Children but no younger adults	323 (9)	258 (9)	65 (7)
Relationship to head of household (%)			
Head	1,783 (49)	986 (36)	797 (89)
Spouse or partner	655 (18)	641 (23)	14 (2)
Parent or parent-in-law	912 (25)	880 (32)	32 (4)
Other relative	169 (5)	130 (5)	39 (4)
Nonrelative	45 (1)	32 (1)	13 (1)
Missing	93 (3)	91 (3)	2 (<1)
Total number of older people	3,657	2,760	897

[a]Sample: women age 60 years or more, men age 65 years or more on January 1, 2000.

[b]The number of observations is given at the bottom of each column, except for the number of household assets and percentage with at least one luxury asset, for which there are 3,492, 2,696, and 863 reports for both sexes, women, and men, respectively.

TABLE 8-2 Percentage Distribution of Households with Resident Members of Pensionable Age According to the Age Composition of Their Other Resident Members and of All Their Other Members, January 1, 2000

	All Other Household Members				
Other Resident Members	Alone or with Older People Only	With Younger Adults	With Younger Adults and Children	With Children Only	Total
Alone or with older people	3	2	1	<1	6
With younger adults	0	6	2	0	8
With younger adults and children	0	0	77	0	77
With children only	0	0	7	2	9
Total	3	7	87	2	N = 3,657

tween households in which older people living with children do so in the absence of any adult involvement (i.e., the child's parent has died or abandoned the child) and households in which younger adult members, although nonresident, return periodically and provide at least some social and economic support for both older person and child. One would expect to find a high proportion of skipped-generation households in South African census data simply because, as Merli and Palloni (this volume, Chapter 4) note, many children "lose a parent" to migration.

As we explain elsewhere (Hosegood and Timaeus, 2005), the limitations of the de facto approach were one reason why the ACDIS data system was designed to enumerate both resident and nonresident household members. (The other major reason was to enable ACDIS to track nonresident and occasionally resident individuals longitudinally). Given the different approach that it adopts to data collection, one would expect to find fewer skipped-generation households in ACDIS than in the census. Both perspectives on the household are valid. However, it is wrong to assume that households in which only older adults and children are usually resident only became common recently as a result of high AIDS mortality. By allowing us to look at both residents and all household members, ACDIS makes it clear that, in rural KwaZulu-Natal at any rate, most de facto skipped-generation households have younger adult members and result from high levels of circulatory labor migration rather than the death of younger adults.

Older People's Experience of Adult Mortality Within Their Households

Over the 2-year period of follow-up, 316 older people (8 percent) resident on January 1, 2000, died. They include seven older women and seven older men who died of AIDS with or without tuberculosis. By the end of the follow-up period, an additional 528 older people were resident in the study area. These people were either below pensionable age in 2000 or only moved into a household in the study area after the start of the surveillance.

Mortality at younger ages in this area is high. Of the 3,180 older people residing in the same household after 2 years, 20 percent had experienced the death of at least one younger adult in their household and 12 percent had experienced one or more deaths of adult household members from AIDS. Household size decreased by 18 percent in households that had a younger adult death, compared with 8 percent in other households with an older person resident.

Changes in the Living Arrangements of Older People

Table 8-3 documents changes in household membership between the beginning of 2000 and the beginning of 2002 for households with older

TABLE 8-3 Percentage Distribution According to Age of the Other Members in 2002 in Households with Residents of Pensionable Age by Age of the Other Members in 2000

3a Households in Which a Younger Adult Member (Ages 18-59) Died in 2000-2001

| | Membership of Household in 2002 | | | | | |
Membership of Household in 2000	Alone or Only with Older People	With Younger Adults	With Younger Adults and Children	With Children Only	Ended Membership/ Died	Number of Older Residents
Alone or only with older people	0	0	0	0	0	0
With younger adults	20	57	0	0	23	30
With younger adults and children	0	2	81	3	14	571
With children only	0	0	0	0	0	0
Was not yet a member/age less than 60	1	4	91	3	0	69
All households with older residents	1	4	79	3	13	670

3b Households in Which No Younger Adult Members (Ages 18-59) Died in 2000-2001

| | Membership of Household in 2002 | | | | | |
Membership of Household in 2000	Alone or Only with Older People	With Younger Adults	With Younger Adults and Children	With Children Only	Ended Membership/ Died	Number of Older Residents
Alone or only with older people	74	0	0	0	26	113
With younger adults	5	75	1	0	20	241
With younger adults and children	0	3	84	1	12	2,609
With children only	12	7	19	52	10	84
Was not yet a member/age less than 60	4	11	83	2	0	459
All households with older residents	4	9	74	2	11	3,506

3c All Households with Resident Members of Pensionable Age

Membership of Household in 2000	Membership of Household in 2002					
	Alone or Only with Older People	With Younger Adults	With Younger Adults and Children	With Children Only	Ended Membership/ Died	Number of Older Residents
Alone or only with older people	74	0	0	0	26	113
With younger adults	6	73	1	0	20	271
With younger adults and children	0	3	84	1	12	3,180
With children only	12	7	19	52	10	84
Was not yet a member/age less than 60	4	10	84	2	0	528
All households with older residents	3	8	75	2	11	4,176

TABLE 8-4 Percentage Distribution According to Age of the Other Residents in 2002 in Households with Residents of Pensionable Age by Age of the Other Residents in 2000

Residential Composition Household in 2000	Residential Composition of Household in 2002					
	Alone or Only with Older People	With Younger Adults	With Younger Adults and Children	With Children Only	Ended Membership/ Died	Number of Older Residents
Alone or only with older people	81	0	1	0	18	233
With younger adults	9	69	0	0	22	302
With younger adults and children	1	3	83	2	12	2,790
With children only	6	4	22	59	9	323
Was not yet a member/age less than 60	9	11	72	8	0	527
All households with older residents	7	8	66	7	11	4,175

residents. Households that experienced the death of a younger adult household member are shown separately from those that did not. Older people who were already living alone with children are not represented in the first of these two groups, although in some instances younger adult members may have joined the household and then died during the 2-year period under consideration. Table 8-4 presents data on changes of residence during 2000 and 2001 for all households with a resident older member.

Comparison of the changes in household type shown in Table 8-3 suggests that older people experiencing younger adult deaths in their households are more likely to undergo substantial changes in their living arrangements than older people living in unaffected households. Younger adult deaths were more likely to change the structure of the households of older people living in households without children than of those living in households with a child as well as adult members.

The death of a young adult left 15 additional older people in households that included children but had no younger adult members. Another 15 such households were created by people leaving or joining households. But these new skipped-generation households were matched by an equal number of shifts out of this type of household. During the 2 years, 38 percent of all those living initially in households with a child but no younger adult members either moved to join another household that had a younger adult member, were joined by a younger adult, or saw the children leave the household. Moreover, the de facto data in Table 8-4 show that the number of older people who were residing with only children and other older people dropped by 11 percent during the 2 years. While older people in skipped-generation households were more likely to have had their living arrangements change than other older people, no increase occurred in the proportion of older people living alone with children.

DISCUSSION

The ACDIS data reveal the high level of younger adult mortality that older people are facing in rural South Africa, even in most their immediate social sphere, with 20 percent of them experiencing such a death in their households in the 2-year period considered. Given the relatively short period of follow-up, longer term changes in the living arrangements of older people experiencing a death in their household late in the period have not been observed. However, as one might suspect, living in a household in which a younger adult dies raises the likelihood that the older person's household no longer contains young adults at the end of the period of follow-up.

Neither the ACDIS data nor the census data provide any evidence that the increase in adult mortality resulting from the HIV/AIDS epidemic is raising greatly the prevalence of skipped-generation households. Data from other African countries also suggest that the majority of older people continue to live in extended, multigenerational households. Recent Demographic and Health Survey data from 16 countries in sub-Saharan Africa show that fewer than 5 percent of older people were living with children and no adults (Zimmer and Dayton, 2003). Even in Uganda, a country with a relatively mature HIV epidemic, the proportion of skipped-generation households was less than 2 percent in 1995 (Ntozi and Zirimenya, 1999).

In discussing the results of their modeling of the living arrangements of older people in South Africa, Merli and Palloni (this volume, Chapter 4) also note that the household composition is not evolving in the way anticipated. They suggest that the lack of increase in older people living with grandchildren in skipped-generation households "may be because the epidemic has not worked its way through with sufficient force, because individuals and groups react in ways that conceal the trail left by HIV/AIDS, or because we may be unable to distinguish the effects associated with HIV/AIDS from those triggered by migration, which mimics the effects of HIV/AIDS on the availability of kin, or those induced by modernization, which changes preferences for coresidence."

These suggestions echo issues we identified in the first two sections of this paper. Even prior to the HIV epidemic in South Africa, older people played an enormously important role in the care of children and the maintenance of rural households. However, it remains fairly unusual for a household with young children and older people not to include any of the children's parents, aunts, or uncles (i.e., the older person's adult children). In South Africa, low marriage rates, extensive labor migration, and the costs involved in establishing independent dwellings have acted to slow the trend toward nuclearization of family life usually observed in the course of development and encouraged younger adults to remain members of their parental household (Bongaarts and Zimmer, 2002). Most families would acknowledge their responsibility toward those older people who are in need of care and support themselves. Thus, it is rare to find young children caring for older people alone without the assistance of adults. Of course, there are older people in South Africa who have no surviving relatives in the next generation or who have lost touch with or quarreled with them all. Usually though, it is only in such extreme circumstances that the relatives of older people and children who find themselves coping alone after the death of an adult would not seek to alter the arrangement. This can be achieved by sending adults to help or placing the children (or the older person, or both) in another household. Thus, in Umkhanyakude, 9-10 percent of older people coreside with their grandchildren or other young children while their adult children are absent. However, less than 30 percent of these de facto skipped-generation households had no younger adult members. Moreover, only half the latter households survived for 2 years, indicating that they are vulnerable to dissolution and the dispersal of their members to other households or to change through younger adults joining the household (Hosegood, McGrath, Herbst, and Timaeus, 2004; Ford and Hosegood, 2005).

The old age pension may also encourage younger adults and children to live with, and if necessary care for, older people in South Africa. The pension may act as a "magnet" that ensures that households with older people are attractive for adult as well as child dependents. Therefore, even after the death of the older person's own adult children, other relatives may be eager to ensure that they do not live alone. In many South African households, older people may be "burdened" by the young rather than vice versa, although in others the pension may just mean that the cost of caring for an older person is reduced.

Although we emphasize that it is rare for older people to live with children without younger adults as coresident or nonresident members of the household, we do not wish to minimize the difficulties faced by older people and children who find themselves, even temporarily, in this situation. In part the severity of these difficulties will depend on the age of the older people with whom children live. The grandmothers of most children under age 18 in South Africa will be fairly young and may be able to provide them with considerable economic, financial, and emotional care. In households containing frail older people, however, the primary direction of caregiving may be from the child or children to the older person.

This study has not examined indicators of well-being for older people and other members of households. However, we believe that for policy makers and programs to target skipped-generation households may be a very poor way of identifying the most vulnerable households. Given the importance of labor migration in South Africa, one would need to examine patterns of residence and caregiving in some detail to determine the extent to which older people and children live alone for considerable periods of time without significant assistance from younger adults and how well they are able to cope with the demands that this places on them.

The impact of HIV/AIDS on older people is receiving increasing research attention. However, there remains a serious lack of empirical data that can be used to examine a broad range of outcomes. Few surveys collect data on the morbidity, nutritional status, or mental health of older people. There are also limited data with which to assess wider impacts of the HIV epidemic on older people, such as stigmatization and isolation following AIDS deaths in their households, increased financial insecurity and increased workloads, and deterioration in the availability and quality of health and welfare services.

We have sought to highlight aspects of life in South Africa that influence the demographic, health, and economic characteristics of older people, as well as those that influence the impact of HIV/AIDS on them. Our population-based data from rural KwaZulu-Natal demonstrate that HIV/AIDS is very much part of many older peoples' lives today. However, we also suggest that adaptive strategies are being adopted by many households to protect dependent individuals, including older people. The existence of a substantial noncontributory old age pension in South Africa is undoubtedly of huge benefit both to those older people whose lives have been affected by AIDS and those who have not. In addition, the fluid nature of households, the limited involvement of most of them in agricultural production, and the stretching of household groups due to migration—all of which developed in response to the political economy of apartheid—give social networks and living arrangements in South Africa a degree of flexibility that benefits many older people when adverse advents occur, such as the death of an adult child.

REFERENCES

Adamchak, D.J., Wilson, A.O., Nyanguru, A., and Hampson, J. (1991). Elderly support and intergenerational transfer in Zimbabwe: An analysis by gender, marital status, and place of residence. *South African Journal of Gerontology, 31*, 505-513.

Barnett, T., and Whiteside, A. (1999). HIV/AIDS and development: Case studies and a conceptual framework. *European Journal of Development Research, 11*(2), 200-234.

Barnett, T., and Whiteside, A. (2000). *Guidelines for studies of the social and economic impact of HIV/AIDS.* (Best Practice Collection). Geneva, Switzerland: Joint United Nations Programme on HIV/AIDS.

Berk, M.L., Schur, C.L., Dunbar, J.L., Bozette, S., and Shapiro, M. (2003). Short report: Migration among persons living with HIV. *Social Science and Medicine, 57*, 1091-1097.

Bongaarts, J., and Zimmer, Z. (2002). Living arrangements of the elderly in the developing world: An analysis of DHS household surveys. *Journal of Gerontology Series B: Psychological Sciences and Social Sciences, 57*(3), S145-S157.

Bradshaw, D., Bourne, D., Schneider, M., and Sayed, R. (1995). Mortality patterns of chronic diseases of lifestyle in South Africa. (Medical Research Council Technical Report). In J. Fourie and K. Steyn (Eds.), *Chronic diseases of lifestyle in South Africa.* Cape Town, South Africa: Medical Research Council.

Burman, S. (1995). Child care by the elderly and the duty of support in multigenerational households. *Southern African Journal of Gerontology, 4*(1), 13-17.

Campbell, C. (1994). Intergenerational conflict in township families: Transforming notions of respect and changing power relations. *Southern African Journal of Gerontology, 3*(2), 37-42.

Case, A. (2001). *Does money protect health status? Evidence from South African pensions.* (NBER Working Paper No. 8495). Cambridge, MA: National Bureau of Economic Research.

Case, A., and Ardington, C. (2004). *ACDIS monograph: Socioeconomic factors.* Mtubatuba, South Africa: Africa Centre for Health and Population Studies.

Case, A., and Deaton, A. (1998). Large cash transfers to the elderly in South Africa. *Economic Journal, 108*(450), 1330-1361.

Case, A., Hosegood, V., and Lund, F. (2003). Child support grant study findings. *Children First, 51,* 45-49.

Case, A., Hosegood, V., and Lund, F. (2005). The reach of the South African child support grant: Evidence from KwaZulu-Natal. *Development Southern Africa, 22*(4), 467-482.

Dayton, J., and Ainsworth, M. (2002). *The elderly and AIDS: Coping strategies and health consequences in rural Tanzania.* (Working Paper No. 1). New York: The Population Council.

Dorrington, R., Bourne, D., Bradshaw, D., Laubscher, R., and Timaeus, I.M. (2001). *The impact of HIV/AIDS on adult mortality in South Africa.* Tygerberg, South Africa: Burden of Disease Unit, Medical Research Council.

Dorrington, R., Moultrie, T.A., and Timaeus, I.M. (2004). *Estimation of mortality using the South African census 2001 data* (Monograph No. 11). Cape Town, South Africa: Centre for Actuarial Research, University of Cape Town. Available: http://www.commerce. uct.ac.za/care/Monographs/Monographs/Mono11.pdf [accessed February 2005].

Drew, R.S., Makufa, C., and Foster, G. (1998). Strategies for providing care and support to children orphaned by AIDS. *AIDS Care, 10*(Suppl. 1), 9-15.

Du Toit, B.M. (1994). Does the road get lonelier? Aging in a coloured community in South Africa. *Journal of Aging Studies, 8*(4), 357-374.

Ellis, M., and Muschkin, C. (1996). Migration of persons with AIDS: A search for support from elderly parents? *Social Science and Medicine, 43*(7), 1109-1118.

Ferreira, M. (2000). Growing old in the new South Africa. *Ageing International,* (Spring), 32-46.

Ferreira, M., Keikelame, M.P., and Mosaval, Y. (2001). *Older women as carers to children and grandchildren affected by AIDS: A study towards supporting the carers.* Cape Town, South Africa: Institute of Ageing in Africa, University of Cape Town.

Ferreira, M., Møller, V., Prinsloo, F.R., and Gillis, L.S. (1992). *Multidimensional survey of elderly South Africans, 1990-1991: Key findings.* (Monograph No. 1). Cape Town, South Africa: Human Sciences Research Council and HSRC/UCT Centre for Gerontology, University of Cape Town.

Ford, K., and Hosegood, V. (2005). AIDS mortality and the mobility of children in KwaZulu Natal, South Africa. *Demography, 42*(4), 757-768.

Foster, G., Shakespeare, R., Chinemana, F., Jackson, H., Gregson, S., Marange, C., and Mashumba, S. (1995). Orphan prevalence and extended family care in a periurban community in Zimbabwe. *AIDS Care, 7*(1), 3-17.

Gafos, M. (2003). *An analysis of the associations between migration, mortality, and health care usage in the adult population of Hlabisa District, KwaZulu Natal in South Africa.* Unpublished MSc thesis, London School of Hygiene and Tropical Medicine.

Gillis, L.S., Welman, M., Koch, A., and Joyi, M. (1991). Psychological distress and depression in urbanizing elderly black persons. *South African Medical Journal, 79*(8), 490-495.

Guest, E. (2001). *Children of AIDS: Africa's orphan crisis.* Pietermaritzburg, South Africa: University of Natal Press.

HelpAge International. (2000). *Ageing issues in Africa: A summary.* London, England: Author.

HelpAge International. (2003). *HIV/AIDS and ageing: A briefing paper.* London, England: Author. Available: http://www.helpage.org/images/pdfs/briefing%20papers/HIV% 20AIDS%20position%20paper.pdf [accessed December 2004].

Hosegood, V., and Timaeus, I.M. (2005). Household composition and dynamics in KwaZulu Natal, South Africa: Mirroring social reality in longitudinal data collection. In E. van der Walle (Ed.), *African households: Census data* (pp. 58-77). New York: M.E. Sharpe.

Hosegood, V., McGrath, N., Herbst, K., and Timaeus, I.M. (2004). The impact of adult mortality on household dissolution and migration in rural South Africa. *AIDS, 18*(11), 1585-1590.

Hosegood, V., Vanneste, A.M., and Timaeus, I.M. (2004). Levels and causes of adult mortality in rural South Africa. *AIDS, 18,* 1-19.

Human Sciences Research Council. (2002). *Nelson Mandela HSRC study of HIV/AIDS: Full report.* Pretoria, South Africa: Human Sciences Research Council Press. Available: http://www.hsrcpublishers.co.za/user_uploads/tblPDF/2009_00_Nelson_Mandela_HIV_Full_Report.pdf [accessed April 2005].

Hunter, N., and Rushby, J. (2002). *Annotated bibliography of recent research on the living conditions of the main target groups of social security grants.* (Research Report No. 53). Durban, South Africa: School of Development Studies.

Izzard, W. (1985). Migrants and mothers: Case-studies from Botswana. *Journal of Southern African Studies, 11*(2), 258-280.

Johnson, P. (1989). The structured dependency of the elderly: A critical note. In M. Jeffreys (Ed.), *Growing old in the twentieth century* (pp. 62-72). London, England: Routledge.

Kahn, K., and Tollman, S.M. (1999). Stroke in rural South Africa: Contributing to the little known about a big problem. *South African Medical Journal, 89*(1), 63-65.

Karim, Q.A., and Karim, S.S.A. (1999). Epidemiology of HIV infection in South Africa. *Aids, 13*(6), 4-7.

Kinsella, K., and Ferreira, M. (1997). *Ageing trends: South Africa.* Washington, DC: Department of Commerce, Bureau of the Census. Available: http://www.census.gov/ipc/prod/ib-9702.pdf [accessed December 2004].

Knodel, J., and VanLandingham, M. (2001). *Return migration in the context of parental assistance in the AIDS epidemic: The Thai experience.* (Population Studies Center Report No. 01-492). Ann Arbor: University of Michigan.

Knodel, J., Watkins, S.C., and VanLandingham, M. (2003). AIDS and older persons: An international perspective. *Journal of Acquired Immune Deficiency Syndrome, 33*(Suppl. 2), 153-165.

Knodel, J., Saengtienchai, C., Im-em, W., and VanLandingham, M. (2001a). The impact of AIDS on parents and families in Thailand. A key informant process. *Research on Ageing, 23*(6), 633-670.

Knodel, J., Saengtienchai, C., Im-em, W., and VanLandingham, M. (2001b). Older people and AIDS: Quantitative evidence of the impact in Thailand. *Social Science and Medicine, 52,* 1313-1327.

Leliveld, A. (1997). The effects of restrictive South African migrant labor policy on the survival of rural households in Southern Africa: A case study from rural Swaziland. *World Development, 25*(11), 1839-1849.

Levy, J.A., Ory, M.G., and Crystal, S. (2003). HIV/AIDS interventions for midlife and older adults: Current status and challenges. *Journal of Acquired Immune Deficiency Syndrome, 33*(Suppl. 2), 59-67.

Madhavan, S. (2004). Fosterage patterns in the age of AIDS: Continuity and change. *Social Science and Medicine, 58*(7), 1443-1454.

May, J. (2003a). *Chronic poverty and older people in South Africa.* (Working Paper No. 25, School of Development Studies). Durban, South Africa: Chronic Poverty Research Centre. Available: http://www.chronicpoverty.org/pdfs/JMay.pdf [accessed May 2005].

May, J. (2003b). *Extent, distribution, and nature of poverty among the elderly in South Africa.* Manchester, England: Chronic Poverty Research Centre.

Mazur, R.E. (1998). Migration dynamics and development in rural South Africa: Demographic and socioeconomic perspectives. In *Research in rural sociology and development, no. 7* (pp. 197-225). Greenwich, CT: JAI Press.

Mohatle, T., and de Graft Agyarko, R. (1999). *Contributions of older people to development: The South African study.* London, England: HelpAge International.

Møller, V., and Ferreira, M. (2003). *Getting by: Benefits of noncontributory pension income for older South African households.* Cape Town, South Africa: Institute of Ageing in Africa, University of Cape Town. Available: http://idpm.man.ac.uk/ncpps [accessed June 2005].

Møller, V., and Sotshongaye, A. (1996). My family eats this money too: Pension-sharing and self-respect among Zulu grandmothers. *South African Journal of Gerontology, 5*(2), 9-19.

Moultrie, T.A., and Timaeus, I.M. (2002). *Trends in South African fertility between 1970 and 1998: An analysis of the 1996 census and the 1998 demographic and health survey.* (Technical report). Tygerberg, South Africa: Medical Research Council. Available: http://www.mrc.ac.za/bod/trends.pdf [accessed March 2004].

Moultrie, T.A., and Timaeus, I.M. (2003). The South African fertility decline: Evidence from two censuses and a demographic and health survey. *Population Studies, 57*(3), 265-283.

Murray, C. (1980). Migrant labour and changing family structure in the rural periphery of Southern Africa. *Journal of Southern African Studies, 6*(2), 139-156.

Nhongo, T.M. (2004). *Impact of HIV/AIDS on generational roles and intergenerational relationships.* Paper presented at the National Research Council Workshop on HIV/AIDS and Family Well-Being, January 28-30, Namibia, South Africa.

Noumbissi, A., and Zuberi, T. (2001). *Household structure and aging in South Africa: A research note.* Presented at the African Census Analysis Project Virtual Conference on African Households, An Exploration of Census Data, November 21-24. Available: http://www.pop.upenn.edu/africahh/NoumbissiZuberi.pdf [accessed April 2005].

Noumbissi, A., Bawah, A.A., and Zuberi, T. (2005). Parental survival and residential patterns. In E. van der Walle (Ed.), *African households. Census data.* New York: M.E. Sharpe.

Ntozi, J.P.M., and Nakayiwa, S. (1999). AIDS in Uganda: How has the household coped with the epidemic? In I.O. Orubuloye, J.C. Caldwell, and J.P.M. Ntozi (Eds.), *The continuing HIV/AIDS epidemic in Africa: Response and coping strategies* (pp. 155-180). Canberra, Australia: Health Transition Centre, Australian National University.

Ntozi, J.P.M., and Zirimenya, S. (1999). Changes in household composition and family structure during the AIDS epidemic in Uganda. In I.O. Orubuloye, J.C. Caldwell, and J.P.M. Ntozi (Eds.), *The continuing HIV/AIDS epidemic in Africa: Responses and coping strategies* (pp. 193-209). Canberra, Australia: Health Transition Centre, Australian National University.

Nyambedha, E.O., Wandibba, S., and Aagaard-Hansen, J. (2003). Changing patterns of orphan care due to HIV epidemic in western Kenya. *Social Science and Medicine, 57,* 301-311.

Preston-Whyte, E. (1978). Families without marriage: A Zulu case study. In J. Argyle and E. Preston-Whyte (Eds.), *Social system and tradition in Southern Africa: Essays in honour of Eileen Krige* (pp. 55-85). Cape Town, South Africa: Oxford University Press.

Preston-Whyte, E. (1988). Women-headed households and development: The relevance of cross-cultural models for research on black women in Southern Africa. *Africanus, 18,* 58-76.

Rugalema, G. (1999). It is not only the loss of labor: HIV/AIDS, loss of household assets and household livelihood in Bukoba district, Tanzania. In G. Mutangadura, H. Jackson, and D. Mukurazita (Eds.), *AIDS and African smallholder agriculture.* Harare, Zimbabwe: Southern Africa HIV and AIDS Information and Dissemination Service.

Sagner, A. (2000). Ageing and social policy in South Africa: Historical perspectives with particular reference to the Eastern Cape. *Journal of Southern African Studies, 26*(3), 523-553.

South Africa Department of Health. (2005). *National HIV and syphilis antenatal seroprevalence survey in South Africa, 2004.* Pretoria: Author. Available: http://www.doh. gov.za/docs/reports/2004/hiv-syphilis.pdf [accessed December 2004].

South Africa Department of Social Development. (2001). *Mothers and fathers of the nation: The forgotten people?* (Vol. 1, main report—Ministerial Committee on Abuse, Neglect, and Ill-treatment of Older Persons). Pretoria: Author. Available: http://www.welfare. gov.za/Documents/2001/March/elder.htm [accessed March 2005].

Spiegel, A. (1987). Dispersing dependents: A response to the exigencies of labour migration in rural Transkei. In J. Eades (Ed.), *Migrants, workers, and the social order* (pp. 113-129). London, England: Tavistock.

Timaeus, I.M. (1999). Mortality in sub-Saharan Africa. In J. Chamie and R.L. Cliquet (Eds.), *Health and mortality: Issues of global concern* (pp. 108-131). New York: Population Division, United Nations and Population and Family Study Centre.

Townsend, N. (1997). Reproduction in anthropology and demography. In D. Kertzer and T. Fricke (Eds.), *Anthropological demography: Toward a new synthesis* (pp. 96-114). Chicago, IL: University of Chicago Press.

U.S. Census Bureau. (2005). *International database.* Available: http://www.census.gov/ipc/www/idbsum.html (accessed August 26, 2005).

Van der Waal, C.S. (1996). Rural children and residential instability in the Northern Province of South Africa. *Social Dynamics, 22*(1), 31-54.

Walker, A.R. (2001). Changes in public health in South Africa from 1876. *Journal of the Royal Society of Health, 121*(2), 85-93.

Weltz, T., and Hosegood, V. (2003, December). *Population-based HIV surveillance in the Hlabisa DSS, South Africa.* Presented at Forum 7, Global Forum for Health Research, Geneva, Switzerland.

Wilkinson, D., Connolly, C., and Rotchford, K. (1999). Continued explosive rise in HIV prevalence among pregnant women in rural South Africa. *Aids, 13*(6), 740.

Wilson, A.O., and Adamchak, D.J. (2001). The grandmothers' disease: The impact of AIDS on Africa's older women. *Age and Ageing, 30,* 8-10.

Women's Budget Initiative. (2003). *What's available? A guide to government grants and other support available to individuals and community groups.* Cape Town, South Africa. Available: http://www.internationalbudget.org/resources/library/govtfunds.pdf [accessed June 2005].

World Health Organization. (2002). *The impact of AIDS on older persons in Africa.* Geneva, Switzerland: Author.

Yamano, T., and Jayne, T.S. (2004). Measuring the impact of working-age adult mortality on small-scale farm households in Kenya. *World Development, 32*(1), 91-119.

Zimmer, Z., and Dayton, J. (2003). *The living arrangements of older adults in sub-Saharan Africa in a time of HIV/AIDS.* (Report No. 169). New York: The Population Council.

9

Interactions Between Socioeconomic Status and Living Arrangements in Predicting Gender-Specific Health Status Among the Elderly in Cameroon

Barthélémy Kuate-Defo

INTRODUCTION

The most influential factor historically in the aging of human populations has been fertility reductions. All populations with declining fertility become older, and the speed of aging increases as mortality declines. For the first time in history, many societies in Africa now have the opportunity to age. Accompanying this broad demographic process, however, are other changes—shifting disease patterns and emerging health threats, macroeconomic strains, emergent technologies, changing work patterns and social norms, and cultural practices within and between societies. These dramatic changes in fertility responses and unprecedented mortality reductions in Africa since the 1950s ensure that the population of this continent is bound to age quite rapidly half a century later.

The secular decline in fertility rates historically has been shown to be the most important factor of population aging, via a sustained increase in the ratio of older to younger people. The fall of mortality rates from a combination of advances in public health (e.g., immunization campaigns), medical technology, and standard of living (e.g., better nutrition) has resulted in improvements in life expectancy. Recent estimates suggest that the aggregate proportions of the elderly population in sub-Saharan Africa will grow rather modestly as a result of continued high fertility in many countries, but the size of the elderly population is expected to increase by 50 percent, from 19.3 to 28.9 million people from 2000 to 2015 (National Research Council, 2001).

These fertility and unprecedented mortality reductions, along with declines in deaths from infections and parasitic diseases, have resulted in increases in life expectancy throughout the world, leading to increasing numbers and proportions of elderly people. This demo-epidemiological transition has been attributed to public health measures, advances in medical science, and health care. Irrespective of reasons, people are living longer and many of them are having more years of healthy, active, and independent life, especially in developed countries.

In contrast, there is a dearth of information and research on the health status and functional limitations of the older populations of many developing countries in general (Gorman, 2002; National Research Council, 2001; Palloni, Pinto-Aguirre, and Pelaez, 2002; Restrepo and Rozental, 1994) and notably in African countries. In this region of the world, population aging coincides with increasing social inequalities, poverty, unemployment, violence, malnutrition, and the devastating and differentiated effects of the rampant HIV/AIDS epidemic on individuals, families, communities, and nations.

The causes and consequences of aging in this region within and between countries are complex, multifactorial, and intertwined. Their study is difficult and demands an interdisciplinary approach, given the complexity of the interactions among social, economic, and environmental variables and their effect on health status and functional limitations. The projected increase in the number of older people poses new challenges to researchers, policy makers, and planners. This paper addresses the following questions: Is the population in Africa living healthier, longer lives or are added years accompanied by disabilities and generally poor health? How do changing family structures and socioeconomic conditions affect the prevalence of poor health and limited activity among the elderly?

Since current and prospective policy responses are likely to differ among countries in Africa, a number of natural experiments are needed to enable countries to learn from each other's experiences. This study examines self-reported health and physical functional status among older people in a transitional environment—the rural and semirural societies of Cameroon—and compares their determinants in men and women. Such an investigation is important as a contrast to the general tendency to focus on urban areas of less developed countries and sub-Saharan Africa. Although differences in health between the richest and the poorest segments of the populations in many societies are clearly identifiable, differences among the rural, semirural, and urban areas of Africa may not be so obvious. In addition to variations in life expectancy, population health, and adult mortality, self-ratings of poor health and disability are likely to be lower in semirural areas than in most urban settings, and the average rate of self-reporting of good health and functional status is usually lower in rural than in urban areas. Furthermore, some differences in social influences (e.g., education, social norms and practices) on perceived health among urban, semirural, and rural dwellers are most likely to be present.

With no study to my knowledge in Africa that has focused simultaneously on the health and functional status of rural and semirural segments of the elderly, research in this area is needed. There is a growing consensus among public health researchers and policy makers that more information is required on the mechanisms that produce gender differences in health outcomes in different social settings (Arber and Ginn, 1993; MacIntyre, Hunt, and Sweeting, 1996). This study explores the health differences between older women and men living in 75 urban and rural localities of Cameroon, with the ultimate aim of extending the information and knowledge base to prevent social exclusion and promote the health of older women and men in Africa. This paper seeks to examine the extent and nature of gender inequalities in health in later life and the extent to which these inequalities can be explained by differences in socioeconomic characteristics and the living arrangements of older women and men. The ultimate goal is to provide local health researchers, professionals, and community organizations with information needed to plan gender-sensitive interventions to promote the health and quality of life of older women and men. More specifically, I consider the following research questions:

1. What explains gender differences in health and functional status among older people?

2. By what mechanisms and to what extent do high socioeconomic status and better living arrangements lead to better health and functional status?

3. To what extent and by what mechanisms are the effects of socioeconomic status and living arrangements on health and functional status of older people dependent on gender?

There are several plausible ways in which certain aspects of gender inequality, socioeconomic status, and living arrangements may influence health and functional status at older ages. For many of these influences, however, empirical studies are lacking that can confirm the importance of particular intermediate variables. The socioeconomic status and living arrangements of older women and men and their possible connections with health and disability may be understood only in particular sociocultural contexts, given the relative position of women and men in different societies (Anker, Buvinic, and Youssef, 1983). This is because indicators of socioeconomic status and living arrangements tend to be heavily context-dependent and also because particular aspects of female versus male status may have contradictory effects on health and disability in different sociocultural contexts.

This paper is devoted to the centrality of health and functional status by focusing on gender, socioeconomic status, and living arrangement differentials in informing health, social, and economic policy formulation. The first section presents the data and methods used for analysis. The next section presents the results. The final section summarizes the main findings and discusses their implications.

DATA AND METHODS OF ANALYSIS

The Data

The study uses data from the first round of the Cameroon Family Life and Health Survey (CFHS), conducted in 1996-1997. This is a survey of representative and randomly selected individuals age 10 and older in 75 urban and rural localities in Cameroon. Each locality uses probability samples in which all households with individuals age 10 and older have a nonzero chance of inclusion, designed to produce comparable locality-level estimates for the population under study. The CFHS employs a self-weighted proportional sampling design, with the proportions of randomly sampled households in all 75 localities forming the Bandjoun region in the sample equal to the same proportions in the general population. The sample was drawn so as to be representative in each of the following age- and sex-specific groups: adolescent boys ages 10-19, adolescent girls ages 10-19, men ages 20-49, women ages 20-49, men age 50 and above, and women age 50 and above. After a household has been selected, one individual among all respondents in that household was randomly selected and interviewed until the sample size required for a given locality was attained. A total sample of 2,381 individuals was interviewed, of whom 631 were age 50 and older. Further details regarding sampling methodology and the survey have been published elsewhere (Kuate-Defo, 1998, 2005; Kuate-Defo and Lepage, 1997). The postulated risk and protective factors used in this study are presented in Table 9-1.

The survey was carried out in the prefecture of Bandjoun, in the western part of Cameroon. This area is representative of the system of beliefs, customs, and social structure of the population of Cameroon. In an area of approximately 274 sq km, this region combines the features of a highly modernized environment with a typical traditional Cameroonian society. The urban and semiurban localities of Bandjoun have one of the country's universities, three public hospitals, two private hospitals in operation since the early 1950s, about a dozen public health centers, several traditional healers attracting people from various social strata, several high schools and professional schools, infrastructures for communication and transportation, and entertainment sites. In the rural areas, there are over 70 tradi-

TABLE 9-1 Sample Proportions of People Age 50 and Older in the Cameroon Family Life and Health Survey, 1996-1997

Variables	Total Sample (N = 613)		Men (N = 270)		Women (N = 343)	
	N	%	N	%	N	%
Outcome Variables						
Self-Rated Health						
Excellent/very good/good/fair	474	77.3	227	84.1	247	72.0
Poor	139	22.7	43	15.9	96	28.0
Physical Functional Limitations						
No	309	50.4	167	61.9	142	41.4
Yes	304	49.6	103	38.1	201	58.6
Poor Health and Functional Limitations						
No	506	82.5	238	88.1	268	78.1
Yes	107	17.5	32	11.9	75	21.9
Exposure Variables						
Gender						
Female	343	56.0	—	—	—	—
Male	270	44.0	—	—	—	—
Level of Education						
None	452	73.7	133	49.3	319	93.0
Some education	161	26.3	137	50.7	24	7.0

Economic Activity Status					
Paid work	162	26.4	108	40.0	54	15.7
Unpaid work	111	18.1	54	20.0	57	16.6
Retired/at home	253	41.3	70	25.9	183	53.4
Unemployed	87	14.2	38	14.1	49	14.3
Marital Status					
Single/widowed/divorced	218	35.6	31	11.5	187	54.5
Married polygamous	211	34.4	109	40.4	102	29.8
Married monogamous	184	30.0	130	48.1	54	15.7
Age at First Marriage (continuous variable)	Mean = 23.2	SD = 8.68	Mean= 29.15	SD = 9.26	Mean = 18.33	SD = 3.71
Kinship Size					
Less than 6	348	56.8	150	55.6	198	57.7
6 or more	265	43.2	120	44.4	145	42.3
Age Cohort (in years)					
50-64	301	49.1	128	47.4	173	50.4
65-74	196	32.0	90	33.3	106	30.9
75-96	116	18.9	52	19.3	64	18.7
Main Region of Residence					
Djaa/Pete/Yom	213	34.7	135	39.4	78	28.9
Djiomghouo/Famleng/Tsela	129	21.0	72	21.0	57	21.1
Demdeng/Sedembom/Haa	164	26.8	88	25.7	76	28.1
Tsela/Famla II/Bagang Fodji	107	17.5	48	14.0	59	21.9

tional chiefdoms with traditional authorities and practices, an extensive practice of polygamy and other gender-related practices, agricultural production, and extensive farming. The geographical distribution of the population reflects one of the highest population densities (a population of over 120,000 inhabitants, thus a density of about 438 inhabitants per sq km) and the highest fertility levels (a total fertility rate close to 7) in the country. The entire region is accessible in all seasons of the year.

Measurements of Self-Rated Health and Functional Limitations

In this study, self-rated health was assessed among 631 individuals residing in 75 urban and rural localities in Cameroon, through a question asked about perceived general health: "Would you say that in general your health is: Excellent, Very Good, Good, Fair, or Poor?" From this item, the study used a dichotomous outcome measure coded 1 if poor and 0 if excellent, very good, good, or fair. Thus, health status for all persons age 50 or older is based on an overall assessment of individual health on a 5-point scale (5 = very good, 4 = quite good, 3 = average, 2 = quite poor, 1= poor).

This measure is one of the most frequently used health status measures in population-based epidemiological research and has been a powerful predictor of morbidity and mortality. It has been demonstrated in previous studies that the reliability of self-rated health has been as good as or even better than that of the multiitem health scales. A review of 27 community studies concluded that even such a simple global assessment appears to have high predictive validity for mortality, independent of other medical, behavioral, or psychosocial risk factors (Idler and Benyamini, 1997). Several subsequent studies have also demonstrated the usefulness of capturing the health status of the elderly persons and their determinants by focusing on such a simple operational measure of health. For most studies, odds ratios for subsequent mortality ranged from 1.5 to 3.0 among individuals reporting poor health compared with those reporting excellent health.

Self-reported health has been demonstrated in longitudinal studies to predict the onset of physical disability and functional or activity limitations (Farmer and Ferraro, 1997; Ferraro, Farmer, and Wybraniec, 1997; Idler and Benyamini, 1997; Idler and Kasl, 1995; Mor et al., 1989; Wilcox, Kasl, and Idler, 1996). While the majority of the elderly are capable of maintaining their autonomy, a sizeable proportion increasing at each age becomes frail and in need of support and care at home or in institutions.

I consider a dependent variable measuring the coexistence of poor health and disability. I do so because not all of those who are ill have functional limitations, and vice versa. What is important is the ability to cope with daily life in spite of chronic morbidity and the degree to which the elderly may need assistance to continue to do this even at decreased levels of activity.

Such functional activity is widely measured by indices of activities of daily living. In this study, functional status was measured among 631 individuals age 50 and over by asking the following questions: "Do you have any activity limitation in fulfilling your activities of daily life? If yes, what is the nature of that limitation? Is the limitation in activity at home, at work, elsewhere, and during leisure/travel?" From answers to these three questions, the researchers created a dichotomous outcome measure coded 1 if any functional limitation was reported and 0 otherwise. We also created a third outcome variable measuring the simultaneous reporting of poor health and functional limitations coded 1 if an elderly person reported as being in poor health also had a limitation in activity and 0 otherwise.

Methods of Analysis

The methods of data analysis in this paper include the description of variables, followed by an examination of the association between each risk or protective factor and the three outcome variables (bivariate analyses), as well as the study of the interrelationships between the different risk or protective factors in predicting the outcomes (multivariate analyses). Since the primary goal is to evaluate the effect of a postulated risk or protective factor on each outcome, I investigate what this effect is before and after controlling for other factors so as to determine whether such an effect is direct or mediated through other postulated risk or protective factors. A mediating factor is a link in the causal chain leading from the postulated risk factor to the outcome and is partly determined by that risk factor.

To illustrate the general strategy, consider three postulated risk factors (V1, V2, and V3) of poor health or disability (or both) among older people. The overall effect of each risk factor (or group of risk factors) V1 is evaluated first (Model A). In the second step, another putative factor or a set of factors V2 is added (Model B) and its effect assessed in the presence of V1, which would then constitute a proper confounding factor. The unconfounded effect of V2 would then be obtained from this equation. The magnitude of the remaining effect of V1 in Model B would reflect only the part that is not mediated through V2. Model B is then extended to add another postulated risk factor V3 in Model C and its effect assessed in the presence of both confounding variables, V1 and V2. Any residual effect of V1 would be the part that is not mediated through either V2 or V3. Similarly, any residual effect of V2 would not be mediated through V3. In interpreting the results, it is worth noting that some if not most of the effect of V1 will be captured by the other two factors (V2 and V3). It would be incorrect to interpret that V1 has no effect after adjustment for confound-

ing variables, since in Model C the overall effect of V1 will be underesti-
mated due to the presence of mediating factors. The strategy may be extended to situations with several variables in each hierarchical level of model
building.

I use general health status and physical functional status and not more
refined cause-specific or level of severity measures because differences in
reporting of such fine-tuned measures can obscure underlying events by
misclassifying outcomes. Empirically, we measure socioeconomic status using two indicators given their pertinence in the study context: level of educational attainment and economic activity status. Living arrangements are
empirically assessed using three indicators: marital status by type of union,
timing of first marriage in the life cycle, and family size support network.
The effects of gender, socioeconomic status, and living arrangements on
self-reported health and physical functional limitations are estimated with
logistic regression models. The general logistic regression model used can
be described as follows:

$$Y_i = \alpha + \beta X_i + \vartheta Z_i + \lambda W_i + \eta C_i$$

where Y_i is the value of individual i on the outcome Y. Since all three outcomes considered in this study are dichotomous (i.e., poor health, functional limitations, poor health with functional limitations), Y_i equals the
logit (or log-odds), α the overall constant or intercept, X_i the value of the
gender of individual i and β the vector of gender effects, Z_i the vector
of socioeconomic status indicators and ϑ the vector of associated parameters, W_i the vector of living arrangements factors and λ its vector of parameters, and C_i the vector of control variables and η the vector of their
corresponding parameters. These models estimate the odds ratios of poor
health (versus excellent/very good/good/fair health), functional limitations,
and poor health with functional limitations, according to gender and various indicators of socioeconomic status and living arrangements. I use this
common statistical technique for studying dichotomous outcomes, which
assumes that, for all individuals in the sample, these outcomes are independent. This procedure is appropriate because in the 1996-1997 CFHS survey, only one person per household was included in the sample, so that
outcomes for family or household members are not correlated, and there is
no room for the health or functional status of one unit in the sample to be
dependent on attributes shared by other members, such as sanitary conditions in the household. Thus, the single-level regression models fitted here
correctly ignore any hierarchical data structure and produce correct standard errors, so that the effects of factors associated with poor health and
disability in the elderly cannot appear significant when in fact they are not.

Thus, one attractive feature of the CFHS-1996-1997 is that the survey data are self-weighted.

RESULTS

Descriptive Analyses

The sample consisted of 631 individuals age 50 years and over (44 percent men, 56 percent women) and 319 individuals age 65 and over (45.8 percent men, 54.2 percent women). Perceived health was missed in just 16 (2.5 percent) individuals age 50 or older and 6 (1.9 percent) individuals age 65 or older, and functional limitations were missed in 14 (2.2 percent) individuals age 50 or older and 5 (1.6 percent) individuals age 65 or older. The rest of the analyses focuses on individuals age 50 years and over, unless otherwise stated. Gender-specific sample characteristics are shown in Table 9-1.

Overall, 22.7 percent of individuals reported their health as being poor, 49.6 percent reported limitations in activity, and 17.5 percent reported having both poor health and functional limitations. Of the 304 individuals who reported limitations, 164 (26 percent) reported being limited in activity at home, 231 (36.6 percent) reported being limited in activity at work, 46 (7.3 percent) reported being limited in activity outside the home, and 194 (30.7 percent) reported having functional limitations for leisure or travel activities.

The two socioeconomic status variables considered in the analyses show important gender disparities. Overall, the level of education of this semirural population is quite low, and 73.7 percent of the sample is illiterate. These data indicate that the numbers and proportions of people who are unemployed or retired are highest among the elderly. The female disadvantage among the elderly is sizeable, since fully 93 percent of older women have no education compared with almost half of older men. Similarly, unemployment is substantially higher for women than for men, and fully 60 percent of men age 50 and over are still working outside the home. But one must keep in mind that most women who reported being "at home" are actually farmers, notably in typical rural and periurban areas of Africa and western Cameroon. Hence, they are probably responsible for providing food and material resources to their family through the output of their agricultural labor.

The three variables capturing living arrangements in the elderly also depict important differences by gender. About one-third of the sample is married monogamous, married polygamous, or single/widowed/divorced, respectively. When analyses are separated by gender, the proportion of older women who are widowed (the main category in the single/widowed/divorced group) is almost five times higher than the proportion of their male counterparts. In contrast, the proportion of older women who are married monogamous (15.7 percent) is only about one-third the proportion of older men in monogamous marriages (48.1 percent). The pattern of age at marriage behaves as expected, with older women being married quite young compared with older men. Irrespective of gender, there is stability in the sample proportions for kinship size (roughly 42-44 percent of the sample having at least six persons in their kinship network).

The age distribution shows that almost half of the sample analyzed is between ages 50 and 65, and only 19 percent of respondents are age 75 and over; the oldest person in the sample was 96 years old. The sample proportions by gender show no differences worthy of notice.

The distribution of respondents by region of residence indicates that about one-third of the sample lives in the urban or semiurban areas of Djaa, Pete, and Yom. The urban regions are considered as the reference category in the analyses, and there are slightly more older men (39.4 percent) than women (28.9 percent) in urban centers.

Differentials by Health and Functional Status of the Elderly

Table 9-2 displays the significance of the differences in the percentages of respondents reporting poor health, functional limitations, and both poor health and functional limitations. Notwithstanding a few nonsignificant differences in kinship size and region of residence, all other differences in postulated risk and protective factors of poor health and activity limitations are statistically significant.

In particular, these bivariate analyses show that significantly higher proportions of female respondents report being in poor health, having functional limitations, or both than male respondents. Higher percentages of older respondents with no education report poor health, functional limitations, or both, than their educated counterparts. These differences are statistically significant for all outcomes, except that the results for older women with functional limitations do not vary with educational attainment. In general, older persons who are retired or who stay at home and to some extent those who are unemployed report significantly more poor health, activity limitations, or both than their counterparts who are in the labor force.

Single, widowed, or divorced elderly people tend to report significantly more poor health and functional limitations than those in monogamous marriages, and women tend to be at a disadvantage compared with men. Significantly higher proportions of older persons who are in polygamous marriages report poor health (20.4 percent), functional limitations (51.7 percent), or both (16.6 percent) than older people married in monogamous unions (13.6, 38.6, and 10.3 percent, respectively). A similar pattern is detected along gender lines, although the general tendency is that older women in all marital states report more poor health and functional limitations than older men. Kinship size of six or more is an advantage for older men, who tend to report lower prevalence of poor health, activity limitations, or both; in contrast, no significant differences in health or functional status by kinship size are found among older women.

In general, the age-specific percentages of older people reporting poor health, limitations in activity, or both consistently show significant dose-response patterns: the older the respondent, the higher the proportions reporting these conditions for the total sample as well as for the male and female samples.

Multivariate Findings

In this section, I regress individual health and functional status on gender, socioeconomic status, living arrangements, and biodemographic putative factors.

Covariates of Poor Health

Table 9-3a presents the estimated odds ratios for the effects of postulated covariates on the probability of reporting poor health, functional limitations, or both. Poor perceived health is associated with low socioeconomic status (i.e., no/lower educational attainment, no labor force participation), being single/widowed/divorced or married in polygamous unions, and being older. The strongest risk factors for poor health are living as single, widowed, or divorced (e.g., odds ratio of 3.06 in Model 5 and 1.89 at the 5 percent significance level in the full model—Model 12), whereas the protective factors for poor health are younger ages (e.g., odds ratios of 0.50 in Model 6 and 0.58 in the Model 12) and working status (e.g., odds ratios of 0.49 in Model 4 and 0.57 in Model 12).

The data show the existence of significant gender differences in self-reported health: Model 1 predicts that older women are more than twice as likely to report being in poor health as older men ($p < 0.01$). The male health advantage persists even after controlling for level of educational attainment, although its magnitude and explanatory power is somewhat attenuated (odds ratio of 0.58, $p < 0.05$). Moreover, when economic activity status is included in the regression equation, the significance of the gender differences in self-reported health is eliminated (Model 7), whereas the significance of the negative association between work and poor health (odds ratios varying between 0.49 and 0.57 at the 5 percent level of significance in Models 4, 7, 10, 11, 12) remains until a control for functional limitations is introduced in the fitted model (Model 13). Put together, these results sub-

TABLE 9-2 Bivariate Analyses of Differences in Health Status by Gender, Socioeconomic Status, Living Arrangements, and Other Putative Covariates

Variables	Percentage with Poor Health		
	Total	Men	Women
Gender	$p < 0.01$		
Female	28.0	—	—
Male	15.9	—	—
Level of Education	$p < 0.01$	$p < 0.05$	$p < 0.05$
None	25.7	18.0	28.8
Some education	14.3	13.9	16.7
Economic Activity Status	$p < 0.01$	$p < 0.01$	$p < 0.01$
Paid work	13.6	13.0	14.8
Unpaid work	13.5	9.3	17.5
Retired/at home	32.0	21.4	36.1
Unemployed	24.1	23.7	24.5
Marital Status	$p < 0.01$	$p < 0.05$	$p < 0.01$
Single/widowed/divorced	32.6	19.4	34.8
Married polygamous	20.4	18.3	22.5
Married monogamous	13.6	13.1	14.8
Age at First Marriage (continuous variable)			
Kinship Size	NS	$p < 0.05$	NS
Less than 6	24.1	20.0	27.3
6 or more	20.8	10.8	29.0
Age Cohort (in years)	$p < 0.01$	$p < 0.05$	$p < 0.01$
50-64	16.6	11.7	20.2
65-75	28.1	17.3	34.0
75-96	29.3	21.1	39.1
Main Region of Residence	$p < 0.05$	NS	NS
Djaa/Pete/Yom	26.3	19.2	30.4
Demdeng/Sedembom/Haa	25.6	18.4	31.8
Djiomghouo/Famleng/Tsela	20.9	14.0	26.4
Tsela/Famla II/Bagang Fodji	13.1	10.2	16.7

stantiate that gender differences in self-reported health among the elderly in Cameroon are entirely explained by their socioeconomic status.

The data show that there appears to be a dose-response gradient in the odds ratios for poor health across levels of socioeconomic indicators. In Model 2, the data show that older people with no education are more than twice as likely to report being in poor health as their educated counterparts ($p < 0.01$). Model 3 shows that gender inequality entirely explains differences in self-reported health and education, and Model 4 indicates that economic activity status fails to mediate the effects of education on self-reported health. As regards labor force activity, older persons who are work-

Percentage with Physical Functional Limitations			Percentage with Poor Health and Physical Functional Limitations		
Total	Men	Women	Total	Men	Women
P < 0.01			P < 0.01		
58.6	—	—	21.9	—	—
38.1	—	—	11.9	—	—
P < 0.01	P < 0.01	NS	P < 0.01	P < 0.05	P < 0.05
55.8	47.4	59.2	20.6	15.0	22.9
32.3	29.2	50.0	8.7	8.8	8.3
P < 0.01	P < 0.01	P < 0.01	P < 0.01	P < 0.05	P < 0.01
34.0	25.9	50.0	9.9	8.3	13.0
40.5	35.2	45.6	8.1	7.4	8.8
63.2	50.0	68.3	26.5	18.6	29.5
50.6	55.3	46.9	17.2	15.8	18.4
P < 0.01	P < 0.05	NS	P < 0.01	P < 0.05	P < 0.05
56.9	41.9	59.4	24.3	16.1	25.7
51.7	42.2	61.8	16.6	14.7	18.6
38.6	33.8	50.0	10.3	8.5	14.8
NS	P < 0.05	NS	P < 0.10	P < 0.01	NS
50.6	42.0	57.1	19.5	16.7	21.7
48.3	33.3	60.7	14.7	5.8	22.1
P < 0.01	P < 0.01	P < 0.01	P < 0.01	P < 0.05	P < 0.01
40.5	27.3	50.3	11.6	7.0	15.0
56.1	44.4	66.0	21.9	15.6	27.4
62.1	53.8	68.8	25.0	17.3	31.3
P < 0.05	NS	P < 0.01	P < 0.05	NS	NS
58.2	38.5	69.6	21.6	14.1	25.9
47.0	44.7	48.9	20.1	17.1	22.7
45.0	36.8	51.4	14.0	7.0	19.4
42.1	30.5	56.3	9.3	6.8	12.5

ing are significantly less likely to report being in poor health. This result is robust to all controls for socioeconomic status, living arrangements, age, and region of residence. However, when the activity limitations are included in the model, no statistically significant difference is found between workers and nonworkers. This finding may suggest that the observed significant advantage of workers compared with nonworkers may be a reflection of the healthy worker effect. Healthy elderly people may be more able to work than their unhealthy counterparts and may be more attractive in the job market, where they can travel and use their skills to compete successfully within the limited opportunity structures offered by the local and national

TABLE 9-3a Odds Ratios for Influences of Gender, Socioeconomic Status, and Living Arrangements on Self-Rated Health of Older Cameroonians

Variables	Model 1	Model 2	Model 3	Model 4	Model 5	Model 6
Gender						
Female	1.00		1.00			
Male	0.49*		0.58§			
Level of Education						
None		1.00	1.00	1.00		
Some education		0.48*	0.66	0.56§		
Economic Activity Status						
Paid/unpaid work				0.49§		
Retired/at home				1.38		
Unemployed				1.00		
Marital Status						
Single/widowed/divorced					3.06*	
Married polygamous					1.62¶	
Married monogamous					1.00	
Age at First Marriage					1.11	
Kinship Size						
Less than 6					1.00	
6 or more					0.85	
Age Cohort (in years)						
50-64						0.50*
65-96						1.00
Main Region of Residence						
Djaa/Pete/Yom						1.00
Demdeng/Sedembom/Haa						0.72
Djiomghouo/Famleng/Tsela						1.03
Tsela/Famla II/Bagang/Fodji						0.45§
Functional Limitations						
No						
Yes						
-2Loglikelihood	643.45	646.90	641.14	624.74	634.08	635.38
Model Chi-square	12.86	9.41	15.17	31.57	22.23	20.93
(df)	(1)	(1)	(2)	(3)	(4)	(4)

* p < 0.01 (two-tailed test); § p < 0.05 (two-tailed test); ¶p < 0.10 (two-tailed test).

economies. In instances in which labor force participation is endogenously determined, it is obvious that there will be associations between poor health and unemployment, irrespective of the labor market environment and individual education and acquired professional skills.

The data demonstrate that older widowed, single, or divorced respondents are at least three times as likely to report being in poor health as those in monogamous marriages, while those in polygamous marriages are more

Model 7	Model 8	Model 9	Model 10	Model 11	Model 12	Model 13
1.00	1.00	1.00		1.00	1.00	1.00
0.73	0.54§	0.48*		0.71	0.61	0.59
1.00			1.00	1.00	1.00	1.00
0.67			0.68	0.76	0.94	1.02
0.51§			0.52§	0.54§	0.57§	0.67
1.34			1.34	1.34	1.31	1.23
1.00			1.00	1.00	1.00	1.00
	2.38*		2.31*	2.07*	1.89§	2.02§
	1.52		1.45	1.40	1.37	1.26
	1.00		1.00	1.00	1.00	1.00
	1.20		1.21	1.22	1.22	1.42§
	1.00		1.00	1.00	1.00	1.00
	0.83		0.85	0.83	0.90	0.90
		0.47*			0.58§	0.72
		1.00			1.00	1.00
		1.00			1.00	1.00
		0.76			0.83	0.96
		1.11			1.16	1.34
		0.50§			0.54§	0.60
						0.27*
						1.00
623.09	629.68	623.00	613.59	612.48	601.08	565.16
33.22	26.63	33.30	42.72	43.83	55.23	91.15
(4)	(5)	(5)	(7)	(8)	(12)	(13)

than 1.5 times as likely to assess their health as poor compared with those in monogamous marriages (model 5). The health disadvantage of elderly widows is robust to all controls, implying that this group is one of the most vulnerable segments of the elderly population. A comparison of Models 5 and 8 in Table 9-3a shows that gender inequality explains the effect of polygamous marriage on self-rated health. It is possible, as discussed above,

that women in polygamous marriages are more likely to have low self-esteem and to report self-assessments of nonphysical health as poor.

The age at first marriage appears significant only in the model including functional status as a covariate. The result indicates that the younger the age at marriage, the higher the odds of self-assessing one's health as poor once functional limitations are taken into account. In contrast, differences by kinship size are trivial.

While there is an apparent and positive dose-response effect of age on poor health, the significance of that effect is eliminated with a control for activity limitation (Model 13), which is itself significantly associated with poor health (p < 0.01). Regional differences in self-reported health are also found, even after all postulated risk and protective factors are controlled (Models 6, 9, and 12), but they are eliminated when functional status is taken into account. Therefore, a number of influences on self-reported health are mediated by the functional status of the respondents, including labor force participation, age cohort, and region of residence.

A useful way of looking at the interactions of gender with socioeconomic status and living arrangements in predicting health and functional status is to carry out separate analyses by gender for those postulated factors. Table 9-3b presents the gender-specific estimated odds ratios for the effects of the postulated covariates on the probability of reporting poor health, functional limitation, or both.

There are no gender differences in the effects of education, and working status has protective effects on older men but not women (Models 1 and 4). This gender difference in the effect of employment is explained entirely by kinship size (Model 6). It is possible that within the social setting typical of most rural and semirural areas like western Cameroon, the influential power of older men and the control that they have over family resources within the kinship allows them to seek assistance and use labor from the family network to ease their health burden and its consequences. In fact, the data substantiate that larger kinship size has protective effects on the health of older men only and that these effects are indeed robust (Models 2 and 5-8).

The analysis also reveals that the health disadvantage associated with widowhood noted earlier is restricted to older women, even after all measured factors are controlled, including functional limitations (Models 2 and 5-8). Similarly, the younger the age at which older women entered into marriage, the higher their odds of reporting being in poor health, even after accounting for activity limitations (Model 8). Put together, these findings demonstrate that older women who married young or who are widowed are the most vulnerable to poor health status.

The age effects tend to be stronger for older women than older men, with younger generations reporting less poor health than older generations. As conjectured for both men and women, functional status entirely explains these age effects on self-rated health. Regional differences are also trivial in most instances, except for women (see Model 3).

Overall, there is a strong association between poor health and low socioeconomic status (measured by no education and nonparticipation in the labor force), unfavorable living arrangements (captured by being single/widowed/divorced or married in polygamous unions), and being older and female. The data confirm the existence of gender differences in self-reported health, functional limitations, and the combination of the two. These gender differences in self-reported health among the elderly in Cameroon are entirely explained by the superior socioeconomic position of men versus women, and that gender inequality explains differences in self-rated health by level of educational attainment. Older people who are working are significantly better off than those who are not working, controlling for socioeconomic status, living arrangements, age, and region of residence. But this work status difference disappears in the presence of a control for activity limitations. Age at first marriage is also found to predict health status: the younger the age at marriage, the higher the odds of poor health. Regional differences in self-rated health exist, but they appear to be determined by activity limitations. Kinship size appears to predict the health status of older men, which may reflect the power differentials in access to family resources (human and material) in their favor. Similarly, the health disadvantage associated with widowhood is limited to older women who also tend to report poor health associated with early marriage. Since no interaction terms are present in the models, the estimated odds ratios represent adjusted estimates that control for all other measured covariates. I refer to these estimates as the "gold standard estimates" of effects, because I consider them to be the best estimates that can be obtained that control for all the potential confounders in the models.

Covariates of Activity Limitations

Table 9-4a presents the odds ratios of covariates of functional limitations. As in the case with self-rated health, gender differences exist in functional limitations, with older women at least twice as likely to have activity limitations as older men. Unlike the case with self-rated health, the effects of gender remain robust to all controls, so that the most complete model (Model 12) shows an odds ratio of 0.44 for older men ($p < 0.01$). This finding implies that there are inherent gender differences in functional limitations, which may be explained by the cumulative consequences of reproductive activities and other harsh farming-related activities that women engage in for family survival.

The effects of socioeconomic status are also robust. Older persons with no education are about twice as likely to report activity limitations as their

TABLE 9-3b Odds Ratios for Gender-Specific Influences of Socioeconomic Status and Living Arrangements on Self-Rated Health of Older Cameroonians

Variables	Model 1 Men	Model 1 Women	Model 2 Men	Model 2 Women	Model 3 Men	Model 3 Women
Level of Education						
None	1.00	1.00				
Some education	0.73	0.57				
Economic Activity Status						
Paid/unpaid work	0.43¶	0.57				
Retired/at home	0.88	1.64				
Unemployed	1.00	1.00				
Marital Status						
Single/widowed/divorced			1.45	3.13*		
Married polygamous			1.43	1.69		
Married monogamous			1.00	1.00		
Age at First Marriage			1.28	1.90*		
Kinship Size						
Less than 6			1.00	1.00		
6 or more			0.47§	1.15		
Age Cohort (in years)						
50-64					0.54¶	0.44*
65-96					1.00	1.00
Main Region of Residence						
Djaa/Pete/Yom					1.00	1.00
Demdeng/Sedembom/Haa					0.63	0.83
Djiomghouo/Famleng/Tsela					0.97	1.20
Tsela/Famla II/Bagang/Fodji					0.51	0.48¶
Functional Limitations						
No						
Yes						
-2Loglikelihood	230.55	391.20	230.31	387.15	230.92	391.47
Model Chi-square	6.20	15.49	6.45	19.54	5.84	15.22
(df)	(3)	(3)	(4)	(4)	(4)	(4)

* $p < 0.01$ (two-tailed test); § $p < 0.05$ (two-tailed test); ¶ $p < 0.10$ (two-tailed test).

educated peers. Similarly, older people who are working are less likely to report having functional limitations; in contrast, those "at home" or retired are more likely to have functional limitations. As the gender-specific models show, the disadvantage associated with being "at home" is mainly a female disadvantage (see Table 9-4b, Models 1, 4, 6, and 7).

Living arrangements are also important predictors of activity limitations. Again, the groups at a disadvantage in terms of marital status are widowed/single/divorced older people and those living in polygamous mar-

Model 4		Model 5		Model 6		Model 7		Model 8	
Men	Women	Men	Women	Men	Women	Men	Women	Men	Women
1.00	1.00			1.00	1.00	1.00	1.00	1.00	1.00
0.94	0.77			0.81	0.61	0.98	0.73	1.29	0.72
0.45¶	0.60			0.49	0.53	0.52	0.59	0.70	0.60
0.83	1.59			0.96	1.53	0.89	1.55	0.89	1.34
1.00	1.00			1.00	1.00	1.00	1.00	1.00	1.00
		1.55	2.60§	1.24	2.59§	1.39	2.23§	1.45	2.34§
		1.39	1.62	1.38	1.44	1.35	1.39	1.21	1.33
		1.00	1.00	1.00	1.00	1.00	1.00	1.00	1.00
		1.26	1.85*	1.20	1.98*	1.22	1.94*	1.05	1.95*
		1.00	1.00	1.00	1.00	1.00	1.00	1.00	1.00
		0.51¶	1.28	0.52¶	1.10	0.53¶	1.20	0.54¶	1.17
0.60	0.48*	0.64	0.54§			0.67	0.58§	0.82	0.69
1.00	1.00	1.00	1.00			1.00	1.00	1.00	1.00
1.00	1.00	1.00	1.00			1.00	1.00	1.00	1.00
0.67	0.92	0.60	0.83			0.62	0.91	0.61	1.07
0.95	1.25	0.91	1.28			0.89	1.30	0.77	1.62
0.55	0.56	0.47	0.49			0.50	0.56	0.52	0.61
								0.18*	0.31*
								1.00	1.00
226.81	380.15	225.49	377.14	225.98	373.49	222.50	366.56	202.25	350.86
9.95	26.55	11.27	29.56	10.78	33.20	14.26	40.13	34.50	55.83
(7)	(7)	(8)	(8)	(7)	(7)	(11)	(11)	(12)	(12)

riages (Models 3 and 6). However, as Model 8 shows, gender inequality in many domains of family and social organization and practices tends to be unfavorable to widowed/single/divorced respondents (especially women), and polygamy is less likely to promote women's status. As in Tables 9-3a and 9-3b, one finds that gender explains at least in part the effect of polygamy on the odds of reporting activity limitations (see Models 3 and 8). Any residual effect of polygamy on the probability of reporting functional limitations is captured by socioeconomic status (see Models 8 and 11).

TABLE 9-4a Odds Ratios for Influences of Gender, Socioeconomic Status, and Living Arrangements on Functional Limitations: Total Sample

Variables	Model 1	Model 2	Model 3	Model 4	Model 5	Model 6
Gender						
Female	1.00					
Male	0.43*					
Level of Education						
None		1.00			1.00	
Some education		0.43*			0.50*	
Economic Activity Status						
Paid/unpaid work		0.56§			0.54§	
Retired/at home		1.51¶			1.36	
Unemployed		1.00			1.00	
Marital Status						
Single/widowed/divorced			1.94*			1.63§
Married polygamous			1.64§			1.55§
Married monogamous			1.00			1.00
Age at First Marriage			0.98			0.98
Kinship Size						
Less than 6			1.00			1.00
6 or more			0.94			1.06
Age Cohort (in years)						
50-64				0.49*	0.59*	0.50*
65-96				1.00	1.00	1.00
Main Region of Residence						
Djaa/Pete/Yom				1.00	1.00	1.00
Demdeng/Sedembom/Haa				0.56§	0.61§	0.56§
Djiomghouo/Famleng/Tsela				0.67¶	0.69¶	0.71
Tsela/Famla II/Bagang/Fodji				0.55§	0.68	0.59§
-2Loglikelihood	824.28	793.68	833.89	820.79	779.31	809.21
Model Chi-square	25.47	56.06	15.86	28.97	70.44	40.55
(df)	(1)	(3)	(4)	(4)	(7)	(8)

* p < 0.01 (two-tailed test); § p < 0.05 (two-tailed test); ¶ p < 0.10 (two-tailed test).

As in the case of self-rated health, age at first marriage is a significant predictor of functional limitations at older ages. As expected, the inverse relationships between age cohort and functional limitations are consistently strong in all models (p < 0.01) and show a direct connection between growing older and developing functional limitations. Finally, the effects of region of residence emerge strongly, with respondents from all rural regions reporting fewer functional limitations than urban and semiurban dwellers from Pete, Djaa, and Yom.

Table 9-4b shows the gender-specific odds ratios of covariates of functional limitations, so their interactions with gender can be assessed. The robustness of the protective effects of education on functional status played

Model 7	Model 8	Model 9	Model 10	Model 11	Model 12
1.00	1.00	1.00		1.00	1.00
0.42*	0.35*	0.43*		0.52§	0.44*
1.00			1.00	1.00	1.00
0.51*			0.44*	0.51*	0.63§
0.59§			0.57§	0.60§	0.58§
1.47¶			1.50¶	1.51¶	1.36
1.00			1.00	1.00	1.00
	1.37		1.34	1.12	0.97
	1.50¶		1.47¶	1.40	1.32
	1.00		1.00	1.00	1.00
	1.03		1.01	1.35¶	1.33¶
	1.00		1.00	1.00	1.00
	0.92		1.01	0.98	1.06
		0.46*			0.54*
		1.00			1.00
		1.00			1.00
		0.58§			0.59§
		0.72			0.72
		0.63¶			0.68
790.95	816.87	795.77	790.22	784.61	768.48
58.81	32.89	53.98	59.54	65.15	81.28
(4)	(5)	(5)	(7)	(8)	(12)

out to the advantage of older men only (Models 1, 4, 6, and 7). Working status is advantageous for older men, while being "at home" or retired is a risk factor of activity limitations among older women (Models 1, 4, 6, and 7). Again, these findings are robust across a range of specifications of models.

As before, age at first marriage is negatively associated with activity limitations for older women, but not for older men. Age effects are also present across gender categories, which shows that the link between disability and age is independent of gender. Regional differences in functional limitations are statistically noticeable only among elderly women. Overall, there are significant interactions among gender, socioeconomic status, and

TABLE 9-4b Odds Ratios for Gender-Specific Influences of Socioeconomic Status and Living Arrangements on Functional Limitations of Older Cameroonians

Variables	Model 1		Model 2		Model 3	
	Men	Women	Men	Women	Men	Women
Level of Education						
None	1.00	1.00				
Some education	0.43*	0.85				
Economic Activity Status						
Paid/unpaid work	0.31*	1.02				
Retired/at home	0.812	2.39*				
Unemployed	1.00	1.00				
Marital Status						
Single/widowed/divorced			1.20	1.46		
Married polygamous			1.42	1.61		
Married monogamous			1.00	1.00		
Age at First Marriage			1.05	1.50§		
Kinship Size						
Less than 6			1.00	1.00		
6 or more			0.65	1.16		
Age-Cohort (in years)						
50-64					0.40*	0.52*
65-96					1.00	1.000
Main Region of Residence						
Djaa/Pete/Yom					1.00	1.00
Demdeng/Sedembom/Haa					0.82	0.46*
Djiomghouo/Famleng/Tsela					1.36	0.44*
Tsela/Famla II/Bagang/Fodji					0.78	0.59
-2Loglikelihood	334.32	449.85	349.64	462.74	343.91	444.74
Model Chi-square	24.67	15.45	9.35	2.56	15.07	20.56
(df)	(3)	(3)	(4)	(4)	(4)	(4)

* $p < 0.01$ (two-tailed test); § $p < 0.05$ (two-tailed test); ¶ $p < 0.10$ (two-tailed test).

living arrangements in predicting functional status, just as in the case of self-reported health.

In sum, gender differences in activity limitations are apparent, with older women being at least twice as likely to report functional limitations as older men. Here, these differences remain robust to controls to all postulated risk and protective factors. The robustness of this finding suggests that the association between gender and functional limitations does not reflect a methodological artifact but rather suggests a depletion process and the trajectory of health underlying the relationship for women but not for

Model 4		Model 5		Model 6		Model 7	
Men	Women	Men	Women	Men	Women	Men	Women
1.00	1.00			1.00	1.00	1.00	1.00
0.58¶	0.95			0.43*	0.84	0.54§	0.88
0.33*	0.91			0.35*	1.02	0.36*	0.92
0.79	1.99§			0.91	2.35*	0.88	1.99§
1.00	1.00			1.00	1.00	1.00	1.00
		1.24	1.01	0.87	1.24	0.95	0.89
		1.33	1.34	1.37	1.45	1.33	1.23
		1.00	1.00	1.00	1.00	1.00	1.00
		0.99	1.51§	1.08	1.52§	1.02	1.53§
				1.00	1.00	1.00	1.00
				0.79	1.13	0.82	1.32
0.53§	0.54*	0.45*	0.48*			0.60¶	0.50*
1.00	1.00	1.00	1.00			1.00	1.00
1.00	1.00	1.00	1.00			1.00	1.00
0.91	0.49*	0.80	0.43*			0.88	0.46*
1.37	0.47*	1.34	0.44*			1.36	0.47*
0.86	0.70	0.69	0.54¶			0.77	0.65
328.23	433.87	336.83	441.56	327.79	448.25	322.62	431.11
30.75	31.43	22.15	23.74	31.19	17.05	36.37	34.19
(7)	(7)	(8)	(8)	(7)	(7)	(11)	(11)

men. The effects of socioeconomic status are also quite robust, showing that low socioeconomic status is associated with functional limitations, just like substandard living arrangements in the study context (being widowed/single/divorced elderly or living in polygamous marriages), especially for women. As for self-assessed health, age at first marriage is a robust predictor of functional limitations at older ages. The strong protective effects of education on functional status are advantageous to older men only, and similarly for working status. Here again, young age at first marriage is associated with activity limitations among older women.

Covariates of Poor Health with Functional Limitations

Tables 9-5a and 9-5b show the odds ratios of influences on the combination of self-rated health and functional limitations.

Gender differences in poor health with activity limitations are expected, since this outcome results from the previous ones, which have shown that, at least in the unadjusted models, gender effects do exist. As in the case of self-reported health, these gender differences are entirely explained by socioeconomic status (Model 7, Table 9-5a) and not by living arrangement

TABLE 9-5a Odds Ratios for Influences of Gender, Socioeconomic Status, and Living Arrangements on Poor Health with Functional Limitations of Older Cameroonians

Variables	Model 1	Model 2	Model 3	Model 4	Model 5	Model 6
Gender						
Female	1.00					
Male	0.48*					
Level of Education						
None		1.00			1.00	
Some education		0.44*			0.54¶	
Economic Activity Status						
Paid/unpaid work		0.48§			0.51¶	
Retired/at home		1.58			1.53	
Unemployed		1.00			1.00	
Marital Status						
Single/widowed/divorced			2.76*			2.41*
Married polygamous			1.71¶			1.66¶
Married monogamous			1.00			1.00
Age at First Marriage			1.01			0.99
Kinship Size						
Less than 6			1.00			1.00
6 or more			0.72			0.82
Age Cohort (in years)						
50-64				0.44*	0.51*	0.49*
65-96				1.00	1.00	1.00
Main Region of Residence						
Djaa/Pete/Yom				1.00	1.00	1.00
Demdeng/Sedembom/Haa				0.56¶	0.64	0.59¶
Djiomghouo/Famleng/Tsela				0.98	1.06	1.07
Tsela/Famla II/Bagang Fodji				0.40§	0.51¶	0.43§
-2Loglikelihood	556.83	531.61	551.63	543.67	517.82	533.07
Model Chi-square	0.84	36.07	16.05	24.00	49.86	34.61
(df)	1 (1)	(3)	(4)	(4)	(7)	(8)

* p < 0.01 (two-tailed test); § p < 0.05 (two-tailed test); ¶ p < 0.10 (two-tailed test).

covariates (Model 8, Table 9-5a) or age cohort and the socioeconomic contextual variable, which is the region of residence (Model 9, Table 9-5a).

The influences of socioeconomic status on poor health with functional limitations are present (Model 2, Table 9-5a) as before and show the protective effects of education and work on health and functional status. But those effects are somewhat attenuated after controlling for age and region of residence ($p < 0.10$, Model 5, Table 9-5a; Model 4, Table 9-5b for men only) and are eliminated in the most complete model (Model 12,

Model 7	Model 8	Model 9	Model 10	Model 11	Model 12
1.00	1.00	1.00		1.00	1.00
0.85	0.44*	0.48*		0.67	0.60
1.00			1.00	1.00	1.00
0.48§			0.47§	0.53¶	0.66
0.49§			0.50§	0.52¶	0.56
1.55			1.58	1.57	1.53
1.00			1.00	1.00	1.00
	2.10§		1.92§	1.73¶	1.54
	1.58		1.46	1.40	1.36
	1.00		1.00	1.00	1.00
	1.37¶		1.23	1.38¶	1.35
	1.00		1.00	1.00	1.00
	0.71		0.74	0.73	0.79
		0.42*			0.54§
		1.00			1.00
		1.00			1.00
		0.59¶			0.65
		1.07			1.11
		0.45§			0.50¶
531.25	545.76	533.34	524.41	523.29	511.26
36.42	21.92	34.33	43.26	44.39	56.41
(4)	(5)	(5)	(7)	(8)	(12)

TABLE 9-5b Odds Ratios for Gender-Specific Influences of Socioeconomic
Status and Living Arrangements on Poor Health with Functional
Limitations of Older Cameroonians

	Model 1		Model 2		Model 3	
Variables	Men	Women	Men	Women	Men	Women
Level of Education						
None	1.00	1.00				
Some education	0.53¶	0.36				
Economic Activity Status						
Paid/unpaid work	0.46	0.51				
Retired/at home	1.23	1.69				
Unemployed	1.00	1.00				
Marital Status						
Single/widowed/divorced			1.88	1.98		
Married polygamous			1.75	1.32		
Married monogamous			1.00	1.00		
Age at First Marriage			1.32	1.54¶		
Kinship Size						
Less than 6			1.00	1.00		
6 or more			0.30*	1.05		
Age Cohort (in years)						
50-64					0.37*	0.43*
65-96					1.00	1.00
Main Region of Residence						
Djaa/Pete/Yom					1.00	1.00
Demdeng/Sedembom/Haa					0.40	0.69
Djiomghouo/Famleng/Tsela					1.31	0.94
Tsela/Famla II/Bagang/Fodji					0.49	0.43¶
-2Loglikelihood	188.20	342.50	185.30	353.52	185.19	346.58
Model Chi-square	8.34	17.79	11.24	6.78	11.35	13.71
(df)	(3)	(3)	(4)	(4)	(4)	(4)

* $p < 0.01$ (two-tailed test); § $p < 0.05$ (two-tailed test); ¶ $p < 0.10$ (two-tailed test).

Table 9-5a). This implies that some effects of socioeconomic status operate
at least in part through demographic attributes and the socioeconomic context of the communities in which older people live.

The health disadvantage of widowhood remains strong, and to some
extent older people in polygamous marriages tend to report being in poor
health with functional limitations. As in Tables 9-3a and 9-3b, gender explains the effects of being in polygamous marriages on the odds of reporting
poor health with activity limitations (see Models 3 and 8, Table 9-5a). Age
at first marriage is also significantly associated with poor health with functional limitations. The age cohort effects also remain strong and unaltered

Model 4		Model 5		Model 6		Model 7	
Men	Women	Men	Women	Men	Women	Men	Women
1.00	1.00			1.00	1.00	1.00	1.00
0.76	0.44			0.63	0.37	0.80	0.42
0.54	0.50			0.58	0.49	0.68	0.50
1.28	1.53			1.42	1.62	1.49	1.52
1.00	1.00			1.00	1.00	1.00	1.00
		2.17	1.48	1.47	1.57	1.75	1.22
		1.72	1.16	1.69	1.09	1.68	0.96
		1.00	1.00	1.00	1.00	1.00	1.00
		1.24	1.56¶	1.29	1.60¶	1.26	1.54¶
		1.00	1.00	1.00	1.00	1.00	1.00
		0.34§	1.20	0.34§	1.20	0.35§	1.13
0.46§	0.49§	0.46§	0.48§			0.55§	0.53§
1.00	1.00	1.00	1.00			1.00	1.00
1.00	1.00	1.00	1.00			1.00	1.00
0.45	0.75	0.38	0.70			0.40	0.75
1.36	0.94	1.23	0.96			1.29	0.94
0.56	0.49	0.45	0.44¶			0.50	0.50
180.92	333.37	176.00	342.98	179.72	336.86	172.90	329.91
15.62	26.92	20.54	17.31	16.82	23.43	23.64	30.38
(7)	(7)	(8)	(8)	(7)	(7)	(11)	(11)

by various controls, but the regional disparities noted in previous models are somewhat attenuated.

As in previous models, the younger the age at first marriage, the higher the odds of reporting poor health with functional limitations (Models 8 and 11, Table 9-5a) but the significance of such a relationship is largely restricted to older women (Models 2 and 5-7, Table 9-5b). Since early marriage is associated with high fertility, which in turn is strongly correlated with short birth intervals in highly fertile populations, such as those of western Cameroon, it is likely that the effects of age at marriage on poor health and functional limitations at older ages operate through the parity effect and maternal depletion syndrome, which has been well documented in the literature on women's health in Cameroon and elsewhere (Kuate-Defo, 1997).

Kinship size appears to have a protective effect on older men but not on older women. The larger the kinship size, the lower the odds of reporting being in poor health with activity limitations among older men: those with kinship size of six or more are at least three times less likely to report these conditions than those with kinship size under six (Models 2 and 5-7, Table 9-5b).

The odds ratios of poor health with activity limitations increase with age, even after all other postulated risk and protective factors are taken into account. Irrespective of gender, there is strong evidence that the younger the generation, the lower the odds of being in poor health with functional limitations, even after all controls are introduced in models for men and women (p < 0.05, Model 7, Table 9-5b). Therefore, functional limitations explain the age-health relationship found above, but age appears to have a direct relationship with the combination of poor health and functional limitations for the elderly in western Cameroon.

Finally, when they are present, regional differences in poor health with functional limitations appear to show a disadvantage for urban and semiurban residents (Models 4-6 and 9, Table 9-5a), but after all controls are introduced, only residents of Tsela, Famla II, and Bagang Fodji have some significant advantage vis-à-vis those from Pete, Djaa, and Yom. When the analyses are separated by gender, only older women from Tsela, Famla II, and Bagang Fodji are at an advantage (Models 3 and 5, Table 9-5b), which is purged by controls for socioeconomic status. Hence, it is likely that regional differences in poor health with activity limitations are largely explained by differences in the socioeconomic context of each region.

There is evidence that gender differences in poor health with activity limitations are present but are fully captured by differences in the socio-economic standing of older men versus women. The influences of socio-economic status on poor health and functional limitations are mediated at least partly through age and the socioeconomic context of communities of residence. The disadvantage associated with widowhood is unaltered, and gender inequality explains the deleterious effects of living in polygamous unions on self-assessed health and functional status. Age at first marriage is strongly associated with poor health with functional limitations among older women, and the age effects remain unaffected by controls for other covariates. Older men who belong to a larger kinship are less likely to report poor health with functional limitations. Poor health with functional limitations increases with age, even after controlling for all postulated risk and protective factors, and this finding applies to both older men and women. Finally, only older women who are residents of Tsela, Famla II, and Bagang Fodji have some significant advantage vis-à-vis those from Pete, Djaa, and Yom, and socioeconomic standing explains their relative advantage. The data also show that residing in the Tsela, Famla II, and Bagang Fodji neighborhoods is associated with decreased odds of poor health of 45 to 55 percent, compared with living in the highest development localities of Djaa, Pete, and Yom. Similar findings emerge concerning functional limitations. Together, these results suggest that living in urban areas may not be sufficient to provide better health status in contexts similar to the study sites investigated.

SUMMARY AND DISCUSSION

This study has demonstrated that it is possible to lengthen life expectancy while maintaining the quality of life in Africa. The results extend previous findings on the health advantages stemming from socioeconomic status and living arrangements to semirural areas of Africa. These factors appear to exert independent effects on self-rated health and functional limitations in most instances. Overall, there are significant interactions among gender, socioeconomic status, and living arrangements in predicting poor health, functional limitations, or both. A number of interactions were tested in models for the total sample as well as gender-specific models, but none reached significance levels. However, after adjusting for all other measured covariates, the models fail to show significant interactions of several measures of socioeconomic status and living arrangements in predicting poor health and disability, but that does not mean that such links are nonexistent. For example, it is likely that decisions about work, retirement, and unemployment are not independent of considerations of living arrangements for the elderly, just as it is the case for younger age groups.

The effects of socioeconomic status on perceived health were quite similar among men and women. Although a robust relationship between education and health status has been demonstrated in previous research (for a review, see Robert, 1999), the processes that explain the link are not well understood, especially in developing countries (Zimmer, Liu, Hermalin, and Chuang, 1998). This study advances such understanding in two notable ways. First, the study found differences in the relationship of education and self-rated health and education and functional limitations among older people. Second, it found that gender inequality entirely explains the education differences in self-rated health.

The importance of socioeconomic differences in health status is well documented in the health literature, and this study provides empirical evidence on the robustness of these differences in the African context. Related to diversity is the fact that the health of elderly populations in all countries varies according to socioeconomic position (National Research Council,

2001). The magnitude of these differences, as well as their causes, varies over time within and among societies.

To develop policies effectively, one must have an understanding of these causes, which in turn requires a fuller understanding of the determinants of socioeconomic differences in health and functioning. Policy responses to such differences will ideally cover a wide range of determinants, including the provision of, access to, and response to medical care and social services. Therefore, an underlying need in any research agenda is to include a link to socioeconomic position in the collection of population and health data on elderly individuals. Economic activity status captures the extent to which an older person is unemployed, working, retired, or housewife. In the multivariate analyses, work was measured broadly to include both paid and unpaid work.

As life expectancy increases, the postretirement life period is expected to get longer; greater health and other needs demand appropriate income for the elderly, who may increasingly be forced to compete in the labor market against younger, more skilled, and highly educated people in order to secure an income. This study confirms that the aging population that is unemployed or retired is numerically and proportionally more important as it grows older, as previous studies have found (e.g., Møller and Devey, 2003). Statistically significant differences in self-rated health by level of education are entirely explained by gender inequality, which is likely to operate in turn through the income or wages advantage of men compared with women.

Evidence of gender differences in self-rated health has been inconsistent, with a male advantage reported in some studies (Gijsbers van Wijk, van Vliet, Kolk, and Everaerd, 1991; Rahman, Strauss, Gertler, Ashley, and Fox, 1994; Zimmer, Natividad, Lin, and Chayovan, 2000), but no advantage in others (Jylhä, Guralnik, Ferrucci, Jokela, and Heikkinen, 1998; Leinonen, Heikkinen, and Jyhhä, 1998; McDonough and Walters, 2001; Zimmer et al., 2000). The evidence from developing measures to test these conjectures remains very limited. Even if measures of self-rated health were reliable and comparable across populations, empirical evidence is likely to be greatly influenced by the cultural and social norms and practices as well as power relations in specific socioeconomic environments.

This study has found that older men are indeed at an advantage compared with older women (odds ratio of 0.49, $p < 0.05$), but that these gender differences in self-rated health in favor of men in Cameroon are entirely explained by the health advantage conferred by their labor force and economic activity status (see Models 1, 3, and 7, Table 9-3a). Similarly, older women tend to report being in poor health with functional limitations more than men, but the female disadvantage again is entirely explained by differences in their socioeconomic status relative to older men. It has been suggested that respondents draw on a number of sources when they make their self-assessment of health, including family history, severity of current illness, possible symptoms of diseases not yet diagnosed, trajectory of health status over time, as well as the availability of external resources (e.g., social support) and internal resources (e.g., perceived control) (Idler and Benjamini, 1997). The findings indicate that irrespective of such sources, gender inequality in health status necessarily operates through a rise in socioeconomic status in Cameroon.

One of the most important findings of this study is that the younger the age at first marriage of an older woman, the higher her odds of reporting being in poor health (Models 2, 5, 6, and 7, Table 9-3b) and having functional limitations (Models 2, 5, 6, and 7, Table 9-4b) as well as the combination of poor health with functional limitations (Models 2, 5, 6, and 7, Table 9-5b), even after all postulated covariates are included in the models. In contrast, age at marriage has a trivial effect on older men's health and functional status. Since early marriage is associated with high fertility, which in turn is strongly correlated with short birth intervals, it is likely that the effects of age at marriage on poor health and functional limitations at older ages operate through the maternal depletion syndrome, which has been well documented in the literature on women's health in Cameroon (Kuate-Defo, 1997).

This finding is also consistent with previous studies, which have demonstrated a relationship between early life conditions and later health and survival (Alter, Oris, Neven, and Broström, 2002; Conde-Agudelo and Belizan, 2000; King, 2003; Lundberg, 1993; Mosley and Gray, 1993). Because early marriage is strongly associated with high fertility and reproductive health problems, these robust findings suggest that women's issues in the areas of child marriage and childbearing are of paramount importance. This concerns the promotion of reproductive health in young girls and their successful transition to adulthood, as well as throughout the life cycle and especially in considering social and health policies for the elderly population.

Indeed, Bledsoe (2002) shows that, in rural Gambia, women view aging as contingent on the cumulative physical, social, and spiritual hardships of personal history, especially obstetric trauma. It is likely that such ill health and disability during old age among women are a result of exacerbated risks across the life course as they assume their reproductive and productive roles. The fact that early marriage is a robust risk factor for poor health and functional limitations among older women suggests that delaying marriage will have large payoffs not only in the short term, to ensure a successful transition to adulthood for girls, but also in the long term, in protecting the health of women and enhancing their quality of life at older ages. Therefore, there is an urgent need for the international community to address more vigorously the problem of early marriage in developing countries and to go beyond rhetoric, following repeated calls for action made by such organizations as UNICEF (2004) to prevent children from bearing children.

The finding that kinship size has a protective effect on the self-rated health of older people (especially men) is also consistent with the finding from a recent study showing that the risk of poor health and mortality is decreased by membership in large patriarchal kin groups (Hammel and Gullickson, 2004). I consider kinship size as a nurturing and enhancement factor in residential patterns that promote health and prevent disability, at least when the older person has some control over the social relations within the kinship. In most African societies the older the men, the stronger their control over familial matters and living arrangements and therefore the bigger their advantage with a larger kinship. The impact of social relations within the kinship is likely to interact with age in predicting health status. Specifically, the type and nature of social relations within the family connections as well as their usefulness will also vary across the lifespan. In contrast to the situation for men, social relations for women are not necessarily positive and may not always contribute to improved coping with illness and disability, especially for those who are caregivers and give social support to family members, in the addition to their traditional roles of reproduction and production in most societies in Africa.

Many researchers have examined the relationship between age and self-reported health, but the evidence is inconsistent (Helweg-Larsen, Kjoller, and Thoning, 2003). About one-third of studies show that older people evaluate their health more positively, another one-third show that the elderly evaluate their health more negatively, and one-third show no relationship between self-reported health and age. Idler (1993) found in a sample of elderly age 65 and older in the United States that older participants rated their health as better than younger participants at any given level of health status. Idler attributed this result to both a cohort effect (i.e., older cohorts may have different perceptions about what constitutes good health), an age effect (i.e., people evaluate their health differently as they age), and a survival effect (i.e., individuals who evaluate their health positively are more likely to survive).

This study shows that younger elderly (under age 65) are significantly less likely to report poor health, before controlling for functional limitations (odds ratio of 0.58, $p < 0.05$). However, when functional limitations are taken into account in the model fitting, the age differences are trivial. Indeed, functional ability is typically highly correlated with self-reported health and declines with age, as expected from biological theory. It has been suggested that if functional ability is not controlled, then self-reported health may appear to decline with age, when in fact this decline can be entirely accounted for by functional ability (Bjorner et al., 1996). The analysis confirms this conjecture (see Model 13, Table 9-3a, and Model 8, Table 9-3b).

The findings of this study allow one to identify opportunities and priorities for further research and appropriate interventions. It has been argued that a sounder theoretical basis for socioeconomic classification would yield better understanding of the determinants involved. One approach to this end is to conceive of three different modes of social stratification: one based on degree of material deprivation, one based on social power relations, and one based on general social standing (National Research Council, 2001). Measures of social deprivation are appropriate for assessing health differences among those living in absolute poverty. Such measures are less appropriate when health follows a social gradient. In such cases, there are clear social inequalities in health among people who are not materially deprived. Other concepts must therefore come into play.

A second approach that does not potentially relate to the whole social gradient is based on power relations in the workplace. Occupations are defined in terms of power and autonomy, a perspective that has its origin in the Marxist concept of class. Such a measure is appropriate for social classification among people of working age and less appropriate for those beyond working age, especially in settings in which aging starts early and the retirement age is 55, as in most sectors of employment in Cameroon until recently. The degree to which occupation continues to provide a reliable indicator of socioeconomic position beyond working age will vary, and additional measures of socioeconomic classification will be needed. This is especially the case for older women, particularly those who are single, widowed, or divorced, which is why I explicitly consider marital status as a predictor in the analyses.

A third approach—general social standing—has features in common with the concept of status based on patterns of consumption and lifestyle. The status group shares the same level of prestige or esteem and, in addition to common forms of consumption and lifestyle, limits its interactions with members of other groups. This approach fits the typical way of life in semirural Cameroon, where the study's data come from, given the social organization of the society and interactions by membership groups in terms of adult roles and responsibilities, sociotraditional ranking in the social hierarchy, and so forth.

Among the most important policy concerns relevant to health and longevity in modern economies are the future fiscal viability of pension, health, and social insurance systems, if any, both public and private, and the implications of these systems for savings and investment rates. How long people continue working, paying taxes, and saving will feature prominently in the consequences of population aging. Many people already work less than half a lifetime because of extended periods of schooling and training in early life, earlier retirement, and enhanced longevity, posing a challenge to the sustainability of systems designed to support older people. In all age groups, but particularly among older people, there is a substantial amount of self-care, as well as varying levels of alternative and complementary health care practices, including self-medication with herbs and the use of alternative practitioners, that may have an impact on health outcomes. These issues also deserve consideration in the context of health research among the elderly, but they were beyond the scope of this study.

This study suggests that a fuller understanding of the appropriate determinants of socioeconomic differences in health and functioning generally requires longitudinal, representative population surveys. Such surveys are essential for establishing causal associations and assessing the magnitude of causes operating in all directions. In other words, longitudinal data are important for determining the degree to which levels of health and functioning determine social and economic position, as well as for assessing the magnitude and nature of these determinants of health and functional status. Both personal behaviors and many public health measures bear on health status. Health promotional activities aimed at older persons may or may not involve direct contact with the formal health care system; examples of such activities include education programs and provision of good preventive nutrition, safe transportation to enhance mobility, and adequate housing. Effective national and regional policies for health promotion among older people require that important deficits in these areas be identified. Community-based population and health surveys may be the only means of acquiring accurate information on such issues as cigarette and alcohol consumption, perceived health status, levels of mobility, and social interaction. Coordination of public and clinic policies relevant to health promotion and disease prevention among the elderly is essential if these policies are to have the desired positive effects on the health status of older people. Again, the most effective means of obtaining the information necessary for such cross-national research is representative household surveys of older people, like the CFHS panel surveys, which so far have been fielded in 140 localities in western and northwestern Cameroon. Because of the higher rates of morbidity and disability that occur with increasing age, older people make substantial use of formal health services. Such services consume an enormous amount of resources. Again, cross-national comparative research is one important avenue for addressing this issue by examining international variations in organization, financing, delivery, and evaluation of elder health services.

Given the current state of knowledge in African countries, one cannot prevent the majority of the diseases and impairments of old age, but to make a start it is necessary to study the epidemiology of these conditions and measure their risk and protective factors. A further extension of this study will involve the epidemiology of the specific diseases with increasing prevalence in the elderly populations of Africa, including but not limiting to hypertension. In addition, it would be necessary to study the aggravating factors that change disease to impairments and impairments to handicaps in the elderly.

ACKNOWLEDGMENTS

This work was supported in part by the Rockefeller Foundation's Intervention Research grant RF 97045 no. 90 to the author; supplemental support was provided by the National Research Council of the National Academy of Sciences of the United States and the PRONUSTIC Research Laboratory at the University of Montreal. I thank two anonymous referees for their suggestions and comments.

REFERENCES

Alter, G., Oris, M., Neven, M., and Broström, G. (2002). *Maternal depletion and mortality after the childbearing years in the nineteenth century East Belgium.* (Early Life Conditions, Social Mobility, and Longevity Working Paper Series 7). Presented at the Social Science History Association, October 24-27, St. Louis, MO.

Anker, R., Buvinic, M., and Youssef, N.H. (Eds.). (1983). *Women's roles and population trends in the third world.* London, England: Croom Helm.

Arber, S., and Ginn, J. (1993). Gender and inequalities in health in later life. *Social Science and Medicine, 36,* 33-46.

Bledsoe, C. (2002). *Contingent lives: Fertility, time and aging in West Africa.* (with contributions by Fatoumatta Banja). Chicago, IL: University of Chicago Press.

Bjorner, J.B., Kristensen, T.S., Orth-Gomer, K., Tibblin, G., Sullivan, M., and Westerholm, P. (1996). *Self-rated health: A useful concept in research, prevention, and clinical medicine.* Stockholm, Sweden: Forskningsrådsnämnden.

Conde-Agudelo, A., and Belizan, J. (2000). Maternal morbidity and mortality associated with interpregnancy interval: Cross sectional study. *British Medical Journal, 321,* 1255-1259.

Farmer, M.M., and Ferraro, K.F. (1997). Distress and perceived health: Mechanisms of health decline. *Journal of Health and Social Behavior, 39,* 298-311.

Ferraro, K.F., Farmer, M.M., and Wybraniec, J.A. (1997). Health trajectories: Long-term dynamics among black and white adults. *Journal of Health and Social Behavior, 38,* 38-54.

Gijsbers van Wijk, C.M., van Vliet, K.P., Kolk, A.M., and Everaerd, W.T. (1991). Symptom sensitivity and sex differences in physical morbidity: A review of health surveys in the United States and the Netherlands. *Women's Health, 17,* 91-124.

Gorman, M. (2002). Global ageing: The nongovernmental organization role in the developing world. *International Journal of Epidemiology, 31,* 782-785.

Hammel, E.A., and Gullickson, A. (2004). Kinship structures and survival: Maternal mortality on the Croatian-Bosnian border 1750-1898. *Population Studies, 58*(2), 145-159.

Helweg-Larsen, M., Kjoller, M., and Thoning, H. (2003). Do age and social relations moderate the relationships between self-rated health and mortality among adult Danes? *Social Science and Medicine, 57,* 1237-1247.

Idler, E.L. (1993). Age differences in self-assessments of health: Age changes, cohort differences, or survivorship? *Journal of Gerontology: Social Sciences, 48,* S289-S300.

Idler, E.L., and Benyamini, Y. (1997). Self-rated health and mortality: A review of twenty-seven community studies. *Journal of Health and Social Behavior, 38*, 21-37.

Idler, E.L., and Kasl, S. (1995). Self-ratings of health: Do they also predict change in functional ability? *Journal of Gerontology: Social Sciences, 50B*, S344-S353.

Jylhä, M., Guralnik, J.M., Ferrucci, L., Jokela, J., and Heikkinen, E. (1998). Is self-rated health comparable across cultures and genders? *Journal of Gerontology Series B: Psychological Sciences and Social Sciences, 53*, S144-S152.

King, J.C. (2003). The risk of maternal nutritional depletion and poor outcomes increases in early or closely spaced pregnancies. *Journal of Nutrition*, (Suppl.), 1732S-1736S.

Kuate-Defo, B. (1997). Effects of socioeconomic disadvantage and women's status on women's health in Cameroon. *Social Science and Medicine, 44*(7), 1023-1042.

Kuate-Defo, B. (1998). Enquête sur vie familiale, sexualité et santé reproductive au Cameroun (EFSR) 1996-1997: Collecte et exploitation des données de Bandjoun. Yaoundé/Montreal, EFSR-FRHS Working Paper Series No. 3.

Kuate-Defo, B. (2005). Facteurs associés à la santé perçue et fonctionnelle des personnes âgées d'Afrique avec référence au Cameroun. *Cahiers Québécois de Démographie, 34*(1).

Kuate-Defo, B., and Lepage, Y. (1997). Enquête sur vie familiale, sexualité et santé reproductive au Cameroun (EFSR) 1996-1997: Méthodologie de sondage. Yaoundé/Montreal, EFSR-FRHS Working Paper Series No. 2.

Leinonen, R., Heikkinen, E., and Jyhhä, M. (1998). Self-rated health and self-assessed change in health in elderly men and women: A five-year longitudinal study. *Social Science and Medicine, 46*, 591-597.

Lundberg, O. (1993). The impact of childhood living conditions on illness and mortality in adulthood. *Social Science and Medicine, 36*, 1047-1052.

MacIntyre, S., Hunt, K., and Sweeting, H. (1996). Gender differences in health: Are things really as simple as they seem? *Social Science and Medicine, 42*, 617-624.

McDonough, P., and Walters, V. (2001). Gender and health: Reassessing patterns and explanations. *Social Science and Medicine, 52*, 547-559.

Møller, V., and Devey, R. (2003). Trends in the living conditions and satisfaction among poorer older South Africans: Objective and subjective indicators of quality of life in the October household survey. *Development Southern Africa, 20*(4), 457-476.

Mor, V., Murphy, J., Materson-Allen, S., Willey, C., Razmpour, A., Jackson, M.E., Greer, D., and Katz, S. (1989). Risk of functional decline among well elders. *Journal of Clinical Epidemiology, 42*, 895-904.

Mosley, H., and Gray, R. (1993). Childhood precursors of adult morbidity and mortality in developing countries: Implications for health programs. In National Research Council, J. Gribble and S. Preston (Eds.), *The epidemiological transition: Policy and implications for developing countries* (pp. 69-100). Washington, DC: National Academy Press.

National Research Council. (2001). *Preparing for an aging world: The case for cross-national research*. Panel on a Research Agenda and New Data for an Aging World, Committee on Population and Committee on National Statistics. Division of Behavioral and Social Sciences and Education. Washington, DC: National Academy Press.

Palloni, A., Pinto-Aguirre, G., and Pelaez, M. (2002). Demographic and health conditions of ageing in Latin America and the Caribbean. *International Journal of Epidemiology, 31*, 762-771.

Rahman, O., Strauss, J., Gertler, P., Ashley, D., and Fox, K. (1994). Gender differences in adult health: An international comparison. *Gerontologist, 34*, 463-469.

Restrepo, H., and Rozental, M. (1994). The social impact of aging populations: Some major issues. *Social Science and Medicine, 39*(9), 1323-1338.

Robert, S. (1999). Socioeconomic position and health: The independent contribution of community socioeconomic context. *Annual Review of Sociology, 25*, 489-516.

UNICEF. (2004). *Children having children: State of the world's mothers 2004.* New York: Author.

Wilcox, V.L., Kasl, S.V., and Idler, L. (1996). Self-rated health and physical disability in elderly survivors of a major medical event. *Journal of Gerontology: Social Sciences, 51B,* S96-S104.

Zimmer, Z., Liu, X., Hermalin, A., and Chuang, Y. (1998). Educational attainment and transitions in functional status among older Taiwanese. *Demography, 35*(3), 361-375.

Zimmer, Z., Natividad, J., Lin, H., and Chayovan, N. (2000). A cross-national examination of the determinants of self-rated health. *Journal of Health and Social Behavior, 41,* 465-481.

10

Survey Measures of Health: How Well Do Self-Reported and Observed Indicators Measure Health and Predict Mortality?

Randall Kuhn, Omar Rahman, and Jane Menken

INTRODUCTION

The costs and difficulties associated with assessing the health of a population have led to an ongoing search for indicators of health status that can be readily collected from large numbers of individuals with minimal expenditure of resources, including time, money, training, and logistics. Measuring health can be demanding in terms of interviewer time and skill, respondent comprehension, and logistic and analytic complexity. Set against the potentially higher costs and returns of physical health testing or the collection of biomarkers, there are simple self-reported and objective indicators that are relatively easy and inexpensive to collect.

If these low-cost measures are valid, they could prove beneficial in sub-Saharan Africa for assessing the overall burden of disease and the effectiveness of health systems. They could help address emerging concerns relating to adult health as processes of population aging gather pace and as HIV/AIDS continues to affect health and mortality at all ages, both directly and through socioeconomic pathways.

Yet data to compare health indicators are rare. Rarer still is follow-up information to assess how well these measures predict subsequent mortality—the ultimate measure of poor health—in developing countries. In fact, the only developing country data set containing both multiple measures of health and prospective mortality follow-up comes from the Matlab study site in rural Bangladesh. Analysis of this data set is included in this volume for two reasons. First, measures that prove useful in one developing country context merit consideration for application in other regions. Second, Matlab partners with community studies in sub-Saharan Africa that are part of the INDEPTH network (the International Network of field sites with continuous Demographic Evaluation of Populations and Their Health in developing countries); they provide the opportunity to replicate this study inexpensively and reasonably quickly in African contexts and in a comparative framework.

In this paper we consider five measures of health—three self-reported and two objectively observed—and address three questions:

- How interrelated are these indicators? Can the same information on individual health be obtained with a smaller set of questions or observations, thereby reducing costs?
- How well does each serve as a predictor of mortality? Here we assume that the poorer the health of an individual, the greater the risk of dying in a defined period (in this case, 5 years) after health is measured. The greater the predictive power, under this assumption, the better the measure is as a gauge of individual health.
- Does the predictive power of the indices vary by age or gender? Here we ask whether, for example, self-reported poor health is related to subsequent mortality similarly across age and gender.

The study is based on health measures collected in the 1996 Matlab Health and Socioeconomic Survey (MHSS). The MHSS was carried out with funding from the U.S. National Institute on Aging as a collaboration among researchers based at the International Centre for Health and Population Research in Dhaka, Bangladesh (ICDDR,B), and at several institutions in the united States. ICDDR,B began its Health and Demographic Surveillance System (HDSS) in Matlab in the early 1960s and, for over 40 years, has visited every household at least monthly to collect accurate information on vital events. The HDSS served as the sampling frame for the MHSS (Rahman et al., 1999). Information on MHSS respondents was therefore automatically collected in the HDSS each month of the 5 years subsequent to the survey. We first consider, using MHSS data alone, the extent to which each of the health measures provides information independent of the others. Next, the combined MHSS/HDSS data are used to test how well each health indicator serves as a predictor of mortality in the follow-up period. We then rank these measures in terms of mortality predictive power and discuss the prevalence of the poor health by age and gender they reveal. Finally, we discuss two issues regarding the usefulness of these simple and inexpensive to collect measures: international comparability and comparability of the indices to more specific information on health obtainable through other means, such as biomarkers. As part of this discussion, we propose a research agenda for measuring health and evaluating health measures in sub-Saharan Africa that takes advantage of INDEPTH. INDEPTH sites, including Matlab, routinely record mortality in their Demographic Surveillance System records, and improved measurement of adult health is one of its current goals.

SIMPLE-TO-OBSERVE HEALTH INDICATORS

The indicators examined in this study are

- *self-reported health* (SRH), whereby respondents are asked to classify their current health status as good, fair, or poor;
- an index based on *self-reported activities of daily living*;
- an index of self-reported *major acute and chronic morbidity conditions*;
- an index of physical disability based on *observed activities of daily living*; and
- current nutritional status as measured by *body mass index*.

Each of these indicators has been collected and studied in health surveys. While these measures are significantly related to one another, each may capture unique dimensions of ill health. They vary widely in terms of data collection time and field costs, yet none requires extensive field training or expensive or delicate equipment.

Because SRH is so easy and inexpensive to collect, there is great interest in determining its validity. Studies, primarily in more developed countries with literate populations and advanced medical systems, have demonstrated that it is a good predictor of mortality and functional ability, even after controlling for other objective health measurements (Appels, Bosma, Grabauskas, Gostautas, and Sturman, 1996; Borawski, Kinney, and Kahana, 1996; Idler and Benyamini, 1997; Idler and Kasl, 1991, 1995; Kaplan and Camacho, 1983; Mossey and Shapiro, 1982; Schoenfeld, Malmrose, Blazer, Gold, and Seeman, 1994; Sugisawa, Liang, and Liu, 1994; Wolinsky and Johnson, 1992). This predictive power may be related to its multifaceted nature, whereby SRH incorporates multiple dimensions of health (physical disability, functional or activity limitations, chronic and acute morbidity), self-assessment of severity, awareness of comorbidity, and past health trajectory (Idler and Benyamini, 1997).

SRH may not be comparable across populations (Angel and Guarnaccia, 1989; Ferraro and Kelley-Moore, 2001; Jylhä, Guralnik, Ferrucci, Jokela, and Heikkinen, 1998; Rahman, Strauss, Gertler, Ashley, and Fox, 1994; Zimmer, Natividad, Lin, and Chayovan, 2000), especially across developed and developing countries. Specifically, due to lower levels of education and formal contact with the health care system, individuals in the developing world may have less knowledge about their own acute and chronic morbidity conditions, which may affect their subjective reports of their health. High levels of family support and lower expectations of independence of movement in developing countries may lead to a weaker relationship between physical disability or functional limitations and SRH. Efforts are under way to develop means of calibrating responses to SRH questions by giving respondents anchoring health vignettes (Salomon, Tandon, and Murray, 2004).

Inconsistent gender differences in SRH have been reported: some studies show a female disadvantage (Gijsbers van Wijk, van Vliet, Kolk, and Everaerd, 1991; Rahman et al., 1994; Zimmer et al., 2000) while others find no disadvantage (Jylhä et al., 1998; Leinonen, Heikkinen, and Jylhä, 1998; McDonough and Walters, 2001; Zimmer et al., 2000). More importantly, several studies in the developed world show gender differences in the association between SRH and mortality, with a stronger association for men (Bath, 2003; Benyamini, Blumstein, Lusky, and Modan, 2003; Deeg and Bath, 2003; Deeg and Kriegsman, 2003; Idler, 2003; Spiers, Jagger, Clarke, and Arthur, 2003). Rather than reflecting a health disadvantage for women, these studies suggest, women's higher reports may reflect their "greater sensitivity" to health conditions.

There are relatively few studies for developing countries (Frankenberg and Jones, 2003; Rahman et al., 1994; Yu et al., 1998; Zimmer et al., 2000). In several nations in which allocation of resources is perceived to be biased in favor of men, men are less likely to report poor SRH; however, women have lower adult mortality rates. Rather than evidence of a sex difference in reporting, most studies have found that women's higher rates of poor SRH actually reflect measurable sex differences in morbidity and disability.

In Bangladesh, women's life expectancy only recently reached equality with men's. Female respondents to the MHSS were 50 percent more likely to report poor SRH than men. Women also reported greater disability and morbidity on more detailed self-reports, and they were observed to have higher levels of physical dysfunction than men (Rahman and Barsky, 2003; Rahman and Liu, 2000). Rahman and Barsky found, when controls for observed disability, self-reports of disability and morbidity, and their interactions were introduced, that no sex difference in SRH remained, so that the SRH differences were not due to women's complaining more for a given level of health as measured in other ways. Body mass index (BMI) was found to be a strong predictor of survival over a 20-year follow-up period in a study that included only women. Their BMI was measured in an ICDDR,B study in the late 1970s, and they were followed subsequently in the HDSS until they died or migrated away (Duffy and Menken, 1998; Menken, Duffy, and Kuhn, 2003). In this group, average BMI was only

18.5, and very few had a BMI greater than 25; the log-odds of survival increased linearly with BMI. No comparable information is available for men.

This analysis seeks to investigate relationships among these measures of health further, with particular emphasis on age and gender differences and to examine how well they predict mortality.

DATA AND METHODS

Setting

Matlab is a rural area about 55 km from the Dhaka, the capital of Bangladesh. ICDDR,B has long maintained a research station that sponsors the HDSS and extensive research on the health of a population of over 200,000 people. It also provides health services that supplement the government system of health care. The overwhelming majority of older individuals live with adult children (mostly sons), and alternative sources of support—financial and otherwise—outside the family are scarce. Bangladesh per capita income in 2000 was US$370/year. The predominant occupation for rural men is agriculture, with labor force participation rates remaining very high even for older men. Women are largely restricted by convention to activities in the home, with relatively little opportunity to venture outside the homestead, although these restrictions have decreased in recent years. Given the high level of poverty and the scarcity of health providers (4,671 persons/physician, 3,312 persons/hospital bed), contact with the formal health care system is thought to be relatively infrequent. National life expectancy in 2000 was 58 for both men and women; at age 50 it was approximately 30 years, again, with no significant gender differences. Approximately 10 percent of the population was over age 50 (Bangladesh Bureau of Statistics, 2002).

The 1996 Matlab Health and Socioeconomic Survey

The MHSS is a multistage, multisample household survey that collected information from 11,150 individuals age 15 and over in 4,538 households. While designed for comparability to similar nationally representative family life surveys, such as the Indonesian and Malaysian Family Life Surveys, MHSS eschewed a nationally representative sample in favor of a sample based entirely in Matlab because of the availability of the HDSS (Rahman et al., 1999). Matlab HDSS data have been used extensively in the demographic literature, and the HDSS is considered to be one of the few high-quality (i.e., complete, accurate, and up-to-date) demographic data sources in the developing world (Fauveau, 1994). In particular, age reporting is considered to be highly accurate, a feature not found in other South Asian data sources (Menken and Phillips, 1990).

As part of a collaborative study funded by the U.S. National Institute on Aging, investigators at the Harvard School of Public Health, the University of Colorado at Boulder, ICDDR,B, and Independent University, Bangladesh, MHSS respondents were tracked through the HDSS from 1996 through 2000. The matching resulted in an event history database that identifies whether a respondent died in a particular calendar year and whether he or she was censored from the HDSS population through migration.

The technique of matching survey data to subsequent surveillance data, often employed using the Current Population Survey and death registration data in the United States, offers some advantages over a panel survey. Foremost among these is cost, since longitudinal analysis requires only matching the survey to subsequent data collected as part of an ongoing system rather than fielding a follow-up study. Furthermore, a surveillance system may date death or censoring more accurately and may be more accurate in distinguishing between these two types of exits from the sample than a periodic panel survey (which collects no information except at the survey points). Panel surveys in other developing countries typically have had attrition rates of 10 percent or more, leading to uncertainty about the cause of attrition and potential bias in assessing mortality. In addition, survey costs can rise considerably as follow-up efforts intensify (Frankenberg and Thomas, 2000). Panel surveys have the advantage of offering far more detailed data on longitudinal changes in health status, nutrition, and morbidity. However, the survey plus surveillance approach offers a crucial opportunity to study the effects of health on subsequent survival. The complementarity of these approaches is obvious. We plan a 10-year follow-up of the MHSS households.

Sampling

The HDSS provided the sampling frame for the MHSS (Rahman et al., 1999). The Matlab surveillance area consists of 8,640 *baris* or residential compounds, of which roughly one-third (31.1 percent) or 2,687 *baris* were randomly selected. The *bari* is the basic unit of social organization in rural Bangladesh and in Matlab in particular (Aziz, 1979; Rahman, 1986). *Baris* usually consist of a cluster of households linked in many instances in a kin network (however, about 16 percent of *baris* consist of only a single household and, even in multihousehold *baris*, kin networks may exist only for subclusters of households). Sampling *baris* rather than households provides a better representation of family networks, a major focus of the MHSS survey. In single-household *baris*, that household was selected for detailed interviews. In all other *baris*, two households were selected. All individuals

TABLE 10-1 Sample Exclusions

	Missing	All Indicators Present
Individual Respondent		
No sampling weight	54	11,096
No HDSS match	165	10,931
Self-Reported Health Indicators		
SRH—general health	0	10,931
ADL—activities of daily living	13	10,918
Major disease	0	10,918
Observed Health Indicators		
ADL—activities of daily living	1,001	9,950
BMI—body mass index	1,304	9,536

SOURCES: 1996 Matlab Health and Socioeconomic Survey and 1996 Health and Demographic Surveillance System.

in these households who were age 50 and over were interviewed. For those below age 50, certain criteria were followed to reduce the interviewing load vis-à-vis large households. Probability weights reflecting this multistage sampling scheme were assigned to each individual and are included in the MHSS public-use data set (Rahman et al., 1999; Rahman, Menken, Foster, and Gertler, 2001).

There were 11,150 individuals age 15 and over in the *bari* sample. People were eliminated from this analysis (see Table 10-1) if the individual probability weight could not be calculated (54) or the MHSS identification number was erroneous and could not be matched in the HDSS (165). Thus we begin with 10,931 respondents who could be followed in the HDSS. Individuals were dropped if information was missing on self-reported activities of daily living, the major disease index, or observed activities of daily living, or if BMI was either missing or out of range. Most nonresponses stem from the fact that there were special teams for collection of observed health indicators and for anthropometric measurement. They visited only subsets of all MHSS households. Very few respondents refused to participate. Thus for the purposes of this study, we focus on 9,536 respondents age 15 and older (4,399 men, and 5,137 women) for whom we have complete information. Rahman and Barsky (2003) found little difference between individuals who had complete information on health indicators and all respondents.

Mortality Analytic Plan

Longitudinal models of mortality subsequent to MHSS fieldwork were estimated to investigate the predictive power of the health measures. Each respondent contributed an observation for each person-year from 1996 to

2000 unless censored by death or out-migration. The logistic hazards model of mortality tested has the following form:

$$Log\left(\frac{\mu_{ik}}{1-\mu_{ik}}\right) = \beta_0 + \beta_1 Female_i + \beta_2 Age_{ik} + \sum_{j=1}^{J} \beta_{2+j} SR_{ij} + ... + m = 1 \sum_{m=1}^{M} \beta_{2+j+m} OBS_{im} + ... + \varepsilon_{ik}$$

where μ_{ik} is the risk that person i who survived to the start of follow-up year k dies in that year, $Female_i$ is 1 if person i is female and 0 if male, Age_{ik} is person i's age at the start of follow-up year k, SR_{ij} is the jth of J self-reported health indicators, and OBS_{im} is the mth of M observed health indicators for person i. The health indicators were recorded once—in the MHSS. Therefore, Age is the only time-varying variable.

Estimation of models incorporates a Huber-White correction for intracluster correlation in the distribution of the probability of mortality across observation years for a given respondent. Results presented in the tables display the relative odds associated with a variable, or the relative change in

$$\frac{\mu}{1-\mu}$$

resulting from a one-unit change in a variable.

Table 10-2 presents the number of MHSS respondents by sex and broad age group and the number of deaths recorded for each sex/age group in the

TABLE 10-2 Respondents, Deaths, Person-Years, and Death Rates

	Respondents	Recorded Deaths	Percentage with Recorded Death	Person-Years	Percentage Dying Per Person-Year
Men					
<50	2,861	26	0.9	12,697	0.2
50+	1,539	197	12.8	7,912	2.5
Total	4,399	223	5.1	20,609	1.1
Women					
<50	3,765	18	0.5	17,136	0.1
50+	1,372	115	8.4	7,387	1.6
Total	5,137	133	2.6	24,523	0.5
Total					
<50	6,626	44	0.7	29,833	0.1
50+	2,910	312	10.7	15,299	2.0
Total	9,536	356	3.7	45,132	0.8

SOURCES: 1996 Matlab Health and Socioeconomic Survey; 1996-2000 Health and Demographic Surveillance System Mortality Files.

HDSS over the subsequent 5 years. Deaths of 10.7 percent of those over age 50 in the MHSS were recorded in the HDSS within the follow-up period, compared with only 0.7 percent of those under age 50 and 3.7 percent overall. These figures, however, do not adjust for out-migration (censoring). Among those over 50 in the MHSS, only 3.2 percent out-migrated during the follow-up period, compared with 15.1 percent of those under age 50 and 11.5 percent of all respondents (not shown). Out-migrants were censored at the end of the last full year of their observation. Those who died contributed a person-year for each year in which they were alive at the start. Those for whom neither death nor out-migration was recorded in the HDSS in the follow-up period each contributed 5 person-years of observation. The number of person-years of observation in which age was under 50, over 50, and all ages at the start of the year is given in Table 10-2 along with the yearly death rates (deaths/person-years). This death rate was 0.8 percent for all ages. While there was a relatively high rate in the older group (2.0 percent), death was a quite rare event in the younger subsample (0.1 percent). For this reason, all mortality analyses were replicated using the Rare Events Logistic Regression package for STATA (King, 2004). In all cases, rare event models resulted in higher coefficient estimates and lower standard errors, so we choose to report the more conservative logistic regression results in our later tables. Table 10-2 also shows lower mortality rates for women than for men; however, as is shown later, with more precise controls for age, sex differences are not significant.

Health Indicators

The five health indicators are defined below. The self-reported and observed activities of daily living (ADL) scores and self-reported indicator of major disease were originally developed by Rahman and Barsky (2003).

SRH was assessed with the simple question "What is your current health status?" Less than 30 seconds were required to administer this question. Responses were healthy, fairly healthy, or in poor health. SRH was coded as 1 if the respondent reported he or she was in poor health, and as 0 for those who reported they were healthy or fairly healthy The latter responses were combined because we were most concerned with poor health. It is important to note, however, that a different coding scheme (i.e., poor or fair versus good health) could affect the results.

Following Merrill, Seeman, Kasl, and Berkman (1997), Rahman and Liu (2000), and Rahman and Barsky (2003), we constructed a series of measures for functional limitations in self-reported ADLs. We used self-report information on 10 ADL items, which were divided into two clusters: (I) limitations in personal care—four items—ability to (a) bathe, (b) dress, (c) get up and out of bed, and (d) use the toilet, and (II) limitations in range of motion—six items—ability to (a) carry a 10 kg weight for 20 yards, (b) use a hand-pump to draw water, (c) stand up from a squatting position on the floor, (d) sit in a squatting position on the floor, (e) get up from a sitting position on a chair or stool without help, and (f) crouch or stoop. Collecting the entire battery of questions required about 5 minutes of interview time.

Because men and women appear to have different norms regarding personal care, in this paper we consider only the second cluster of six range-of-motion questions. Each of the six components of range of motion was scored as 0 (can easily do all the activities in the cluster) or 1 (have trouble with one or more activities in the cluster, resulting in an self-reported ADL score ranging from 0 (no limitation) to 6.

Self-reported chronic morbidity (Rahman et al., 1999), to which we refer as *major disease*, was assessed with a checklist of 14 sentinel conditions (anemia, arthritis, broken bones, cataracts, vision problems, asthma, other breathing difficulty, diabetes, pain or burning on urination, paralysis, tuberculosis, gastric/ulcer problems, edema, and a residual category called other conditions). For each condition, respondents were asked to report whether they had experienced it in the three months prior to the survey, and if so whether it had caused them no difficulty, some difficulty, a great deal of difficulty, or inability to carry out their day-to-day activities. Collection of the full battery of morbidity questions required about 6 minutes of interview time. Those who had experienced one or more of the sentinel conditions that had caused a great deal of difficulty/inability to carry out their day-to-day activities were scored as 1, while those who had none of the sentinel conditions or who experienced only minor chronic disease were scored as 0.

Physical disability was assessed objectively as in prior studies (Merrill et al., 1997; Rahman and Liu, 2000; Rahman and Barsky, 2003) by asking respondents to perform four timed physical tasks: maintaining side by side, semi-tandem and tandem positions (balance); walking 8 feet twice (gait); chair-rises (lower extremity movement); and shoulder rotation (upper extremity movement). Collection of these measures required about 10 minutes of data collection team time, as well as moderately higher equipment and training costs. Each task had a three-level score: 2 (unable to do the activity), 1 (had some difficulty doing the activity), and 0 (could do the activity easily), assigned by an independent observer. The four individual subscales were added to form a scale ranging in value from 0 to 8, with lower scores indicating better performance and 0 indicating the person could perform all activities easily. When this measure was dichotomized, those with scores of 3 or above were considered in poor health.

Height and weight were measured and BMI calculated as (weight in kg)/(height in meters)^2. Collection of these measures required 5 minutes of data collection team time, as well as extra costs for measurement tools and training of specific enumerators to operate scales and measuring sticks. Those with a BMI less than 16 were considered to be severely malnourished and scored as 1, while those with a BMI of 16 or above were scored as 0.

It is worth noting that for self-reported major disease, the summary measure is comprised of heterogeneous categories of symptoms and disease labels that reflect the prevailing morbid conditions in rural Bangladesh. As such they are locally specific, and cross-country comparisons using these summary measures would be difficult to interpret.

RESULTS

Figures 10-1 and 10-2 present, by age group and sex, the percentage estimated by self-reported and observed indicators respectively to be in poor health. Poor health increases with age and the rise begins early in adulthood. In this society, the slowest rise with age is in observed severe malnutrition. There are striking sex differences in poor health according to nearly

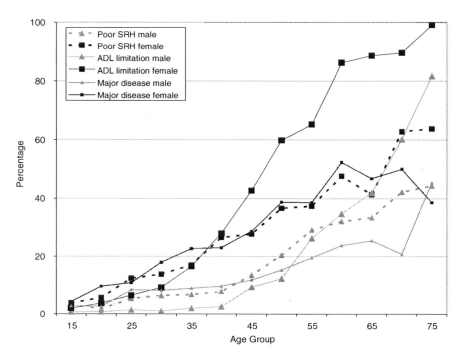

FIGURE 10-1 Self-reported health indicators, by age and sex.
SRH = self-reported health; ADL = activities of daily living.

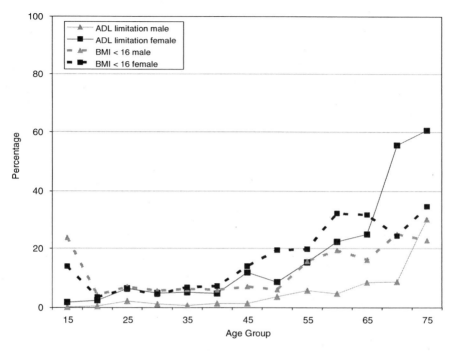

FIGURE 10-2 Observed health measures, by age and sex.
ADL = activities of daily living; BMI = body mass index.

all measures and especially at older ages. At age 40, over 20 percent of women self-reported poor health, no matter how measured, while the corresponding figures for men are about 10 percent. Until about age 40, there was little difference in the proportion severely malnourished, but after that age, women disproportionately were underweight for their height.

Extent to Which the Various Health Indicators Are Interrelated

Bivariate and multiple correlations (when each indicator is estimated from the other four) are shown in Table 10-3. Clearly, while these indicators are related, none is very closely determined by the others. These results are confirmed in a principal component analysis (not shown). In that analysis, the first component, which accounts for close to 50 percent of the variation, shows approximately equal weightings from all five indicators. Yet it is not until four factors are included that the variation accounted for reaches 89 percent. Thus, while the indicators are interrelated, each has a sizeable component unrelated to the others.

TABLE 10-3 Interrelationships Between Health Measures: 1996 Matlab Health and Socioeconomic Survey

All Respondents (n = 9,536)	Dyadic Correlations					Multiple Correlations		
	SRH	SR-ADL	SR-MD	OBS-ADL	OBS-BMI<16	Other Self-Reported	Other Observed	All Others
Self-Reported Health	—	0.441	0.329	0.181	0.158	0.474	0.229	0.483
Self-Reported Activities of Daily Living	0.441	—	0.379	0.271	0.177	0.506	0.310	0.540
Self-Reported Major Disease	0.329	0.379	—	0.164	0.099	0.420	0.184	0.423
Observed Activities of Daily Living	0.181	0.271	0.164	—	0.097	0.284	0.097	0.287
Observed BMI < 16	0.158	0.177	0.099	0.097	—	0.199	0.097	0.204

NOTE: All variables are dichotomous. SRH = self-reported health; SR-ADL = self-reported activities of daily living; SR-MD = self-reported major disease; OBS-ADL = observed activities of daily living; OBS-BMI = observed body mass index.

TABLE 10-4 Subsequent Mortality by Health Status

	Status	Percentage in Category	Percentage Died in 5-year Follow-Up Period
Self-Reported			
SRH	Poor	17.7	10.2
	Not Poor	82.3	1.9
ADL score>0	Yes	20.9	11.8
	No	79.1	1.2
Major disease	Yes	18.4	8.4
	No	81.6	2.3
Observed			
ADL score ≥3	Yes	6.3	16.7
	No	93.7	2.5
BMI < 16	Yes	12.7	9.1
	No	87.3	2.6
Observations	8,432		

NOTE: All descriptive results use individual sample weights. 1,004 individuals who migrated out of the study area between 1996 and 2000 are excluded. SRH = self-reported health; ADL = activities of daily living; BMI = body mass index.

Mortality in the Five Years Subsequent to the MHSS in Relation to the Health Indicators

Health status, as measured by each of the five indicators treated dichotomously, is substantially related to subsequent mortality (Table 10-4). Of those who self-reported poor health, 10.2 percent died versus 1.9 percent of those who self-reported good or fair health. ADL scores, whether self-reported or observed, showed greater differentials in outcome by health status, while major disease and BMI indicators differentiated risk of dying less well. Figure 10-3 works backward from survival outcome. It provides evidence that those who died, compared with those who survived the five-year follow-up period, were much more likely to have been in poor health at the time of the MHSS. Using SRH, 53 percent of those who died had said they were in poor health, compared with only 16 percent of those who survived. For reported ADL limitations, 72 percent of those who died had reported some limitation, compared with 19 percent of those who lived. For observed ADL limitations, less common overall, 31 percent of those who died had been observed to be mobility-impaired, compared with only 5 percent of those who survived. The greatest difference clearly was in the reported ADL measure.[1]

---

[1]Out-migration does not qualitatively affect this differential, as demonstrated by treating all out-migrants first as dying and then as surviving the follow-up period.

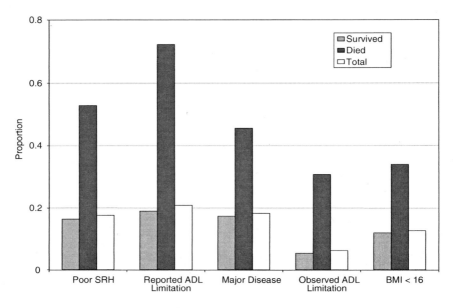

FIGURE 10-3 Health status indicators by subsequent survival.
SRH = self-reported health; ADL = activities of daily living; BMI = body mass index.

Figure 10-4 demonstrates the predictive power of the ADL scores—which characterize people along a continuum rather than a simple dichotomy. The likelihood of dying over the 5-year follow-up period shows a generally monotonic increase with ADL score, whether self-reported or observed. Furthermore, the two measures appear to capture slightly different mortality trajectories. Self-reported ADL shows a greater increase in mortality as it moves from representing people who can do all tasks easily (score = 0) to those who score difficulty with only one or two. It may be that individuals recognize the level or change in level more acutely than can be picked up on the kinds of measures that went into the observed ADL score. Observed ADL scores may capture extreme levels of poor health better: respondents who scored five or more experienced a subsequent mortality risk that approached 30 percent.

Multivariate Models

We turn to multivariate models of mortality to address several questions. First, which indicator adds greatest explanatory power when age and sex are taken into account? Second, does the predictive power of these health measures differ for older and younger adults? Initial models predicting the

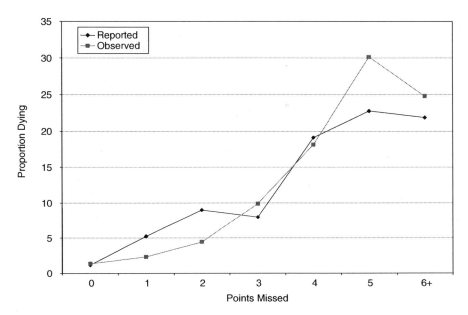

FIGURE 10-4 Proportion dying by self-reported and observed ADL scores.

odds of dying are shown in Table 10-5 for the total sample of person-years, person-years for which the individual was under 50 at the start of the year, and person-years for which the individual was 50 or over at the start. The first line reports on the model in which age is the only predictor. The pseudo-R^2 is .18 for total person-years. Interestingly, age is not a significant predictor of mortality in adults under 50. Adding sex does not significantly improve the predictive power of the model, as shown in line 2. Therefore, once age-in-years is in the model, no sex difference is detected. The remaining lines show the improvement in pseudo-R^2 when a single health indicator is added. For total person-years, SRH adds .01 to the pseudo-R^2 and those with poor SRH have odds of dying 2.28 times the odds of those of the same age and sex who do not report poor SRH. In all three models, poor SRH is significantly associated with increased subsequent mortality. A much larger coefficient is estimated for the young subsample of person-years, in which there is a low baseline level of mortality. The yearly probability of dying for this subsample is 0.12 percent (Table 10-2). Poor SRH in the young group (OR = 5.6), when age and sex are held constant at their means, raises the probability of death from 7 to 41 in 10,000. This is a large effect, especially considering that it results from a single question. For the over-50 subsample, the effect of poor SRH is smaller but highly significant (OR =

TABLE 10-5 Logistic Regression Models of Mortality Adding Age, Sex, and One Health Measure

	All		Age <50		Age 50+	
	Pseudo-R^2 Gain	Odds Ratio^a	Pseudo-R^2 Gain	Odds Ratio^a	Pseudo-R^2 Gain	Odds Ratio^a
Age	0.179^b	1.09***	0.001^b	0.99	0.092^b	1.11***
Female	0.001	0.80	0.001	0.99	0.001	0.09
Adding a single health indicator to model with age and sex						
Self-Reported						
SRH	0.012	2.28***	0.028	5.57*	0.012	2.08***
ADL score	0.024	0.76***	0.048	.51***	0.023	0.79***
Major disease	0.006	1.82**	0.028	5.45*	0.006	1.64**
Observed						
ADL score	0.014	0.78***	0.001	1.17	0.020	0.78***
BMI < 16	0.010	2.28***	0.017	3.63	0.010	2.00***
Observations	45,098		29,807		15,291	

NOTE: Calculations treat all observations for an individual as a cluster and use individual sample weights. SRH = self-reported health; ADL = activities of daily living; BMI = body mass index.

^{a}The odds ratio for female is from the model with age and sex; those for the health indicators are from models with age and sex plus that indicator as predictors.

^{b}This figure is the pseudo-R^2 for the model with age as the single predictor.

* p<.05; ** p<.01; *** p<.001.

2.1) and the probability of death, again estimated at the means of age and sex, rises from 1 to 2 percent. While each indicator is significant in the total and age 50 and over models, only the self-reports—whether of general health or ADLs or major disease—add predictive power for younger people.

Stepwise regressions were carried out (Table 10-6) in which age and sex were entered first and then health indicators entered in the order of the magnitude of their additional predictive power. For total person-years and the over-50 subsample, observed ADLs entered first, followed by self-reported ADLs, BMI, and SRH. The index of major disease did not enter at all. For the under-50 subsample, *only* self-reported ADLs served to predict mortality, whereas for those over 50, all indicators except major disease increased the fit to the data.

Finally, the complete models, in which age, sex, and the four indicators that were significant in any of the Table 10-6 models are included, are shown in Table 10-7. For the total person-years and over-50 models, mortality increases significantly with age, with each additional year associated with a 6-7 percent increase in the odds of dying. Controlling for age and health, the odds of dying for a woman in the same samples are less than half (.44-.46) those of a man. The sizable advantage in mortality controlling for health that women have is substantial enough that, despite having substantially worse health on all observed and self-reported health indicators, their mortality (adjusted only for age and shown in Table 10-4) was not significantly different from men's.

This disjunction between sex differences in health and mortality introduces the possibility that, as in other studies, women may overreport poor health and greater disability. If this were the case, the inclusion of interactions between sex and each of the significant health measures included in Table 10-7 would show significant negative interactions between health measures and the female main effect, indicating that the health measure was a worse predictor of health for women. Yet when sex–health measure interactions were entered, either individually or as a group, none approached statistical significance (models not shown, see Kuhn, Rahman, and Menken, 2004).

The absence of any significant interactions between the respondent's sex and the predictive power of SRH measures is an extremely robust finding. The effects do not even approach significance, and these results do not change when nonsignificant interaction terms for sex and observed health measures are dropped (models not shown). Women's adjusted risk of mortality, controlling for other factors, is much lower than men's. Women's low baseline mortality risks are multiplied by risks due to poor health, which are more common among women; the result is overall equality in mortality of men and women. The process is not driven by a less substantial relationship between women's poor health and women's survival, but by the fact

TABLE 10-6 Stepwise Logistic Regression Models of Mortality Adding Health Measures to Age and Sex

By Entry Order	All		Age <50		Age 50+	
	Pseudo-R^2 Gain	Odds Ratio	Pseudo-R^2 Gain	Odds Ratio	Pseudo-R^2 Gain	Odds Ratio
Observed ADL Score	0.014	1.28***	—	—	0.020	1.29***
Reported ADL Score	0.017	1.26***	0.048	1.94***	0.015	1.21***
BMI < 16	0.006	1.91***	—	—	0.006	1.72**
SRH	0.003	1.51*	—	—	0.002	1.42*
Major Disease	—	—	—	—	—	—
Final Pseudo-R^2	0.220		0.050		0.135	
Observations	45,098		29,807		15,291	

NOTE: The gain and odds ratio come from the model in which the indicator first entered (see note to Table 10-4). SRH = self-reported health; ADL = activities of daily living; BMI = body mass index.

* p<.05; ** p<.01; *** p<.001.

TABLE 10-7 Logistic Regression Model of Mortality with Age, Sex, and Health Measures as Predictors

	All		Age <50		Age 50+	
	Odds Ratio	S.E.	Odds Ratio	S.E.	Odds Ratio	S.E.
Age	1.06***	0.01	0.97	0.04	1.07***	0.01
Female	0.44***	0.07	0.62	0.34	0.46***	0.08
Self-Reported						
SRH	1.51*	0.28	3.00*	1.64	1.42*	0.25
ADL score	1.21***	0.04	1.83***	0.08	1.17***	0.04
Observed						
ADL score	1.18***	0.04	1.47	0.60	1.21***	0.03
BMI < 16	1.81**	0.33	2.46	1.39	1.65**	0.28
Observations	45,098		29,807		15,291	
Pseudo-R^2	0.220		0.084		0.135	

NOTE: Major disease is excluded because it was not significant in any model. SRH = self-reported health; ADL = activities of daily living; BMI = body mass index.
* p<.05; ** p<.01; *** p<.001.

that the same poor health multiplier effect is applied to a lower baseline mortality effect. This result holds in rare events logistic regression models and probit regression models, both of which also apply the very realistic assumption that mortality risks are multiplicative in nature, not additive. These models were also run using a linear probability model in order to estimate the size of interaction effects if mortality risks were indeed additive. Interactions between sex and SRH were found to be highly nonsignificant in these models as well.

Discussion

This analysis demonstrates both the multidimensional nature of the relatively simple and low-cost health measures in the MHSS and their substantial value and validity in a low-income setting such as Bangladesh. We believe this is the only study to examine subsequent mortality in relation to these multiple measures of health. Each measure is a significant predictor of subsequent mortality, particularly for elders. With the exception of major disease, each appears to capture, at least in part, a different dimension of health from the others. These findings support the notion that individuals can effectively assess their own health status even in settings of poor education and low levels of interaction with modern health systems.

Furthermore, the measures seem equally appropriate for men and women. The higher age-specific prevalence of poor health, whether reported or observed, among women does not appear to result from their overreporting poor health compared with men. The proportional increase of mortality for those whose health was poor versus not poor, whichever the health measure used, did not differ for women and men. At the same level of health, women had lower mortality risks than men; however, these lower risks were combined with much higher rates of poor health. These differences countered one another; as a result, we found no sex differences in overall age-adjusted mortality.

Objective health measures are frequently assumed to be superior to self-reports because they minimize concerns over reporting bias and international comparability. We find, however, that they are not necessarily better predictors of mortality. The self-reported and observed measures were similar in predicting mortality at older ages, while self-reports were the *only* significant predictors of mortality at younger ages.

The marginal time and financial costs of collecting each measure vary substantially. Cost estimates based on the MHSS are given in Table 10-8, along with the improvement in mortality prediction found when each health measure was added to the model based on age and sex (repeated from Table 10-5). For comparison, we consider the high expected costs of drawing and analyzing a blood sample. For the second round of the MHSS, we have proposed a battery of seven biomarker analyses.[2] The estimated costs are included in Table 10-8. Self-reported measures take less survey time than observational tests or drawing a blood sample and incur no additional capital costs; in addition, they can be collected by less skilled interviewers. The observed indicators cost at least 2.5 times more to collect than the self-reports. The current cost of collecting biomarkers is extremely high, but is likely to decrease in the future for two reasons. First, as collection is standardized, less expensive technology may be developed. Second, with continuing research, a small set of essential indicators is likely to be agreed upon.

These results raise questions regarding a minimal set of survey-based health measures that ensures precision and accordance with international standards. The least expensive measure, a single SRH question requiring $0.01 per respondent, adds significantly in predicting subsequent mortality for respondents of all ages. In fact, it predicts mortality better than a number of more complex health indicators.

---

[2]The battery includes blood cholesterol (total cholesterol, high density lipoprotein, low density lipoprotein, triglycerides); glycosolated hemoglobin; complete blood count (white blood cell count and morphology); homocysteine and related cofactors (e.g., folate); c-reactive protein; serum albumin; and serum creatinine. Because HIV prevalence is so low in Bangladesh, testing is not planned for MHSS2.

TABLE 10-8 Cost of Health Measures and Increase in Pseudo-R²

	Marginal Cost ($)				Increase in Pseudo-R² (%)		
	Time	Labor	Capital	Total	All	Under 50	Age 50+
Self-Reported							
SRH	0:20	0.01	0	0.01	1.2	2.8	1.2
ADLs	4:40	0.12	0	0.12	2.4	4.8	2.3
Major disease	6:00	0.16	0	0.16	0.6	2.8	0.6
Observed							
ADLs	10:00	0.50	0.05	0.55	1.4	0.1	2.0
Body mass index	5:00	0.30	0.10	0.40	1.0	1.7	1.0
Blood-drawn biomarkers	20:00	22.00	38.00	60.00	–	–	–

NOTE: Taken from Table 10-5; change when each health measure is added to model with age and sex. SRH = self-reported health; ADL = activities of daily living; BMI = body mass index.

The self-reported ADL index, the next least expensive indicator to collect, adds even more to the predictive power of our models. This indicator seems to work at least as well, and possibly better, than observed ADLs and anthropometric measures that are far more demanding of resources. However, as for SRH, it is important to ask whether self-reported ADLs produce results that are truly comparable across different populations and subgroups within populations. The results here indicate they are promising enough to be included in studies in other countries in order to assess their usefulness.

The detailed questions on specific conditions that went into the major disease index were far more complicated to implement than the ADL questions and the index added no explanatory power to the analysis of mortality. It may be that the questions on specific conditions are better predictors than the overall index; we plan to address this issue in further analyses of the MHSS.

The observed ADL index and BMI add significantly in predicting mortality for elders. They are not significant for those under 50. It may be that the activities that go into the MHSS ADL index are not sufficiently difficult to detect disabilities that contribute to higher short-term mortality risk in younger adults. Neither the observed ADL index nor BMI picks up the increase in poor health with age for those under 50, especially for females, that is self-reported. In contrast, SRH and the self-reported ADL index increase with age and are significant mortality predictors, perhaps because younger adults recognize change in their own abilities or differences in comparison with peers even when their disabilities do not put them in a range considered unusual by the observer. We suspect that, unless the set of tasks is changed to detect more subtle disability, observed ADL measures for younger adults should be included in survey data collection only as a baseline for longitudinal follow-up rather than as valid health indicators.

The four measures discussed here—SRH, self-reported and observed ADLs, and BMI—are strong predictors of survival over the next 5 years in the rural Bangladesh context, although the observed measures work best for elders. They are therefore good markers of general health and the effects of the health system and can be used to examine basic gender and socioeconomic differentials in that society. The high prevalence of poor health based on the self-reports, even at low ages, in Bangladesh makes these measures perhaps even more valuable than they would be in more advanced societies. More importantly, compared with complex measures such as biomarkers or disability adjusted life years, these measures can be obtained more frequently and in much larger samples for the same cost. If resources are especially constrained, it may be possible to restrict the set of measures collected further and still be able to capture levels, differentials, and trends in overall health over time.

Given the urgent need to assess health and track its trends over time in sub-Saharan Africa, we strongly recommend including a range of health indicators in data collection—in a way that permits research on indicators in this region. Studies are needed that collect, in selected settings, simple and low-cost health indicators like those examined in this paper; expanded versions of these indicators (e.g., SRH with more categories); other objective measures (e.g., lung capacity, grip strength) that are more costly in terms of survey-team time, equipment, and training; and selected biomarkers that are far more expensive to collect and more difficult to analyze. It would also be appropriate to address issues of comparability of measures across population through techniques such as calibrating vignettes. Simultaneous collection—in a few selected studies—of all of these indicators in comparable manner will permit the kind of "head-to-head" analysis performed here for one country and for the measures included in the MHSS. This research would be most informative if carried out where it is possible to follow respondents for some period of time to observe survival outcomes.

The expected outcomes of this research include

• Identification of measures that provide valid information on prevalence of specific conditions or diseases and those which provide information on overall health.
• Estimates of costs and difficulties of collecting each indicator.
• Cost-benefit analyses, which would help investigators decide on the package of indicators to be included in future data collection.

One obvious locus for this type of research is the INDEPTH network. Its Demographic Surveillance System sites offer crucial advantages. Since the sites carry out continuous longitudinal follow-up of large populations, they provide data on mortality trends prior to collection of the health measures. While few sites have been operating as long as the Matlab HDSS (which is a member of INDEPTH), a number, such as Agincourt in South Africa and Navrongo in Ghana, have been operating for at least 10 years. A set of health indicators measured in a one-time survey would contribute to the assessment of measures described in this paper. INDEPTH sites routinely collect the follow-up data needed to study relationships of health measures to subsequent mortality. In addition, if these measures were included periodically in subsequent DSS rounds, their sensitivity to trends and emerging differentials in health could be assessed.

The issue of comparability between populations could be addressed in two ways—for which DSS sites are again especially appropriate. Following the work on vignettes (see Salomon et al., 2004), calibrating vignettes could be included in at least one DSS round that includes health indicators. These vignettes could be extended to include ADLs as well as other aspects of health for which self-reports are collected. In addition, mortality prediction across sites could be analyzed to determine if, as for men and women in Bangladesh, the increase in the odds of mortality for those in poor health as measured by a specific indicator is the same across countries.

Development of low-cost and informative health status modules could be guided by this research. They could be regularly included in DSS data collection rounds, providing valuable comparable information across sites on health levels and trends over time. These modules could also be included in standalone surveys covering larger geographic areas. Nationally representative surveys could then provide the basis for comparative studies of countries, with data from INDEPTH sites providing greater detail and longitudinal validation.

In addition to tracking changes in health over time in defined populations, DSS sites have demonstrated they are ideal settings for conducting and evaluating health and social interventions intended to improve health either directly (e.g., family planning programs, oral rehydration programs) or indirectly (education of women, micro-credit programs). They offer well-established sampling frames with regular follow-up so that program and control groups can be established and compared over time. Increasingly, programs include direct adult health interventions, such as Agincourt's South African Stroke Prevention Initiative. Regular observation of simple health measures can provide a baseline for assessing differences between experimental and control groups, and follow-up information for assessing the long-term impact of interventions on comparable health status measures. At the same time, repeated observation of health status allows researchers in DSS sites to measure the health impact of programs not aimed directly at health, including education, family planning, and women's status interventions. Finally, such measures facilitate analysis of the health effects of unexpected economic or political crises and other changing social or health patterns.

As societies in sub-Saharan Africa grow older and continue to absorb the consequences of the HIV/AIDS epidemic, it will grow increasingly important to assess their health and health needs on a regular basis and to evaluate the impact of intervention programs. For these reasons, further research on the promising set of simple indicators evaluated here for one developing country setting and on the more detailed and expensive measures discussed here is an essential part of a research agenda on aging in Africa.

ACKNOWLEDGMENTS

This work was supported by NIA grants R01 AG16308, R03 AG19294-01, P30 AG17248, and P01 AG11952-05 to Harvard University and the University of Colorado. The research is based on collaboration among investigators at ICDDR,B: International Centre for Health and Population Research, Harvard University, Brown University, University of Colorado, Independent University, Bangladesh, and RAND. As always, we thank the people of Matlab, Bangladesh, for their commitment to research and participation in the Matlab Health and Socioeconomic Survey and the ICDDR,B Health and Demographic Surveillance System.

REFERENCES

Angel, R., and Guarnaccia, P. (1989). Mind body and culture: Somatization among Hispanics. *Social Science and Medicine, 28,* 1229-1238.

Appels, A., Bosma, H., Grabauskas, V., Gostautas, A., and Sturmans, F. (1996). Self-rated health and mortality in a Lithuanian and a Dutch population. *Social Science and Medicine, 42,* 681-690.

Aziz, K.M.A. (1979). *Kinship in Bangladesh.* Dhaka, Bangladesh: International Centre for Diarrhoeal Disease Research.

Bangladesh Bureau of Statistics. (2002, January). *Statistical pocketbook of Bangladesh, 2000.* Dhaka: Statistics Division, Ministry of Planning, Government of the People's Republic of Bangladesh.

Bath, P.A. (2003). Differences between older men and women in the self-rated health-mortality relationship. *Gerontologist, 43,* 387-395.

Benyamini, Y., Blumstein, T., Lusky, A., and Modan, B. (2003). Gender differences in the self-rated health-mortality association: Is it poor self-rated health that predicts mortality or excellent self-rated health that predicts survival? *Gerontologist, 43,* 396-405.

Borawski, E.A., Kinney, J.M., and Kahana, E. (1996). The meaning of older adults' health appraisals: Congruence with health status and determinants of mortality. *Journals of Gerontology Series: Psychological Sciences and Social Sciences, 51,* S157-S170.

Deeg, D.J.H., and Bath, P.A. (2003). Self-rated health, gender, and mortality in older persons: Introduction to a special section. *Gerontologist, 43,* 369-371.

Deeg, D.J.H., and Kriegsman, D.M.W. (2003). Concepts of self-rated health: Specifying the gender difference in mortality risk. *Gerontologist, 43,* 376-386.

Duffy, L., and Menken, J. (1998). *Health, fertility, and socioeconomic status as predictors of survival and later health of women: A 20-year prospective study in rural Bangladesh.* (Working Paper No. WP-98-11). Population Program, Institute of Behavioral Science, University of Colorado at Boulder.

Fauveau, V. (1994). *Matlab: Women, children and health.* Dhaka, Bangladesh: International Centre for Health and Population Research.

Ferraro, K.F., and Kelley-Moore, J.A. (2001). Self-rated health and mortality among black and white adults: Examining the dynamic evaluation thesis. *Journal of Gerontology Series B: Psychological Sciences and Social Sciences, 56,* S195-S205.

Frankenberg, E., and Jones, N. (2003). *Self-rated health and mortality: Does the relationship extend to a low-income setting?* Minneapolis, MN: Population Association of America.

Frankenberg, E., and Thomas, D. (2000). *The Indonesia family life survey (IFLS): Study design and results from waves 1 and 2.* Santa Monica, CA: RAND.

Gijsbers van Wijk, C.M., van Vliet, K.P., Kolk, A.M., and Everaerd, W.T. (1991). Symptom sensitivity and sex differences in physical morbidity: A review of health surveys in the United States and the Netherlands. *Women Health, 17,* 91-124.

Idler, E.L. (2003). Discussion: Gender differences in self-rated health, in mortality, and in the relationship between the two. *Gerontologist, 43,* 372-375.

Idler, E.L., and Benyamini, Y. (1997). Self-rated health and mortality: A review of 20-seven community studies. *Journal of Health and Social Behavior, 38,* 21-37.

Idler, E.L., and Kasl, S.V. (1991). Health perceptions and survival: Do global evaluations of health status really predict mortality? *Journal of Gerontology, 46,* S55-S65.

Idler, E.L., and Kasl, S.V. (1995). Self-ratings of health: Do they also predict changes in functional ability? *Journals of Gerontology Series B: Psychological Sciences and Social Sciences, 50,* S344-S353.

Jylhä, M., Guralnik, J.M., Ferrucci, L., Jokela, J., and Heikkinen, E. (1998). Is self-rated health comparable across cultures and genders? *Journals of Gerontology Series B: Psychological Sciences and Social Sciences, 53,* S144-S152.

Kaplan, G.A., and Camacho, T. (1983). Perceived health and mortality: A nine-year follow-up of the human population laboratory cohort. *American Journal of Epidemiology, 117,* 292-304.

King, G. (2004). *ReLogit: Rare events logistic regression for STATA* (version 1.1, 10/29/99). Available: -http://gking.harvard.edu/stats.shtml [accessed March 2005].

Kuhn, R., Rahman, O., and Menken, J. (2004). *Relating self-reported and objective health indicators to adult mortality in Bangladesh.* Paper presented at the 2004 annual meeting, Population Association of America, Population Aging Center, Institute of Behavioral Science, University of Colorado at Boulder.

Leinonen, R., Heikkinen, E., and Jylhä, M. (1998). Self-rated health and self-assessed change in health in elderly men and women: A five-year longitudinal study. *Social Science and Medicine, 46,* 591-597.

McDonough, P., and Walters, V. (2001). Gender and health: Reassessing patterns and explanations. *Social Science and Medicine, 52,* 547-559.

Menken, J., and Phillips, J.F. (1990). Population change in a rural area of Bangladesh, 1967-87. *Annals of the American Academy of Political and Social Science, 510,* 87-101.

Menken, J., Duffy, L., and Kuhn, R. (2003). Childbearing and women's survival in rural Bangladesh. *Population and Development Review, 29*(3), 405-426.

Merrill, S.S., Seeman, T.E., Kasl, S.V., and Berkman, L.F. (1997). Gender differences in the comparison of self-reported disability and performance measures. *Journals of Gerontology Series A: Biological Sciences and Medical Sciences, 52,* M19-M26.

Mossey, J.M., and Shapiro, E. (1982). Self-rated health: A predictor of mortality among the elderly. *American Journal of Public Health, 2,* 800-808.

Rahman, M. (1986). *Tradition, development, and the individual: A study of conflicts and supports to family planning in rural Bangladesh.* Asian Population Change Series No. 1. P. Kane and L. Ruzicka (Eds.). Department of Demography, Australian National University, Canberra.

Rahman, M.O., and Barsky, A.J. (2003). Self-reported health among older Bangladeshis: How good a health indicator is it? *The Gerontologist, 43,* 856-863.

Rahman, M.O., and Liu, J. (2000). Gender differences in functioning for older adults in rural Bangladesh: The impact of differential reporting. *Journals of Gerontology Series A: Biological Sciences and Medical Sciences, 55,* M28-M33.

Rahman, M.O., Strauss, J., Gertler, P., Ashley, D., and Fox, K. (1994). Gender differences in adult health: An international comparison. *The Gerontologist, 34,* 463-469.

Rahman, M.O., Menken, J., Foster, A., Peterson, C., Khan, M.N., Kuhn R., and Gertler, P. (1999). *The Matlab health and socioeconomic survey: Overview and user's guide.* (DRU-2018/1). Santa Monica, CA: RAND.

Rahman, O., Menken, J., Foster, A., and Gertler, P. (2001). *Matlab (Bangladesh) health and socioeconomic survey.* Available: http://webapp.icpsr.umich.edu/cocoon/ICPSR-STUDY/02705.xml [accessed May 13, 2005].

Salomon, J.A., Tandon, A., and Murray, C.J.L. (2004, January). Comparability of self-rated health: Cross-sectional multicountry survey using anchoring vignettes. *British Medical Journal*, doi:10.1136/bmj.37963.691632.44.

Schoenfeld, D.E., Malmrose, L.C., Blazer, D.G., Gold, D.T., and Seeman, T.E. (1994). Self-rated health and mortality in the high functioning elderly: A closer look at healthy individuals. (MacArthur Field Study of Successful Aging). *Journals of Gerontology Series A: Biological Sciences and Medical Sciences, 49*, M109-M115.

Spiers, N., Jagger, C., Clarke, M., and Arthur, A. (2003). Are gender differences in the relationship between self-rated health and mortality enduring? Results from three birth cohorts in Melton Mowbray, United Kingdom. *Gerontologist, 43*, 406-411.

Sugisawa, H., Liang, J., and Liu, X. (1994). Social networks, social support, and mortality among older people in Japan. *Journal of Gerontology, 49*, S3-S13.

Wolinsky, F.D., and Johnson, R.J. (1992). Perceived health status and mortality among older men and women. *Journal of Gerontology, 47*, S304-S312.

Yu, E.S.H., Kean, Y.M., Slymen, D.J., Liu, W.T., Zhang, M., and Katzman, R. (1998). Self-perceived health and 5-year mortality risks among the elderly in Shanghai, China. *American Journal of Epidemiology, 147*, 880-890.

Zimmer, Z., Natividad, J., Lin, H., and Chayovan, N. (2000). A cross-national examination of the determinants of self-assessed health. *Journal of Health and Social Behavior, 41*, 465-481.

Appendixes

Appendix A

Workshop Agenda

Workshop on Aging in Africa
Committee on Population
U.S. National Academy of Sciences

and

School of Public Health/Population Program
University of the Witwatersrand, Johannesburg

Venue: Hofmeyr House, University of the Witwatersrand Campus

Monday, July 26

Site visit to MRC/WITS—Agincourt Health and Population Unit and WITS Rural Facility (WRF)

Tuesday, July 27

Morning   Return from WRF

2:00 P.M.   LUNCH

2:45 P.M.   WELCOME AND INTRODUCTIONS

> *Professor Jane Menken, University of Colorado (chair)*
> *Professor Belinda Bozzoli, University of the*
>   *Witwatersrand*
> *Dr. Barney Cohen, The National Academies*
> *Dr. Richard Suzman, National Institutes of Health*

3:15 P.M.   DEMOGRAPHIC OVERVIEW

> Aging in Sub-Saharan Africa: The Changing Demography of
> the Region
>
> *Dr. Victoria Velkoff, U.S. Census Bureau*
> *Dr. Paul Kowal, World Health Organization*
>
> Discussant: *Dr. Eric Udjo, Human Sciences Research Council,*
> *Pretoria*
>
> Q&A and General Discussion

4:15 P.M.   BREAK

4:30 P.M.   INSIGHTS FROM SIMULATION MODELS

> I. Demographic Impacts of the HIV Epidemic and
>   Consequences of Population-Wide Treatment of HIV for the
>   Elderly: Results from Microsimulation
>
> > *Dr. Samuel J. Clark, University of Colorado and*
> > *University of the Witwatersrand*
>
> II. The HIV/AIDS Epidemic, Kin Relations, Living
>   Arrangements, and the Elderly in South Africa
>
> > *Professor M. Giovanna Merli, University of Wisconsin*
> > *Professor Alberto Palloni, University of Wisconsin*
>
> Discussant: *Professor Rob Dorrington, University of Cape*
> *Town*
>
> Q&A and General Discussion

6:00 P.M.   ADJOURN

Wednesday, July 28

9:00 A.M.   FORMAL AND INFORMAL SOCIAL SECURITY SYSTEMS

> I. An Overview of Formal and Informal Social Security Systems in Africa
>
>> *Professor Edwin Kaseke, University of Zimbabwe*
>
> II. Labor Migration and Households: A Reconsideration of the Effects of the Social Pension on Labor Supply in South Africa
>
>> *Professors Dorrit Posel, James Fairburn, and Frances Lund, University of KwaZulu-Natal*
>
> Discussant: *Professor Servaas van der Berg, University of Stellenbosch*
>
> Q&A and General Discussion

10:30 A.M. Break

10:45 A.M.   RURAL/URBAN DIFFERENCES IN AGING AND ADULT HEALTH: INSIGHTS FROM THE IN-DEPTH NETWORK

> I. Health Transitions in Rural Southern Africa: New Understanding, Growing Complexity
>
>> *Dr. Kathleen Kahn, University of the Witwatersrand*
>> *Professor Stephen Tollman, University of the Witwatersrand*
>
> II. The Situation of the Elderly in Poor Urban Settings: The Case of Nairobi, Kenya
>
>> *Dr. Abdhalah Ziraba Kasiira, African Population and Health Research Center (APHRC)*
>> *Dr. Negussie Taffa, APHRC*
>> *Dr. Alex Ezeh, APHRC*
>
> Discussant: *Dr. Ayaga Bawah, Navrongo Health Research Centre*
>
> Q&A and General Discussion

12:15 P.M. LUNCH

1:15 P.M.   EXIT FROM THE LABOR FORCE

Labor Force Withdrawal of the Elderly in South Africa

Professor David Lam, University of Michigan
Professor Murray Leibbrandt, University of Cape Town
Vimal Ranchhod, University of Michigan

Discussant: *Professor Martin Wittenberg, University of Cape Town*

Q&A and General Discussion

2:15 P.M.   MEASUREMENT ISSUES

Relating Self-Reported Health and Objective Health Indicators of Adult Mortality

Professor Jane Menken, University of Colorado

Discussant: *Professor Robert Willis, University of Michigan*

Q&A and General Discussion

3:15 P.M.   BREAK

3:45 P.M.   LIVING ARRANGEMENTS

I. HIV/AIDS and Older People in South Africa

Professor Victoria Hosegood, London School of Hygiene and Tropical Medicine
Professor Ian M. Timaeus, London School of Hygiene and Tropical Medicine

II. Interactions Between Socioeconomic Status and Living Arrangements in Predicting Gender-Specific Health Status Among the Elderly in Cameroon

Professor Barthélémy Kuate-Defo, University of Montreal

Discussant: *Dr. Kalanidhi Subbarao, The World Bank*

Q&A and General Discussion

5:15 P.M.   ADJOURN

Thursday, July 29

9: 00 A.M.   POLICY

From Piecemeal Action to Integrated Solutions: The Need for Policies on Ageing and Older People in Africa

Tavengwa Nhongo, HelpAge International, Nairobi
Karen Peachey, Independent Consultant

Discussant: *Dr. Benoit Kalasa, United Nations Fund for Population Activities, Ethiopia*

Q&A and General Discussion

10:30 A.M.   BREAK

10:45 A.M.   ROUNDTABLE ON DATA NEEDS AND FUTURE RESEARCH DIRECTIONS

Professor Frances Lund, University of KwaZulu-Natal
Dr. Alex Ezeh, APHRC
Dr. Peter Byass, Umeå University
Professor Robert Willis, University of Michigan

Q&A and General Discussion

12:45 P.M. Wrap-up / Points to Be Incorporated in Final Report

> *Professor Jane Menken, University of Colorado,*
> *Boulder*

1:00 P.M Lunch

2:00 P.M. Closed Session

The organizers of the meeting will meet to discuss publication plans for the volume and their consensus statement on future research needs.

> *Professor Jane Menken (chair), University of Colorado*
> *Dr. Alex Ezeh, APHRC*
> *Professor Edwin Kaseke, University of Zimbabwe*
> *Professor Barthélémy Kuate-Defo, University of*
> *   Montreal*
> *Professor David Lam, University of Michigan*
> *Professor Stephen Tollman, University of the*
> *   Witwatersrand*
> *Professor Robert Willis, University of Michigan*

5:30 P.M. Adjourn

Friday, July 30

9:00 A.M. Closed Session [CONT.]

1:00 P.M. Adjourn

Appendix B

About the Contributors

PANEL MEMBERS AND STAFF

Jane Menken is the director of the Institute of Behavioral Science and professor of sociology at the University of Colorado. Prior to her move to Colorado, she held professorships at the University of Pennsylvania and Princeton University, where she was associated with the Population Studies Center and the Office of Population Research. She has developed mathematical models of reproduction and analytic techniques and has carried out studies of the increase in sterility as women age, of fertility determinants in Bangladesh, and of teenage pregnancy and childbearing in the United States. Her recent research has focused on adult health in developing countries and the impact of HIV/AIDS on elders and the family. She is a member of the board of directors of the African Population and Health Research Center and served on several advisory committees at the National Institutes of Health. She has served on numerous committees on the National Research Council since 1977, including the Committee on Population and Demography; the Committee on Population; and the Committee on AIDS Research Needs in the Social, Behavioral, and Statistical Sciences. She has been a Guggenheim Fellow and a fellow at the Center for Advanced Study in the Behavioral Sciences and is a member of the American Academy of Arts and Sciences. She was elected to the National Academy of Sciences in 1990 and the Institute of Medicine in 1995. She has a B.A. in mathematics from the University of Pennsylvania (1960), an M.S. from the Harvard School of Public Health in biostatistics (1962), and a Ph.D. in sociology and demography from Princeton University (1975).

Barney Cohen is director of the Committee on Population at the National Research Council. For the past 14 years he has worked at the National Research Council on numerous domestic and international population-related issues. He has an M.A. in economics from the University of Delaware and a Ph.D. in demography from the University of California at Berkeley.

Alex Ezeh is the executive director of the African Population and Health Research Center, in Nairobi, Kenya. Prior to joining the center in November 1998, he worked at Macro International Inc. for six years, where he provided technical expertise to governmental and nongovernmental institutions in several African countries in the design and conduct of demographic and health surveys. His research interests include health inequity, health consequences of third world urbanization, gender and reproductive outcomes and aging. He has a Ph.D. in demography from the University of Pennsylvania.

Edwin Kaseke is director of the School of Social Work and professor of Social Work at the University of Zimbabwe in Harare. He serves on the editorial board of several journals, including the *Journal of Social Development in Africa*, the *Journal of Social Policy and Administration*, and the *International Social Work Journal*. He is a former member of the executive committee and board member of the International Association of Schools of Social Work. He has consulted for many national and international organizations including International Development Research Centre-Canada, the International Labour Organization, UNICEF, GTZ, the Friedrich Ebert Foundation, and the governments of Swaziland, Namibia, and Zimbabwe. He is the author of books and articles on social security systems and other formal and informal social welfare systems in Africa. He has B.S.W. and Ph.D. degrees from the University of Zimbabwe and an M.S. from the London School of Economics and Political Science.

Barthélémy Kuate-Defo is professor of demography and preventive medicine at the University of Montreal. He is a current member of the Committee on Population. His research interests include the epidemiology of aging, fertility and mortality linkages, sexuality and reproductive health, child health and nutrition, African demography, and event history and multilevel methods. Much of this work has been focused on Cameroon. He is the principal investigator of the ongoing population observatory in social epidemiology and of a large-scale quasi-experimental intervention research on reproductive health promotion and family health during the life course in Cameroon. He has a Ph.D. in population studies from the University of Wisconsin, Madison, as well as M.S. degrees in epidemiology and demography.

David Lam is a professor in the Department of Economics and a research professor in the Population Studies Center at the University of Michigan, Ann Arbor. He previously served as director of Michigan's Population Studies Center and director of the Michigan Center on the Demography of Aging. His research focuses on the interaction of economics and demography in developing countries. He has worked extensively in Brazil and South Africa, where his research analyzes labor markets, income inequality, and links between generations. He has been a visiting professor in the School of Economics at the University of Cape Town in 1997-1998 and 2004-2006. He is principal investigator of the Cape Area Panel Study, a longitudinal survey being conducted in collaboration with researchers at the University of Cape Town. He has an M.A. in Latin American studies from the University of Texas, Austin, and an M.A. in demography and a Ph.D. in economics from the University of California, Berkeley.

Alberto Palloni is H. Edwin Young professor of population and international studies in the Department of Sociology, Population Health Sciences, and the Institute for Environmental Studies at the University of Wisconsin at Madison. He is a member of the American Academy of Arts and Sciences and current president of the Population Association of America. He has been a Guggenheim Fellow and a fellow at the Center for Advanced Study in the Behavioral Sciences at Stanford. His current research interests include the relation between early health status and social stratification, models for the spread of HIV/AIDS, families and households in Africa and Latin America, aging and mortality, and mathematical models. He has a B.A. from the Catholic University of Chile and a Ph.D. from the University of Washington.

Stephen Tollman is founding director of the MRC/Wits Rural Public Health and Health Transitions Research Unit (Agincourt). He heads the Health and Population Division of the School of Public Health, University of the Witwatersrand (Wits) in South Africa, and chairs the university's Population Program Executive. He is currently board chair of the INDEPTH Network of African, Asian, and Latin American demographic and health surveillance sites, and leads the network's multisite initiative in adult health and aging. Much of his published work addresses the profound health, population, and social transitions affecting South Africa and the region, and potential public-sector responses. He holds an M.Med from the University of the Witwatersrand, an M.P.H. from the Harvard School of Public Health, and an M.A. from Oxford University.

Robert J. Willis is professor in the Department of Economics, and research professor in the Survey Research Center and the Population Studies Center of the Institutes for Social Research at the University of Michigan. Previously he held appointments at the University of Chicago, the State University of New York at Stony Brook, and Stanford University. He is director of the Health and Retirement Study, a large-scale, nationally representative longitudinal survey of Americans over the age of 50. His research interests include labor economics, economic demography, economic development and the economics of aging. He has conducted research relating to economic behavior over the entire life-cycle, including theoretical and empirical research on fertility, marriage, divorce and out-of-wedlock childbearing, education and earnings, intergenerational transfers, and the determinants of poverty among elderly widows. Recently, he has begun a new area of research dealing with the relationship between probabilistic thinking and savings and wealth accumulation and other aspects of cognition. He is a past president of the Midwest Economics Association, currently president-elect of the Society of Labor Economists and received the Mindel C. Sheps Award in 2002 from the Population Association of America. He is also a current member of the Committee on Population and has served on a number of past National Research Council committees and panels. He has a B.A. in economics from Dartmouth College and an M.A. and Ph.D. in economics from the University of Washington.

OTHER CONTRIBUTORS

Gloria Chepngeno is a Ph.D. research student in the Division of Social Statistics, University of Southampton. Her current research focus is on the impact of HIV/AIDS on older people. She has an M.A. in population studies from the University of Nairobi, Kenya.

Samuel J. Clark is assistant professor in the Department of Sociology, University of Washington, and research associate at the Institute of Behavioral Science, University of Colorado at Boulder. He also is research officer, MRC/WITS Rural Public Health and Health Transitions Research Unit (Agincourt), School of Public Health, University of the Witwatersrand. He has a Ph.D. in demography from the University of Pennsylvania.

Mark Collinson is field research manager at the MRC/WITS Rural Public Health and Health Transitions Research Unit (Agincourt). He is completing an M.S. in migration and child health in rural South Africa at the University of the Witwatersrand.

Myles Connor is a senior lecturer and senior neurologist in the Division of

Neurology, Department of Neurosciences, University of the Witwatersrand, and at Chris Hani Baragwanath Hospital. He is also coinvestigator on the Southern African Stroke Prevention Initiative.

Michel Garenne is director of research at the French Institute for Research and Development, Paris, and senior scientific advisor at the MRC/WITS Rural Public Health and Health Transitions Research Unit (Agincourt). He has a Ph.D. in demography from the University of Pennsylvania.

Victoria Hosegood is head of population studies at the Africa Center for Health and Population Studies, South Africa, and a lecturer at the London School of Hygiene and Tropical Medicine. Her research interests include African family demography and the impact of HIV/AIDS. She has a Ph.D. in maternal and child health.

Gillian Hundt is professor of Social Sciences in Health, and codirector of the Institute of Health, University of Warwick, United Kingdom. She has a Ph.D. in sociology from the University of Warwick.

Kathleen Kahn is senior lecturer at the Health and Population Division, School of Public Health, University of the Witwatersrand, and senior researcher at the MRC/WITS Rural Public Health and Health Transitions Research Unit (Agincourt).

Abdhalah Ziraba Kasiira is a research officer at the African Population and Health Research Center, Nairobi, Kenya. He has an M.S. in clinical epidemiology and biostatistics.

Paul Kowal is a scientist in the Multi-Country Studies unit within the Department of Evidence and Information for Policy at the World Health Organization. He coordinates the WHO Study on Global Ageing and Adult Health.

Randall Kuhn is director of the Global Health Affairs Program and assistant professor at the Graduate School of International Studies, University of Denver. He has a Ph.D. in demography and sociology from the University of Pennsylvania.

Murray Leibbrandt is professor of economics at the School of Economics, University of Cape Town, and director of the Southern African Labour and Development Research Unit. He has a Ph.D. in economics from Notre Dame University.

M. Giovanna Merli is associate professor in the Department of Sociology at the University of Wisconsin at Madison. She has a Ph.D. in demography from the University of Pennsylvania.

Omar Rahman is professor of demography, and pro-vice chancellor of Independent University, Bangladesh. He has an M.D. from Northwestern University Medical School, an M.P.H in health policy, and a D.Sc. in epidemiology from the Harvard School of Public Health.

Vimal Ranchhod is a doctoral candidate in the Department of Economics, University of Michigan.

Margaret Thorogood is chair of epidemiology, and director of research degrees at the University of Warwick, United Kingdom. Prior to that, she was reader in Public Health and Preventative Medicine at the London School of Hygiene and Tropical Medicine.

Ian M. Timaeus is professor of demography at the London School of Hygiene & Tropical Medicine. His current research interests include adult health and mortality, and AIDS mortality. He has a Ph.D. in faculty of medicine from the London School of Hygiene & Tropical Medicine.

Victoria Velkoff is the chief of the Aging Studies Branch, International Programs Center, U.S. Census Bureau. She has a Ph.D. in sociology from Princeton University. Her research interests include aging issues and adult mortality measurement.

Zewdu Woubalem is a research associate at the African Population and Health Research Center, Nairobi, Kenya. He has a Ph.D. in sociology from Brown University. His research interests include health and health-related issues in sub-Saharan Africa.